Textbook of
Receptor
Pharmacology

Edited by

John C. Foreman, D.Sc., Ph.D.
Department of Pharmacology
University College London
United Kingdom

Torben Johansen, M.D.
Department of Pharmacology
Odense University
Denmark

CRC Press
Boca Raton   New York   London   Tokyo

Acquiring Editor: David Grist
Project Editor: Andrea Demby
Marketing Manager: Susie Carlisle
Direct Marketing Manager: Becky McEldowney
Cover design: Denise Craig
Manufacturing: Sheri Schwartz

Library of Congress Cataloging-in-Publication Data

Textbook of receptor pharmacology / edited by John C. Foreman and
    Torben Johansen.
          p. cm.
      Includes bibliographical references and index.
      ISBN 0-8493-9227-6 (alk. paper)
      1. Drug receptors.   I. Foreman, John C. II. Johansen, Torben.
      [DNLM: 1. Receptors, Drug--agonists.   2. Receptors, Drug-
    -antagonists & inhibitors.   Receptors, Drug--physiology.
    4. Signal Transduction--physiology.   5. Radioligand Assay--methods.
    QV 38 T356 1996]
    RM301.41.T486   1996
    615'.7--dc20
    DNLM/DLC
    for Library of Congress   96-14485
                                                                        CIP

Textbook of

Receptor Pharmacology

Preface

For about three decades now a course in receptor pharmacology has been given for undergraduate students at University College London in their final year of study for the Bachelor of Science degree in Pharmacology. More recently, the course has also been taken by students reading for the Bachelor of Science degree in Medicinal Chemistry. The students following the course have relied for their reading upon a variety of different sources including original papers, reviews, and various textbooks but there has been no single text which brought together the material that is included in the course.

In 1993 and 1995, in Denmark, we organized a course for graduate students in pharmacology from the Nordic and other European countries. It was based upon the final year undergraduate course given at University College London. The generous financial support of the Danish Research Academy and the Nordic Research Academy allowed us to bring together expert teachers in the field. Those teachers, together with some other specialists in the field of receptor pharmacology, have written this textbook. A very important part of the production of this book has been the constructive criticisms and comments of the students who have followed the course. The aim of the book has been to construct a logical introduction to the various approaches that can be taken to the study of drug receptors, which we hope will be of value to both undergraduate students in pharmacology and those graduate students embarking on drug receptor research.

Characterization of drug receptors involves several different approaches: quantitative description of functional studies with agonists and antagonists; quantitative description of the binding of ligands to receptors; the molecular structure and genetics of drug receptors; and the signal transduction systems associated with drug receptors. These four different approaches are the basis of the four main sections of this book.

This is intended as an introductory text on receptor pharmacology. Some prior knowledge is assumed and we hope that readers will wish to follow up some topics in greater depth; therefore, the further reading for each chapter will have material which is intended to provide a background for those who need it, as well as material which extends the coverage in the chapter.

John C. Foreman
Torben Johansen

The Editors

John C. Foreman, B.Sc., Ph.D., D.Sc., M.B., B.S. is Professor of Immunopharmacology, University College London and a Visiting Professor at the University of Tasmania, Hobart, Australia. He also served a Visiting Professorship at Odense University, Denmark in 1991.

Dr. Foreman is also Vice-Dean of the Faculty of Life Sciences, University College London and Senior Tutor of University College London. He was Sub-Dean of the Faculty of Life Sciences and Admissions Tutor for Medicine from 1982 to 1993.

Dr. Foreman was made a Fellow of University College London in 1993 and received the Doctor of Science degree from the University of London in 1993.

Dr. Foreman initially read Medicine at University College London, but interrupted his studies in medicine to take the B.Sc. and Ph.D. in pharmacology before returning to complete the medical degrees M.B.B.S. which he obtained in 1976. After internships at Peterborough District Hospital, he spent two years as Visiting Instructor of Medicine, Division of Clinical Immunology, Johns Hopkins University School of Medicine, Baltimore, Maryland. He then returned to University College London where he has remained on the permanent staff.

Dr. Foreman is a member of the British Pharmacological Society and served as an editor of the *British Journal of Pharmacology* from 1980 to 87. He is also an affiliate member of the American Society of Pharmacology and Experimental Therapeutics, and a member of the Physiological Society, and the British Society for Immunology. Dr. Foreman is an Associate Editor of *Immunopharmacology* and is also on the Editorial Boards of *Inflammation Research, Pharmacology and Toxicology,* and *Skin Pharmacology.*

Dr. Foreman has presented over 60 invited lectures around the world. He is co-editor of the *Textbook of Immunopharmacology,* which is now in its third edition, and has published approximately 150 research papers, as well as reviews and contributions to books. His current major research interests include bradykinin receptors in the human nasal airway and the control of microvascular circulation in human skin by peptides.

Torben Johansen, M.D., Dr. Med. Sci., is Docent in Pharmacology, Department of Pharmacology, Institute of Medical Biology, Faculty of Health Sciences, Odense University, Denmark.

Dr. Johansen obtained his M.D. degree in 1970 from the University of Copenhagen, became a research fellow in the Department of Pharmacology, Odense University in 1970, lecturer in 1972, and then senior lecturer in 1974. Since 1990 he has been Docent in pharmacology. In 1979 he was a visiting research fellow for three months at the University Department of Clinical Pharmacology, Oxford University. In 1980 he did his internship in medicine and surgery at Odense University Hospital. He obtained his Dr. Med. Sci. in 1988 from Odense University.

Dr. Johansen is a member of the British Pharmacological Society, the Danish Medical Association, the Danish Pharmacological Society, and the Danish Society for Clinical Pharmacology.

Dr. Johansen has published more than 60 research papers. His current major research interest is transmembranal ion transport and signaling mechanisms in mast cells.

Acknowledgments

Chapter 10 is based upon a review written by the authors and published in *Annual Reviews of Physiology,* 1994, with the generous agreement of the publishers, Annual Reviews, Inc., Palo Alto, California.

Professor D.H. Jenkinson is grateful to Dr. A. Gibb for reading and commenting upon Chapter 1.

The Editors would like to thank Nicholas Hayes for his assistance with the editorial preparation of the manuscript.

Contributors

Sir James W. Black, Nobel Laureate, F.R.S.
James Black Foundation
King's College School of Medicine
  and Dentistry
London, United Kingdom

Shamshad Cockcroft, Ph.D.
Department of Physiology
University College London
London, United Kingdom

Annette C. Dolphin, Ph.D.
Department of Pharmacology
Royal Free Hospital School of Medicine
London, United Kingdom

Jan Egebjerg, Ph.D.
Molecular and Cellular Biology
Novo-Nordisk, Denmark

John C. Foreman, D.Sc.
Department of Pharmacology
University College London
London, United Kingdom

Steen Gammeltoft, M.D.
Department of Clinical Biochemistry
Glostrup Hospital
Glostrup, Denmark

Alasdair J. Gibb, Ph.D.
Department of Pharmacology
University College London
London, United Kingdom

Dennis G. Haylett, Ph.D.
Department of Pharmacology
University College London
London, United Kingdom

Donald H. Jenkinson, Ph.D.
Department of Pharmacology
University College London
London, United Kingdom

C. Ronald Kahn, M.D.
Research Division
Joslin Diabetes Center
Boston, Massachusetts

Haruo Kasai, M.D.
Department of Physiology
Faculty of Medicine
University of Tokyo
Tokyo, Japan

IJsbrand Kramer, Ph.D.
Department of Pharmacology
University College London
London, United Kingdom

Carl C.H. Petersen, Ph.D.
Department of Cellular
  and Molecular Pharmacology
University of California
San Francisco, California

Ole H. Petersen, M.D., For. Memb. R. Danish Acad. Sci.
The Physiological Laboratory
University of Liverpool
Liverpool, United Kingdom

Ronit Sagi-Eisenberg, Ph.D.
Department of Cell Biology
  and Histology
Sackler School of Medicine
Tel-Aviv University
Tel-Aviv, Israel

Thue W. Schwartz, M.D.
Laboratory for Molecular Pharmacology
Rigshospitalet
København Ø, Denmark

Table of Contents

Section I: Drug-Receptor Interaction

Section II: Molecular Structure of Receptors

Section III: Ligand Binding Studies of Receptors

Section IV: Signal Transduction Systems

Section V: Receptors as Pharmaceutical Targets

Section I

Drug-Receptor Interaction

1 Classical Approaches to the Study of Drug-Receptor Interactions

Donald H. Jenkinson

CONTENTS

0-8493-9227-6/96/$0.00+$.50
© 1996 by CRC Press, Inc.

1.1   INTRODUCTION

SOME HISTORY

The term receptor is used in pharmacology to denote a class of cellular macromolecules that are concerned specifically and directly in chemical signaling between and within cells. Combination of a hormone, neurotransmitter, or intracellular messenger with its receptor(s) results in a change in cellular activity. Hence a receptor has not only to recognize the particular molecules that activate it but also, when recognition occurs, to alter cell function by causing, e.g., a change in membrane permeability, or an alteration in gene transcription.

The concept has a long history. Humans have always been intrigued by the remarkable ability of animals to distinguish between different substances by taste and smell. Writing in ~50 B.C., Lucretius (in *De Rerum Natura*, *Liber IV*) speculated that odors might be conveyed by tiny, invisible "seeds" with distinctive shapes which would have to fit into minute "spaces and passages" in the palate and nostrils. In his words

> Some of these must be smaller, some greater, they must be three-cornered for some creatures, square for others, many round again, and some of many angles in many ways.

The same principle of complementarity between substances and their recognition sites is implicit in John Locke's prediction in his *Essay Concerning Human Understanding* (1690):

> Did we but know the mechanical affections of the particles of rhubarb, hemlock, opium and a man, as a watchmaker does those of a watch, ... we should be able to tell beforehand that rhubarb will purge, hemlock kill and opium make a man sleep...

(Here *mechanical affections* could be replaced in modern usage by *chemical affinities*.)

Prescient as they were, these early ideas could only be taken further when in the early nineteenth century it became possible to separate and purify the individual components of materials of plant and animal origin. The simple but powerful technique of fractional crystallization allowed plant alkaloids such as nicotine, atropine, pilocarpine, strychnine, and morphine to be obtained in a pure form for the first time. The impact on biology was immediate and far reaching, for these substances proved to be invaluable tools for the unraveling of physiological function. To take a single example, J. N. Langley made much use of the ability of nicotine to first activate and then block nerves originating in the autonomic ganglia to map out the distribution and divisions of the autonomic nervous system.

Langley also studied the actions of atropine and pilocarpine, and in 1878 he published (in the first volume of the *Journal of Physiology,* which he founded) an account of the interactions between pilocarpine (which causes salivation) and atropine (which blocks this action of pilocarpine). Confirming and extending the pioneering work of Heidenhain and Luchsinger, Langley showed that the inhibitory action of atropine could be overcome by increasing the dose of pilocarpine. Moreover, the restored response to pilocarpine could in turn be abolished by further atropine. Commenting on these results, Langley wrote

> We may, I think, without too much rashness, assume that there is some substance or substances in the nerve endings or [salivary] gland cells with which both atropine and pilocarpine are capable of forming compounds. On this assumption, then, the atropine or pilocarpine compounds are formed according to some law of which their relative mass and chemical affinity for the substance are factors.

If we replace *mass* by *concentration,* the second sentence can serve as well today as when it was written, though the nature of the law which Langley had correctly inferred must exist was not to be formulated (in a pharmacological context) until almost 60 years later. It is considered in Section 1.5.2 below.

J. N. Langley maintained his interest in the action of plant alkaloids throughout his life. In work with nicotine (which can contract skeletal muscle) and curare (which abolishes this action of nicotine, and also blocks the response of the muscle to nerve stimulation, as first shown by Claude Bernard), he was able to infer in 1905 that the muscle must possess a "receptive substance":

> Since in the normal state both nicotine and curari abolish the effect of nerve stimulation, but do not prevent contraction from being obtained by direct stimulation of the muscle or by a further adequate injection of nicotine, it may be inferred that neither the poison nor the nervous impulse act directly on the contractile substance of the muscle but on some accessory substance.

> Since this accessory substance is the recipient of stimuli which it transfers to the contractile material, we may speak of it as the receptive substance of the muscle.

At the same time, Paul Ehrlich, working in Frankfurt, was reaching similar conclusions, though from evidence of a quite different kind. He was the first to make a thorough and systematic study of the relationship between the chemical structure of organic molecules and their biological actions. This was put to good use in collaboration with the organic chemist A. Bertheim. Together, they prepared and tested more than 600 organometallic compounds incorporating mercury and arsenic. Among the outcomes was the introduction into medicine of drugs such as salvarsan which were toxic to pathogenic microorganisms responsible for, e.g., syphilis, at doses which had relatively minor side effects in humans. Ehrlich also investigated the selective staining of cells by dyes, as well as the remarkably powerful and specific actions of bacterial toxins. All these studies convinced him that biologically active molecules had to become bound in order to be effective, and after the fashion of the time he expressed this neatly in Latin:

Corpora non agunt nisi fixata*

In Ehrlich's words *(Collected Papers, Vol. III, Chemotherapy)*

---

* Literally: *entities do not act unless attached.*

When the poisons and the organs sensitive to it do not come into contact, or when sensitiveness of the organs does not exist, there can be no action.

If we assume that those peculiarities of the toxin which cause their distribution are localized in a special group of the toxin molecules and the power of the organs and tissues to react with the toxin are localized in a special group of the protoplasm, we arrive at the basis of my side chain theory. The distributive groups of the toxin I call the "haptophore group" and the corresponding chemical organs of the protoplasm the "receptor". …Toxic actions can only occur when receptors fitted to anchor the toxins are present.

Nowadays it is accepted that Langley and Ehrlich deserve comparable recognition for the introduction of the receptor concept. It has to be added that in the same years, biochemists studying the relationship between substrate concentration and enzyme velocity had also come to think in terms of an "active site" which could discriminate between different substrates and inhibitors. As often happens, different strands of evidence had converged at almost the same time to point to a single conclusion.

1.2 MODELING THE RELATIONSHIP BETWEEN AGONIST CONCENTRATION AND TISSUE RESPONSE

With the concept of the receptor established, pharmacologists turned their attention to understanding the quantitative relationship between drug concentration, receptor occupancy, and the observed response of a tissue. There are two parts to this. The first is to find the relationship between agonist concentration and the proportion of the receptors occupied by agonist molecules. The second is to understand the dependence of the observed response on the degree of receptor occupancy.

Nowadays the first question can often be studied directly with the aid of radiolabeled drugs, as described in Chapter 5. This method was of course unavailable to the early pharmacologists. Also, the only responses that could then be measured (e.g., the contraction of an intact piece of smooth muscle, or a change in the rate of the heart beat) were indirect, in the sense that many cellular events lay between the initial step (activation of the receptors) and the observed response. For these reasons the early workers had no choice but to devise ingenious indirect approaches, several of which are still important. These approaches are based on "modeling" the two relationships identified above, and then comparing the predictions of the models with the behavior actually observed with isolated tissues. This will now be illustrated.

1.2.1 Relationship Between Drug Concentration and Receptor Occupancy

To begin with, we will consider the simplest possible model for the combination of a drug, A, with its receptor, R:

$$A + R \underset{k_{-1}}{\overset{k_{+1}}{\rightleftharpoons}} AR \qquad (1.1)$$

Here k_{+1} and k_{-1} are the *association rate constant* ($M^{-1}s^{-1}$) and the *dissociation rate constant* (s^{-1}), respectively.

The law of mass action states that the rate of a reaction is proportional to the product of the concentrations of the reactants. Applying it to this simple scheme, and assuming that equilibrium has been reached, we have

$$k_{+1}[\text{A}][\text{R}] = k_{-1}[\text{AR}]$$

where [R] and [AR] are the concentrations of free and occupied receptors, respectively.

It may well seem odd to refer to receptor *concentrations* in this context when the receptors are free to move only in the plane of the membrane (and then perhaps to no more than a limited extent, since many receptors are anchored). However, the model can be formulated equally well in terms of the proportions of a population of binding sites that are either free or occupied by a drug molecule. If we define p_R as the proportion free, equal to $[\text{R}]/[\text{R}]_T$, where $[\text{R}]_T$ represents the total concentration of receptors, and p_{AR} as $[\text{AR}]/[\text{R}]_T$, we have

$$k_{+1}[\text{A}] \; p_R = k_{-1} \, p_{AR}$$

Since we are for the present concerned only with equilibrium conditions and not with kinetics, we can combine k_{+1} and k_{-1} to form a new constant, $K_A, = k_{-1}/k_{+1}$. K_A is a *dissociation equilibrium constant* (see Appendix 1.2A), though often abbreviated to either *equilibrium constant* or *dissociation constant*:

$$[\text{A}]p_R = K_A \, p_{AR}$$

Because, on this simple model, the receptor is either free or combined, we can write

$$p_R + p_{AR} = 1$$

$$\frac{K_A}{[\text{A}]} p_{AR} + p_{AR} = 1$$

Hence*

$$p_{AR} = \frac{[\text{A}]}{K_A + [\text{A}]} \tag{1.2}$$

This is the important ***Hill-Langmuir equation***. A. V. Hill was the first to apply the law of mass action to the relationship between drug concentration and receptor occupancy at equilibrium, and to the rate at which this equilibrium is approached.** The physical chemist. I. Langmuir, showed a few years later that a similar equation (the *Langmuir adsorption isotherm*) applies to the adsorption of gases to the surface of a metal.

In deriving Equation 1.2 we have assumed that the concentration of A does not change as drug receptor complexes are formed. In effect, the drug is considered to be present is such excess that it is scarcely depleted by a combination of a little of it with the receptors: [A] can be regarded as constant.

The relationship between p_{AR} and [A] predicted by Equation 1.2 is illustrated in Figure 1.1. The concentration of A has been plotted using a linear (left) and a logarithmic scale (right). The value of K_A has been taken to be 1 μM. (Note from Equation 1.2 that when $[\text{A}] = K_A$, $p_{AR} = 0.5$, i.e., half of the receptors are occupied).

---

* If you find this difficult, see Appendix 1.2B, at the end of the section.
** Hill had been an undergraduate student in the Department of Physiology at Cambridge where J. N. Langley suggested to him that this would be useful to examine in relation to finding whether the rate at which an agonist acts on an isolated tissue is determined by diffusion or by combination with the receptor.

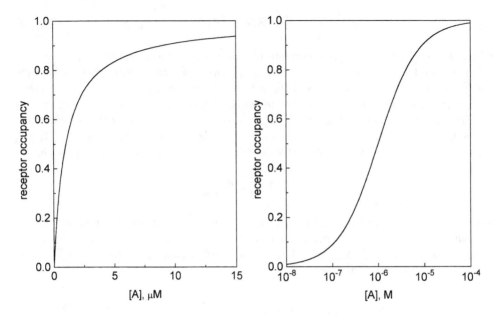

FIGURE 1.1   The relationship between receptor occupancy and drug concentration (left, linear scale; right, log scale), as predicted by the Hill-Langmuir equation. K_A has been taken to be 1 μM for both curves.

With the logarithmic scale, the slope of the line initially increases: the curve has the form of an elongated "S", and hence is said to be *sigmoidal*. In contrast, with a linear (arithmetic) scale for [A], there is no sigmoidicity: the slope declines as [A] increases, and the curve forms part of a rectangular hyperbola.

Equation 1.2 can be rearranged to

$$\frac{p_{AR}}{1 - p_{AR}} = \frac{[A]}{K_A}$$

Takings logs, we have

$$\log\left(\frac{p_{AR}}{1 - p_{AR}}\right) = \log [A] - \log K_A$$

Hence a plot of log $(p_{AR}/(1 - p_{AR}))$ against log [A] should give a straight line of unit slope. Such a graph is described as a **Hill plot**, again after A. V. Hill who was the first to employ it, and is often used when p_{AR} is measured directly with a radiolabeled ligand (see Chapter 5). In practice, the slope of the line is not always unity (as discussed below) and is referred to as the **Hill coefficient** (n_H) or **Hill slope**.

1.2.2   RELATIONSHIP BETWEEN RECEPTOR OCCUPANCY
AND TISSUE RESPONSE

This is the second of the two questions identified at the start of Section 1.2, where it was noted that the earliest pharmacologists had no choice but to use indirect methods. A. J. Clark and A. V. Hill were the pioneers in modeling the complete concentration-response relationship. In the absence, at that time, of any means of obtaining direct evidence on the point, they explored the consequences of assuming (1) that the law of mass action applies, so that Equation 1.2 (derived above) holds, and (2) that the response of the tissue is linearly related to receptor occupancy. Clark went further and made the *tentative* assumption that the relationship might be one of direct proportionality (though he was well aware that this was almost certainly an oversimplification, as we now know it often is).

Should there be direct proportionality, and if the response of a tissue (expressed as a percentage of the maximum response attainable with a large concentration of the drug) is denoted by *y*, the relationship between occupancy* and response becomes

$$\frac{y}{100} = p_{AR} \qquad (1.3)$$

Combining this with Equation 1.2 provides

$$\frac{y}{100} = \frac{[A]}{K_A + [A]} \qquad (1.4)$$

which can be rearranged to

$$\frac{y}{100 - y} = \frac{[A]}{K_A} \qquad (1.5)$$

Taking logs,

$$\log\left(\frac{y}{100 - y}\right) = \log [A] - \log K_A$$

This can be tested by measuring a series of responses *(y)* to different concentrations of A, and then plotting log $(y/(100 - y))$ against log [A] (the Hill plot). If Equation 1.4 holds, a straight line with a slope of 1 should be obtained. A. J. Clark was the first to test this using the responses of isolated tissues, and Figure 1.2 shows some of his results. Equation 1.4 provides a good fit to the experimental values, and the slopes of the Hill plots in *B* are close to unity. While these findings are in keeping with the simple model that has been outlined, they do not amount to proof that it is correct. Indeed, later studies with a wide range of tissues have shown that some concentration-response relationships cannot be fitted by Equation 1.4. In particular, the Hill coefficient is generally, if not always, greater than unity for responses mediated by ligand-gated ion channels (see Chapter 7). Also, it is now known that in many tissues the maximal response (for example, contraction of intestinal smooth muscle) may occur when an agonist such as acetylcholine occupies less then a tenth of the available receptors. By the same token, when an agonist is applied at the concentration (usually termed the $[A]_{50}$ or EC_{50}) needed to give a half-maximal response, receptor occupancy may be as little as 1% in some tissues**, rather than the 50% to be expected were the response to be directly proportional to occupancy.

Pharmacologists have therefore had to abandon (sometimes rather reluctantly and belatedly) their attempts to explain the shapes of the dose-response curves of complex tissues in

---

* Note that no distinction is made here between *occupied* and *activated* receptors: it is tacitly assumed that all the receptors occupied by agonist molecules are in an active state, hence contributing to the initiation of the observed response. As we shall see in Section 1.4.4, this is an oversimplification.
** See Sections 1.6.2 and 1.6.3.

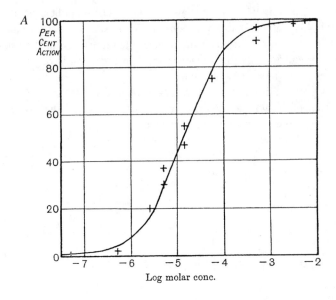

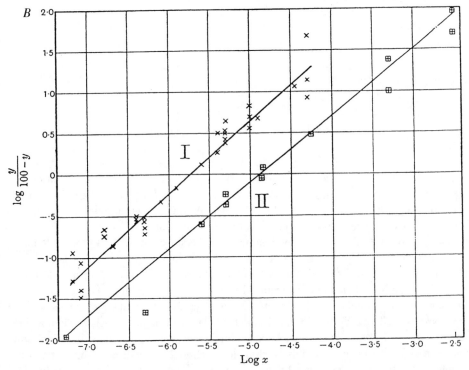

FIGURE 1.2   *A.* Concentration-response relationship for the action of acetylcholine in causing contraction of the frog rectus abdominis muscle. The curve has been drawn using Equation 1.5, a rearranged form of Equation 1.4. *B.* Hill plots for the action of acetylcholine on frog ventricle (I) and rectus abdominis (II). (From A. J. Clark, *J. Physiol.*, 61, 530-547, 1926. With permission.)

terms of the simple models first explored by Clark and by Hill. Nevertheless, as Clark's work showed, the relationship between the concentration of an agonist and the response of a tissue commonly has the same general form seen in Figure 1.1. In keeping with this, concentration-response curves can often be fitted *empirically* by the simple expression

$$y = y_{max} \frac{[A]^{n_H}}{[A]_{50}^n H + [A]^{n_H}} \qquad (1.6)$$

This is usually described as the ***Hill equation*** (see also Appendix 1.2B). Here n_H is the Hill coefficient and y and y_{max} are, respectively, the observed response and the maximum response to a large concentration of agonist. $[A]_{50}$ is the concentration of A at which y is half maximal. Because it is a constant for a given concentration-response relationship, it is sometimes denoted by K. While this is algebraically neater (and moreover was the symbol used by Hill), it should be remembered that K in this context does not necessarily correspond to an equilibrium constant. Employing $[A]_{50}$ in Equation 1.6 serves to remind us that the relationship between [A] and response is here being *described* rather than *explained* in terms of a model of receptor action.

1.2.3 APPENDIXES TO SECTION 1.2

1.2.3.1   Appendix 1.2A. Equilibrium, Dissociation, and Affinity Constants

Confusingly, all these terms are in current use to express the position of the equilibrium between a drug and its receptors. The choice arises because the ratio of the rate constants k_{-1} and k_{+1} can be expressed either way up. In this chapter we take K_A to be k_{-1}/k_{+1}, and it is then strictly a *dissociation equilibrium constant*, which is often abbreviated to either *dissociation constant* or *equilibrium constant*. The inverse ratio, k_{+1}/k_{-1}, gives the *association equilibrium constant* which is always abbreviated to *affinity constant*.

One way to reduce the risk of confusion is to express drug concentrations in terms of K_A. This "normalized" concentration is defined as $[A]/K_A$, and will be denoted here by the symbol ϕ_A. We can therefore write the Hill-Langmuir equation in three different though equivalent ways:

$$p_{AR} = \frac{[A]}{K_A + [A]} = \frac{K_A'[A]}{1 + K_A'[A]} = \frac{\phi_A}{1 + \phi_A}$$

where the terms are as follows

	Abbreviation	*Dimension*
Dissociation equilibrium constant	K_A	M
Affinity constant	K_A'	M^{-1}
Normalized concentration	ϕ_A	Dimensionless

1.2.3.2   Appendix 1.2B. Step-By-Step Derivation of the Hill-Langmuir Equation

We start with the two key equations given in Section 1.2.1:

$$[A]\, p_R = K_A\, p_{AR} \qquad (1)$$

$$p_R + p_{AR} = 1 \qquad (2)$$

From (1), $p_R = \dfrac{K_A}{[A]} p_{AR}$ Remember, if $ax = by$ then $x = \dfrac{b}{a} y$

Next, use Equation 3 to replace p_R in Equation 2 (because we wish to find p_{AR})

$$\frac{K_A}{[A]} p_{AR} + p_{AR} = 1$$

$$p_{AR}\left(\frac{K_A}{[A]} + 1\right) = 1 \qquad\qquad \text{Remember, } ax + x = x\,(a+1)$$

$$p_{AR}\left(\frac{K_A + [A]}{[A]}\right) = 1 \qquad\qquad \text{Remember, } \frac{s}{t} + 1 = \frac{s+t}{t}$$

$$\boxed{p_{AR} = \frac{[A]}{K_A + [A]}} \qquad\qquad \text{Remember if } x\frac{u}{v} = 1 \quad \text{then } x = \frac{v}{u}$$

Rearrangements of the Hill-Langmuir equation.

Cross-multiplying $\qquad\qquad\qquad$ Remember, $y = \dfrac{x}{a + x}$

$$p_{AR}\, K_A + p_{AR} \cdot [A] = [A] \qquad \text{is the same as } \frac{y}{1} = \frac{x}{a+x}, \text{ready for cross-multiplication.}$$

Cross multiplication:

$$\therefore\ (p_{AR} \cdot K_A = [A]\,(1 - p_{AR}) \qquad \text{if } \frac{a}{b} = \frac{c}{d}\cdot \text{ then } a \times d = c \times b$$

$$\boxed{\frac{p_{AR}}{1 - p_{AR}} = \frac{[A]}{K_A}}$$

Taking logs,

$$\boxed{\log\left(\frac{p_{AR}}{1 - p_{AR}}\right) = \log[A] - \log K_A} \qquad \text{Remember, } \log(a/b) = \log a - \log b$$

1.2.3.3   Appendix 1.2C. The Hill Equation and the Hill Plot

In some of his earliest work, published in 1910, A. V. Hill examined how the binding of oxygen to hemoglobin varied with the oxygen partial pressure. He found that the relationship between the two could be fitted by the following equation

$$y = \frac{K'x^n}{1 + K'x^n}$$

Here y is the fractional binding, x is the partial pressure of O_2, K' is an affinity constant, and n is a number which in Hill's work varied from 1.5 to 3.2.

This equation can also be written as

$$y = \frac{x^n}{K_e + x^n} \tag{1.7a}$$

where $K_e = 1/K'$, and as

$$y = \frac{x^n}{K^n + x^n} \tag{1.7b}$$

This final variant is convenient because K has the same dimension as x, and moreover is the value of x for which y is half maximal.

Equation 1.7b can be rearranged and expressed logarithmically as:

$$\log\left(\frac{y}{1-y}\right) = n \log x - n \log K$$

Hence a Hill plot (see earlier) should give a straight line of slope n (the Hill coefficient, often expressed as n_H).

Hill plots are often used in pharmacology, when y may be either the fractional response of a tissue or the amount of a ligand bound to its binding site, expressed as a fraction of the maximum binding, and x is the concentration. It is sometimes found (especially when tissue responses are measured) that the Hill coefficient differs markedly from unity. What might this mean?

One of the earliest explanations to be considered was that n molecules of drug might bind simultaneously to a single binding site, R:

$$nA + R \rightleftharpoons A_nR$$

This would lead to the following expression for the proportion of binding sites occupied by A:

$$p_{A_nR} = \frac{[A]^n}{K + [A]^n}$$

where K is the dissociation equilibrium constant. Hence the Hill plot would be a straight line with a slope of n. However, this model is quite unlikely to apply: there are few examples of chemical reactions in which three or more molecules (e.g., two of A and one of R) have to combine simultaneously. Another explanation has to be sought. One possibility arises when the tissue response measured is indirect, in the sense that a sequence of cellular events links receptor activation to the response that is finally measured. The Hill coefficient may not then be unity (or even a constant) because of a nonlinear and variable relation between the proportion of receptors activated and one or more of the events that follow.

Even if receptor activation is measured relatively directly, for example, by recording the flow of current through the ion channels that are intrinsic to "fast" receptors, the Hill slope is characteristically greater than unity. This is most clearly established for the nicotinic receptors for acetylcholine. In this instance the most likely explanation is that the receptor macromolecule carries two binding sites for the agonist, and both of these have to be occupied for receptor activation, at least in its normal mode. Should the two sites be identical (almost certainly an oversimplification), the proportion of receptors in which both binding sites are occupied by agonist is given by

$$p_{A_2R} = \left(\frac{[A]}{K_A + [A]} \right)^2$$

The Hill coefficient n_H would then be

$$n_H = \frac{2(K_A + [A])}{K_A + 2[A]}$$

This predicts a nonlinear Hill plot. When [A] is small in relation to K_A, n_H approximates to 2. However, as [A] is increased, n_H tends towards unity.

1.2.3.4   Appendix 1.2D. Logits, the Logistic Equation and Their Relation to the Hill Plot

The *logit transformation* of a variable p is defined as

$$\text{logit } [p] = \log_e \left(\frac{p}{1-p} \right)$$

Hence the Hill plot can be regarded as a plot of logit (p) against log concentration (though it is more usual to employ logarithms to base 10 than to base e).

It is worth noting the distinction between the *Hill equation* and the *logistic equation*, which was first formulated in the nineteenth century as a means of describing the time-course of population increase. It is defined by the expression

$$p = \frac{1}{1 + e^{-(a+bx)}} \tag{1.8}$$

This is easily rearranged to

$$\frac{p}{1-p} = e^{a+bx}$$

Hence

$$\text{logit } [p] = \log_e \left(\frac{p}{1-p} \right) = a + bx$$

If we redefine a as $-\log_e K$, and x as $\log_e z$, then

$$p = \frac{z^b}{K + z^b} \tag{1.9}$$

which is a form of the Hill equation (see Equation 1.7a). However, note that Equation 1.9 has been obtained from 1.8 only by transforming one of the variables. It follows that the terms logistic equation (or curve) and Hill equation (or curve) should not be regarded as interchangeable. To illustrate the distinction, if the independent variable in each equation is set to zero, the dependent variable becomes $1/(1 + e^{-a})$ in Equation 1.8 as compared with zero in Equation 1.9.

1.3 THE TIME COURSE OF CHANGES IN RECEPTOR OCCUPANCY

1.3.1 INTRODUCTION

Measuring how quickly a drug combines with its receptors can be surprisingly difficult. At first sight, the simplest approach would seem to be to observe the rate at which the drug acts on an isolated tissue. However, there are two immediate problems. The first is that the exact relationship between the effect on a tissue and the proportion of receptors occupied by the drug generally is not known, and cannot be assumed to be simple. Only rarely does a half-maximal tissue response correspond to half-maximal receptor occupation. We can take as an example the blocking action of tubocurarine on an indirectly stimulated, isolated skeletal muscle, such as the rat phrenic nerve-diaphragm preparation. Because neuromuscular transmission normally has a large safety margin, the twitch response to nerve stimulation begins to fall only when tubocurarine has occupied, on average, more than 80% of the nicotinic acetylcholine receptors located on the superficial muscle fibers.

The second complication is that the rate at which a drug acts on an isolated tissue is often determined not by the combination of the drug with the receptors but by the rate at which the drug diffuses through the tissue. Again taking the action of tubocurarine on the isolated diaphragm as our example, the slow development of the block reflects not the rate of binding to the receptors but rather the failure of neuromuscular transmission in an increasing number of individual muscle fibers, as tubocurarine slowly diffuses between the closely packed muscle fibers into the interior of the preparation. Moreover, as an individual drug molecule diffuses deeper into the tissue it may bind and unbind several times (and for different periods) to a variety of sites (including receptors). This repeated binding and dissociation can greatly slow the diffusion of the drug into and out of the tissue.

For these reasons, kinetic measurements are now often done using single isolated cells (e.g., a neurone or a muscle fiber). Another approach is to work with a cell membrane preparation and examine the rate at which a suitable radioligand combines with, or dissociates from, the receptors that the membrane carries (see Chapter 5). Our next task is to consider what binding kinetics might be expected under such conditions.

1.3.2 INCREASES IN OCCUPANCY

In the following, we continue with the simple model for the combination of a drug with its receptors which was introduced in Section 1.2.1 (Equation 1.1). Assuming as before that the law of mass action applies, the rate at which receptor occupancy (p_{AR}) changes with time should be given by the equation:

$$\frac{d(p_{AR})}{dt} = k_{+1}[A]p_R - k_{-1}p_{AR} \tag{1.10}$$

In words, this states that the rate of change of occupancy is simply the difference between (1) the rate at which drug-receptor complexes are formed, and (2) the rate at which they break down.

At first sight, Equation 1.10 looks difficult to solve because there are no less than four variables: p_{AR}, t, [A], and p_R. However, we know that $p_R = (1 - p_{AR})$. Also, we will assume as before that [A] remains constant throughout: i.e., that so much A is present in relation to the number of receptors that the combination of some of it with the receptors will not appreciably reduce the overall concentration. Hence, only p_{AR} and t remain as variables so that the equation becomes easier to handle.

Substituting for p_R, we have

$$\frac{d(p_{AR})}{dt} = k_{+1}[A](1 - p_{AR}) - k_{-1}p_{AR} \tag{1.11}$$

Rearranging terms,

$$\frac{d(p_{AR})}{dt} = k_{+1}[A] - (k_{-1} + k_{+1}[A]p_{AR}) \tag{1.12}$$

This still looks rather complicated, so we will drop the subscript from p_{AR} and also make the following substitutions for the constants in the equation:

$$a = k_{+1}[A]$$

$$b = k_{-1} + k_{+1}[A]$$

Hence

$$\frac{dp}{dt} = a - bp$$

This can be rearraranged to a standard form which is easily integrated (see Appendix 1.3) in order to find how the occupancy changes with time:

$$\int_{p_1}^{p_2} \frac{dp}{a - bp} = \int_{t_1}^{t_2} dt$$

Integrating,

$$\log_e\left(\frac{a - bp_2}{a - bp_1}\right) = -b(t_2 - t_1)$$

We can now consider how quickly occupancy rises after the drug is first applied at time zero ($t_1 = 0$). Receptor occupancy is initially 0, so that p_1 is 0. Thereafter occupancy increases steadily, and will be denoted $p(t)$ at time t:

$t_1 = 0$	$p_1 = 0$
$t_2 = t$	$p_2 = p(t)$

Hence

$$\log_e \left\{ \frac{a - bp(t)}{a} \right\} = -bt$$

$$\frac{a - bp(t)}{a} = e^{-bt}$$

$$p(t) = \frac{a}{b} \left(1 - e^{-bt} \right)$$

Replacing a and b by the original terms, we have

$$p(t) = \frac{k_{+1}[A]}{k_{-1} + k_{+1}[A]} \left\{ 1 - e^{-(k_{-1} + k_{+1}[A])t} \right\} \qquad (1.13)$$

Recalling that $k_{-1}/k_{+1} = K_A$, we can write

$$p(t) = \frac{[A]}{K + [A]} \left\{ 1 - e^{-(k_{-1} + k_{+1}[A])t} \right\}$$

When t is very great, so that the drug and the receptors are in equilibrium, the term in the large brackets becomes unity. This is because $e^{-\infty} = 0$ so that we can then write

$$p(t) = p(\infty) \left\{ 1 - e^{-(k_{-1} + k_{+1}[A])t} \right\} \qquad (1.14)$$

where

$$p(\infty) = \frac{[A]}{K_A + [A]}$$

The time course predicted by Equation 1.14 is shown in Figure 1.3 for three concentrations of A. Note how the rate at which equilibrium is approached increases as [A] becomes greater. This is because the time course is determined by $k_{-1} + k_{+1}[A]$. This quantity is sometimes replaced by a single constant, so that Equation 1.14 can be rewritten as either

$$p(t) = p(\infty) \left(1 - e^{-\lambda t} \right) \qquad (1.15)$$

or

$$p(t) = p(\infty) \left(1 - e^{-t/\tau} \right) \qquad (1.16)$$

where

$$\lambda = k_{-1} + k_{+1}[A], \ = 1/\tau$$

τ ('tau') is the *time constant*, and has the dimension of *time*. λ ('lambda') is the *rate constant* which is sometimes written as k_{on} (as in Chapter 5) and has the dimension of *time^{-1}*.

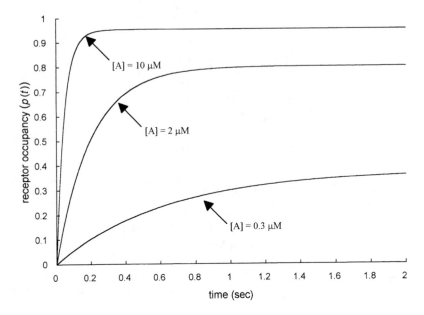

FIGURE 1.3 The predicted time course of the rise in receptor occupancy following the application of a drug at the three concentrations shown. The curves have been drawn according to Equation 1.14, using a value of 2×10^6 M^{-1} sec^{-1} for k_{+1}, and of 1 sec^{-1} for k_{-1}.

1.3.3 FALLS IN OCCUPANCY

Earlier, we had assumed for simplicity that the occupancy was zero when the drug was first applied. It is straightforward to extend the derivation to predict how the occupancy will change with time even if it is not initially zero. We change the limits of integration to

$t_1 = o$	$p_1 = p(o)$
$t_2 = t$	$p_2 = p(t)$

Here $p(0)$ is the occupancy at time zero, and the other terms are as previously defined.

Exactly the same steps as before then lead to the following expression to replace Equation 1.14

$$p(t) = p(\infty) + \{p(0) - p(\infty)\}e^{-(k_{-1} + k_{+1}[A])t} \tag{1.17}$$

We can use this to examine what would happen if the drug is rapidly removed. This is equivalent to setting [A] abruptly to zero, at time zero; p(∞) also becomes zero because eventually all the drug receptor complexes will dissociate. Equation 1.17 then reduces to

$$p(t) = p(0) \ e^{-k_{-1}t} \tag{1.18}$$

This has been plotted in Figure 1.4.

The time constant, τ, for the decline in occupancy is simply the reciprocal of k_{-1}. A related term is the *half-time* ($t_{1/2}$). This is the time needed for the quantity ($p(t)$ in the present example) to reach halfway between the initial and the final value, and is given by

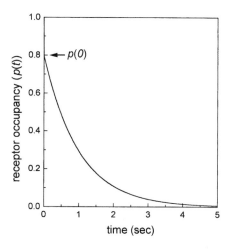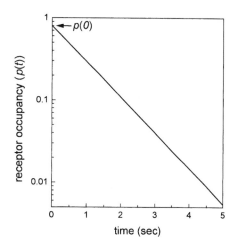

FIGURE 1.4 The predicted time course of the decline in receptor occupancy. The curves have been plotted using Equation 1.18, taking k_{-1} to be 1 s^{-1}, and $p(0)$ to be 0.8. A linear scale for $p(t)$ has been used on the left, and a logarithmic scale on the right.

$$t_{1/2} = \frac{0.693}{k_{-1}}$$

For the example illustrated in Figure 1.4, $t_{1/2} = 0.693$ s. Note that τ and $t_{1/2}$ have the dimension of *time*, as compared with *time*$^{-1}$ for k_{-1}.

It has been assumed throughout this elementary account that so many receptors are present that the average number occupied will rise or fall smoothly with time: events at single receptors have not been considered. When a drug is abruptly removed, the time for which an individual receptor remains occupied will of course vary from receptor to receptor, just as does the lifetime of individual atoms in a sample of an element subject to radioactive decay. It can be shown that the *median* lifetime of the occupancy of individual receptors is given by $0.693/k_{-1}$. The *mean* lifetime is $1/k_{-1}$. The introduction of the single-channel recording method has made it possible to obtain information about the occupancy of single receptors, and this is described in Chapter 7.

1.3.4 Appendix 1.3: Integrating the Rate Equation

A final substitution is helpful:

$$z = a - bp$$

Differentiating this, in order to be able to express dp/dt in terms of dz/dt:

$$\frac{dz}{dt} = -b\frac{dp}{dt}$$

The differential equation we wish to solve

$$\frac{dp}{dt} = a - bp$$

then becomes simply

$$\frac{dz}{dt} = -bz$$

Separating the variables gives

$$\frac{dz}{z} = -b\,dt$$

Integrating

$$\int_{z_1}^{z_2} \frac{dz}{z} = -b\int_{t_1}^{t_2} dt$$

$$\left[\log_e z\right]_{z_1}^{z_2} = -b[t]_{t_1}^{t_2}$$

$$\log_e \frac{z_2}{z_1} = -b(t_2 - t_1)$$

Recalling that $z = a - bp$, we have

$$\log_e\left(\frac{a - b\,p_2}{a - b\,p_1}\right) = -b(t_2 - t_1)$$

1.4. PARTIAL AGONISTS

1.4.1 INTRODUCTION AND EARLY CONCEPTS

The discovery of new drugs commonly requires the syntheses of large numbers of structurally related compounds. If agonists of this kind are tested on a particular tissue, they are often found to fall into two categories. Some can elicit a maximal tissue response, and accordingly are described as *full agonists* in that experimental situation. The others cannot elicit this maximal response, no matter how high the concentration, and are termed *partial agonists*.
    Examples include

Partial agonist	Full agonist	Acting at
Prenalterol	Adrenaline, isoprenaline	β-adrenoceptors
Pilocarpine	Acetylcholine	Muscarinic receptors
Impromidine	Histamine	Histamine H_2 receptors

Figure 1.5 shows concentration response curves which compare the action of the β-adrenoceptor partial agonist prenalterol with that of the full agonist isoprenaline on a range of tissues and responses. In every instance, the maximal response to prenalterol is smaller, though the magnitude of the difference varies greatly.
    A superficial explanation for the inability of a partial agonist to match the response to a full agonist could be that it fails to combine with all the receptors. This can easily be ruled

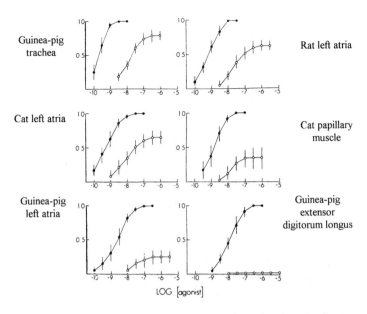

FIGURE 1.5 Comparison of the log concentration-response relationships for β-adrenoceptor-mediated actions, on six tissues, of a full and a partial agonist (isoprenaline (●) and prenalterol (○), respectively). The ordinate shows the response as a fraction of the maximal response to isoprenaline. From T. P. Kenakin and D. Beek, *J. Pharmacol. Exp. Ther.*, 213, 406-413, 1980.

out by testing the effect of increasing concentrations of a partial agonist on the response of a tissue to a fixed concentration of a full agonist. Figure 1.6 illustrates such an experiment for two agonists acting at H_2 receptors. As the concentration of the partial agonist impromidine is raised, the response of the tissue gradually falls from the large value seen with the full agonist alone, and eventually reaches the maximal response to the partial agonist acting on its own. The implication is that the partial agonist is perfectly able to combine with all the receptors, provided that a high enough concentration is applied, but the effect on the tissue is less than would be seen with a full agonist. The partial agonist is in some way less able to elicit a response.

The experiment of Figure 1.7 points to the same conclusion. When low concentrations of histamine are applied in the presence of the partial agonist impromidine, the response is larger than that to impromidine alone. However, the concentration-response curves cross as the histamine concentration is further increased. This is because the presence of impromidine reduces receptor occupancy by histamine (at all concentrations). When the lines intersect, the reduction in the contribution of histamine to the response is no longer fully offset by the contribution from the receptors occupied by impromidine. Beyond this point, the presence of impromidine reduces the response to histamine. Again, the implication is that the partial agonist is capable of combining with all the receptors, but the response is less than with a full agonist. The important question of how this can be understood in terms of events at single receptors is considered in Section 1.4.4 and in Chapter 7.

1.4.2 How to Express the Maximum Response to a Partial Agonist

In 1954 the Dutch pharmacologist E. J. Ariëns introduced the term *intrinsic activity,* which is now usually defined as

$$\text{Intrinsic activity} = \frac{\text{maximum response to test agonist}}{\text{maximum response to a full agonist acting through the same receptors}}$$

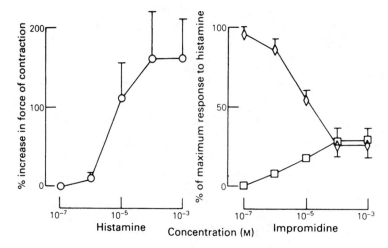

FIGURE 1.6 Interaction between histamine and the H_2-receptor partial agonist impromidine on isolated ventricular strips from human myocardium. The concentration-response curve on the left is for histamine alone, and those on the right show the response to impromidine acting either on its own (□) or in the presence of a constant concentration (10^{-4} μM) of the full agonist histamine (◇). (From T. A. H. English et al., *Br. J. Pharmacol.,* 89, 335-340, 1986. With permission.)

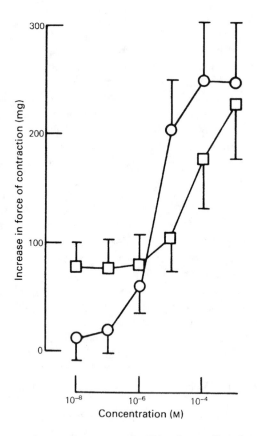

FIGURE 1.7 Log concentration-response curves for histamine applied alone (○) or in the presence (□) of a constant concentration of the partial agonist impromidine (10^{-5} M). Tissue and experimental conditions as in Figure 1.6. (From T. A. H. English et al., *Br. J. Pharmacol.,* 89, 335-340, 1986. With permission.)

For full agonists, the intrinsic activity (often denoted by α) is unity, by definition, as compared with zero for a competitive antagonist. Partial agonists have values between these limits. Note that the definition is entirely descriptive — nothing is assumed about mechanism. Also, "intrinsic" should not be taken to mean that a given agonist has a characteristic activity, regardless of the experimental circumstances. To the contrary, the intrinsic activity of a partial agonist such as prenalterol can vary greatly, not only between tissues as Figure 1.5 illustrates, but also in a given tissue depending on the experimental conditions (see later). Indeed, the same compound can be a full agonist with one tissue and a partial agonist with another. For this reason, the term *maximal agonist effect* is perhaps preferable to *intrinsic activity*.

Similarly, the finding that a pair of agonists can each elicit the maximal response of a tissue (i.e., they have the same intrinsic activity, unity) should not be taken to imply that they are equally able to activate receptors. Suppose that the tissue has many spare receptors (see Section 1.6.3). One of the agonists might have to occupy 5% of the receptors in order to produce the maximal response, whereas the other might require only 1% occupancy. Evidently the second is more effective, despite both being full agonists. A more subtle measure of the ability of an agonist to activate receptors is clearly needed, and it was provided by R. P. Stephenson. He suggested that receptor activation resulted in a "stimulus" or "signal" *(S)* to the cells, and the magnitude of this stimulus was determined by the product of what he termed the **efficacy** *(e)* of the agonist and the proportion, p, of the receptors that it occupies*:

$$S = ep \tag{1.19}$$

An important difference from Ariëns's concept of intrinsic activity is that efficacy, unlike intrinsic activity, has no upper limit — it is always possible that an agonist with a greater efficacy than any existing compound may be discovered. Also, Stephenson's proposal was not linked to any assumption about the exact relationship between receptor occupancy and the response of the tissue. (Ariëns had initially supposed that there was direct proportionality: an assumption later to be abandoned). According to Stephenson,

$$y = f(S_A) = f(e_A\, p_{AR}) = f\left(\frac{e_A[A]}{K_A + [A]} \right)$$

Here y is the response of the tissue, and e_A is the efficacy of the agonist, A; $f(S_A)$ merely means "some function of S_A" (i.e., y depends on S_A in some unspecified way).

In order to be able to compare the efficacies of different agonists acting through the same receptors, Stephenson proposed the convention that the stimulus S is unity for a response that is 50% of the maximum attainable with a full agonist. This is the same as postulating that a partial agonist that has to occupy all the receptors to produce a half-maximal response has an efficacy of unity. We can see this from Equation 1.19; if our partial agonist has to occupy all the receptors (i.e., $p = 1$) in order to produce the half-maximal response, at which point S, too, is unity (by Stephenson's convention), then e must also be 1.

R. F. Furchgott later suggested a refinement of Stephenson's concept. Recognizing that the response of a tissue to an agonist is influenced by the density of receptors as well as by the ability of the agonist to activate them, he wrote

$$e = \varepsilon\, [R]_T$$

---

* No distinction is made here between *occupied* and *activated* receptors. We shall see in Section 1.4.4 that this is of key importance for understanding and comparing the ability of different ligands to activate receptors.

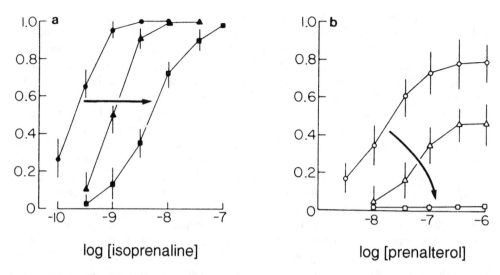

FIGURE 1.8 The effect of carbachol at two concentrations, 1 µM (triangles) and 10 µM (squares), on the relaxations of tracheal smooth muscle caused by a partial agonist, prenalterol, and by a full agonist, isoprenaline. The responses are plotted as a fraction of the maximum to isoprenaline. (From T. P. Kenakin and D. Beek, *J. Pharmacol. Exp. Ther.,* 213, 406-413, 1980. With permission.)

Here $[R]_T$ is the total "concentration" of receptors, and ε (epsilon) is the ***intrinsic efficacy*** (not to be confused with *intrinsic activity*). Thus ε can be regarded as a measure of the contribution of individual receptors to the overall efficacy.

The efficacy of a particular agonist, as defined by Stephenson, can vary between different tissues in the same way as can the intrinsic activity, and for the same reasons. Moreover, the value of both the intrinsic activity and the efficacy of an agonist in a given tissue will depend on the experimental conditions. This is illustrated in Figure 1.8. Relaxations of tracheal muscle in response to isoprenaline and prenalterol were measured first in the absence (circles) and then in the presence (triangles, squares) of a muscarinic agonist, carbachol, which causes contraction and so tends to oppose β-adrenoceptor-mediated relaxation. Hence greater concentrations of the β-agonists are needed, and the curves shift to the right. With isoprenaline, the maximal response can still be obtained, despite the presence of carbachol at either concentration. The pattern is quite different with prenalterol. Its inability to produce complete relaxation becomes even more evident in the presence of carbachol at 1 µM. Indeed, when administered with 10 µM carbachol, prenalterol causes little or no relaxation: its intrinsic activity and efficacy (in Stephenson's usage) have become negligible.

By the same token, reducing the number of available receptors (for example, by applying an alkylating agent — see Section 1.6.1) will always diminish the maximal response to a partial agonist. In contrast, the log concentration-response curve for a full agonist may first shift to the right, and the maximal response will become smaller only after there are no longer any spare receptors (see also Section 1.6.3).

1.4.3 MEASURING EFFICACY

In the following, the term *efficacy* is used only in the specific sense introduced by Stephenson. Three methods for determining efficacy will be outlined. The first two apply only to partial agonists and presuppose that the measurements are made with a tissue that has a large receptor reserve. It is also assumed that a full agonist which is able to produce a maximal response when occupying few of the receptors is available.

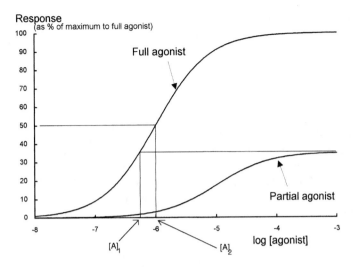

FIGURE 1.9 Estimating the efficacy of a partial agonist by comparing its concentration-response curve with that for a full agonist. See text for further detail.

Method 1

Concentration-response curves are constructed for the full agonist (A) and for the partial agonist [P] whose efficacy is to be determined (Figure 1.9).

Two concentrations are read off the curve for the full agonist. The first, $[A]_1$, causes a half-maximal response. The second, $[A]_2$, elicits the same response as the maximum seen with the partial agonist. Then

$$e_p = \frac{[A]_2}{[A]_1}$$

This can be seen as follows. For a half-maximal response, $S = 1$ (by Stephenson's convention) and $p_{AR} \approx [A]_1/K_A$. This approximation holds because if A occupies few receptors (i.e., $[A] \ll K_A$), then

$$\frac{[A]}{K_A + [A]} \approx \frac{[A]}{K_A}$$

Hence, recalling that $S_A = e_A p_{AR}$, we have

$$1 = e_A \frac{[A]_1}{K_A} \tag{1.20}$$

When the partial agonist occupies all the receptors in order to produce its maximal response, $p_{PR} = 1$. Hence the stimulus (S_P) attributable to P is simply e_P. Assuming that the same tissue response, whether elicited by A or by P, corresponds to the same value of S, we can write

$$S_P = S_A$$

$$\therefore \quad e_P = e_A \frac{[A]_2}{K_A} \tag{1.21}$$

Dividing Equation 1.21 by Equation 1.20, we obtain

$$e_{\mathrm{p}} = \frac{[A]_2}{[A]_1}$$

Method 2

This provides estimates of e_{P} and of K_{P}, the dissociation equilibrium constant for the partial agonist-receptor combination. Exactly the same assumptions and measurements are made as before (see again Figure 1.9). From the concentration-response curves for the full and the partial agonist, the values of [A] and [P] which produce the same response are read off, for several levels of response.
Just as before, we assume that S_{A} equals S_{P}, for the same response.
Therefore

$$e_{\mathrm{A}} \frac{[A]}{K_{\mathrm{A}} + [A]} = e_{\mathrm{p}} \frac{[P]}{K_{\mathrm{p}} + [P]}$$

If A occupies few receptors (so that $[A] \ll K_{\mathrm{A}}$ — see Method 1), we can write

$$e_{\mathrm{A}} \frac{[A]}{K_{\mathrm{A}}} \approx e_{\mathrm{p}} \frac{[P]}{K_{\mathrm{p}} + [P]}$$

$$\Rightarrow \frac{1}{[A]} = \frac{e_{\mathrm{A}} K_{\mathrm{P}}}{e_{\mathrm{p}} K_{\mathrm{A}}} \frac{1}{[P]} + \frac{e_{\mathrm{A}}}{e_{\mathrm{p}} K_{\mathrm{A}}}$$

Hence a plot of 1/[A] against 1/[P] should provide a straight line of slope $e_{\mathrm{A}}K_{\mathrm{P}}/e_{\mathrm{P}}K_{\mathrm{A}}$ and intercept $e_{\mathrm{A}}/e_{\mathrm{P}}K_{\mathrm{A}}$. The ratio of the slope to the intercept should give an estimate of K_{P}. If the partial agonist can produce a response equal to or greater than 50% of that to the full agonist, the value of e_{P} can then be calculated by using K_{P} to work out the proportion of receptors occupied by the partial agonist when it elicits the half-maximal response: the reciprocal of this occupancy gives e_{P} (since S is then unity, by definition). If, however, the partial agonist can produce only a small response, then Method 1 can be applied to estimate e_{P}.

Method 3

This is more general than the others, in the sense that it is applicable to full agonists, at least in principle. Suppose that we have some reliable means of determining the dissociation equilibrium constant for the combination of the agonist with its receptors. One procedure that has been used is Furchgott's irreversible antagonist method, as described in Section 1.6.4. We can then apply the Hill-Langmuir equation to calculate the proportion of receptors occupied at the concentration of agonist which produces a half-maximal response. Because S is now unity, by definition, the reciprocal of this occupancy gives the value of e (from Equation 1.19). This is the basis of Furchgott's estimate of the efficacy of histamine acting on isolated guinea-pig ileum (see Section 1.6.4.).

All these methods have been used in recent years. However, note that each is based on the classical (Hill, Clark, Gaddum) model of receptor action, and on the specific definition of efficacy introduced by Stephenson. It is now appreciated that the classical model is incomplete in important regards, *and this has implications for the interpretation of the results of all three methods.* Indeed, it has only been through the realization that receptor activation is more complex than the early workers had supposed that it has become possible to devise more satisfactory measures of the ability of ligands to activate receptors. Our next task is to consider these.

1.4.4 THE INTERPRETATION OF PARTIAL AGONISM IN TERMS OF EVENTS AT SINGLE RECEPTORS

The concepts of intrinsic activity and efficacy outlined above are essentially descriptive, without reference to mechanism. We now turn to the question of how differences in efficacy are to be explained in terms of the molecular events that underlie receptor activation, and we begin by considering some of the experimental evidence that has provided remarkably direct evidence on the nature of these events.

Just a year after Stephenson's classical paper of 1956, J. del Castillo and B. Katz published an electrophysiological study of the interactions between a set of agonists acting on the nicotinic receptors at the endplate region of skeletal muscle. Their findings could be best explained in terms of the following model for the activation of the nicotinic receptor by an agonist, A:

$$A + R \underset{}{\overset{K_1}{\rightleftharpoons}} AR \underset{}{\overset{K_2}{\rightleftharpoons}} AR^* \text{ (active)} \tag{1.22}$$

Here AR and AR^* refer to two interconvertible forms or *states* of the occupied receptor, inactive and fully active, respectively. Suppose that a very large concentration of the agonist A is applied, so that all the receptors become occupied, i.e., in either the AR or the AR^* state. The position of the equilibrium between AR and AR^* will then determine the magnitude of the maximal response. On this view, a weak partial agonist would be one for which the equilibrium strongly favors AR, with few receptors in the active, AR^*, state. For a full agonist, the reverse would apply.

Note that this scheme *(the del Castillo-Katz model of receptor activation)* is very different from the classical model of Hill, Clark, and Gaddum, in which no clear distinction was made between the *occupation* and the *activation* of a receptor by an agonist.

The next major advance was the introduction by E. Neher and B. Sakmann in 1976 of the single-channel recording method. This allowed the minute electrical currents passing through the ion channel intrinsic to the nicotinic receptor to be measured directly, and so provided for the first time a means of studying the activity of individual receptors *in situ* (see Chapter 7). It was quickly shown that, for a wide range of nicotinic agonists, these currents had exactly the same amplitude. What differed between the agonists was the proportion of time for which the current flowed, i.e., for which the channels were open. This is just what would be expected on the del Castillo-Katz scheme if it is assumed that the active and inactive (AR and AR*) forms of the occupied receptor are the same for different agonists. If A is a weak partial agonist, the receptor is in the AR* (open channel) state for only a small proportion of time, even if all the binding sites for A are occupied.

The next question to consider is the interpretation of efficacy (both in the particular sense introduced by Stephenson and in more general terms) in the context of the model proposed by del Castillo and Katz. This has been examined in particular detail by D. Colquhoun, whose main conclusions will now be outlined. A first requirement is to apply the law of mass action to derive a relationship between the concentration of agonist and the proportion of receptors that are in the active form at equilibrium. This proportion will be denoted by p_{AR^*}.

As in all the derivations in this chapter, there are only two steps to take. The first is to apply the law of mass action to each of the equilibria that exist (two in the present instance — see Equation 1.22). The second is to write an equation that expresses the fact that the proportions of receptors in each state that can be distinguished must add up to 1 (the "conservation rule"). In the del Castillo-Katz scheme in its simplest form there are three such states: R (vacant and inactive), AR (inactive though A is bound), and AR* (occupied and active). The corresponding proportions of receptors in these states are p_R, p_{AR}, and p_{AR*}.

Applying the law of mass action to the two equilibria:

$$[A]p_R = K_1 p_{AR} \tag{1.23}$$

$$K_2 p_{AR*} = p_{AR} \tag{1.24}$$

Also,

$$p_R + p_{AR} + p_{AR*} = 1 \tag{1.25}$$

What we wish to know is p_{AR*}, so we use Equations 1.23 and 1.24 to substitute for p_R and p_{AR} in Equation 1.25, obtaining:

$$\frac{K_1 K_2}{[A]} p_{AR*} + K_2 p_{AR*} + p_{AR*} = 1$$

$$\therefore \quad p_{AR*} = \frac{[A]}{K_1 K_2 + (1 + K_2)[A]} \tag{1.26}$$

This is the expression we require. Though it has the same general form as the Hill-Langmuir equation, there are two important differences: (1) as [A] is increased, p_{AR*} tends not to unity but to $\frac{1}{1+K_2}$. The value of K_2 will determine the maximal response to A, and only if K_2 is very small in relation to unity will all the receptors be activated; and (2) the equation gives the proportion of *active* receptors (p_{AR*}), rather than *occupied* receptors ($p_{occ} = p_{AR} + p_{AR*}$). To obtain the occupancy, we can use Equation 1.24 to express p_{AR} in terms of p_{AR*}:

$$p_{occ} = p_{AR} + p_{AR*} = (1 + K_2) p_{AR*}$$

$$= \frac{(1 + K_2)[A]}{K_1 K_2 + (1 + K_2)[A]}$$

$$= \frac{[A]}{\dfrac{K_1 K_2}{1 + K_2} + [A]} \tag{1.27}$$

This can be rewritten as

$$p_{occ} = \frac{[A]}{K_{eff} + [A]}$$

where K_{eff}, the *effective dissociation equilibrium constant** is defined by

$$K_{eff} = \frac{K_1 K_2}{1 + K_2} \qquad (1.28)$$

Hence, if the relationship between the concentration of an agonist and the proportion of receptors that it occupies is measured directly, e.g., using a radioligand binding method, the outcome should be a simple hyperbolic curve describable by the Hill-Langmuir equation. The apparent dissociation equilibrium constant for the binding will be K_{eff}, which is influenced by K_2 as well as by K_1 (see also Chapter 5).

How can we interpret efficacy in these terms? We first recall Stephenson's concept that the response of a tissue to an agonist is determined by the product, S, of the agonist's efficacy and of the proportion of receptors occupied (see Equation 1.19). To relate this to the del Castillo-Katz scheme, we rewrite Equation 1.27 to obtain a relation between p_{AR*} (which determines the response of the tissue) and total receptor occupancy:

$$p_{AR*} = \frac{1}{1 + K_2} \, p_{occ} \qquad (1.29)$$

From this we can see that the term $\frac{1}{1+K_2}$ is equivalent, in a formal sense at least, to Furchgott's intrinsic efficacy. If all the receptors are occupied, the proportion in the active state is $\frac{1}{1+K_2}$. If the agonist is very effective, i.e., if K_2 is $\ll 1$, the proportion of active receptors becomes close to unity, the upper limit. Consider next a hypothetical partial agonist which, even when occupying all the receptors ($p_{occ} = 1$), causes only half of them to be in the active form (i.e., $p_{AR*} = p_{AR} = 0.5$). From Equation 1.29, we can see that K_2 must be unity for this agonist. On Stephenson's scheme, such an agonist would have an efficacy of unity provided that the response measured is a direct indication of the proportion of activated receptors. This illustrates the close connection between efficacy and the value of K_2. However, as K_2 falls efficacy rises, suggesting that it would be better in this context to use the reciprocal of K_2, rather than K_2 itself. This reciprocal is often denoted by E, because of the relation to efficacy.

Substituting E for $1/K_2$, we can rewrite Equation 1.26 as

$$p_{AR*} = \frac{E[A]}{K_1 + (1 + E)[A]},$$

Equation 1.28 as

$$K_{eff} = \frac{K_1}{1 + E}$$

and Equation 1.29 as

$$p_{AR*} = \frac{E}{1 + E} \cdot p_{occ}$$

---

* Because K_{eff} applies to a scheme that involves more that one equilibrium (see Equation 1.22), it is referred to as a *macroscopic* equilibrium constant, to distinguish it from the *microscopic* equilibrium constants (K_1, K_2) that describe the individual equilibria.

The realization that the ability of an agonist to activate a receptor can be expressed in this way made it of the greatest interest to measure the four rate constants (two each for K_1 and E) that determine the kinetics of agonist action. The single-channel recording technique allows this to be done for ligand-gated ion channels, as described in Chapter 7. Such receptors generally carry two binding sites for the agonist, so that the relatively simple scheme just considered (Equation 1.22) has to be modified (see Equation 7.2 in Chapter 7).

A further complication encountered in such work, and indeed one likely to be met in any detailed study of the relationship between the concentration of an agonist and its action, is the occurrence of ***desensitization***. The response declines despite the continued presence of the agonist. Several factors can contribute. One that has been examined in work with "fast" receptors (ligand-gated ion channels) is that receptors occupied by agonist, and in the active state (AR*), may isomerize to an inactive, desensitized, state, AR_D. This can be represented as:

$$A + R \underset{}{\overset{K_1}{\rightleftharpoons}} AR \underset{}{\overset{K_2}{\rightleftharpoons}} AR^* \underset{}{\overset{K_3}{\rightleftharpoons}} AR_D$$
$$\text{(inactive)} \qquad \text{(inactive)} \qquad \text{(active)} \qquad \text{(inactive)}$$

As discussed in Chapter 7, quantitative studies of desensitization at ligand-gated ion channels have shown that the scheme is an oversimplification, and it is necessary to include the possibility that even the unliganded receptor may exist in a desensitized state (see Equation 7.7 in Chapter 7, and the related text).

Desensitization can occur in other ways. With G-protein-coupled receptors (Chapter 8) it can result from phosphorylation of the receptor by one or more protein kinases which become active following the application of agonist. This may be followed by the loss of some of the receptors from the cell surface.

1.4.5 CONSTITUTIVELY ACTIVE RECEPTORS: INVERSE AGONISTS

The del Castillo-Katz scheme (in common, of course, with the simpler model explored by Hill, Clark, and Gaddum) supposes that the receptors are inactive in the absence of agonist. Recent evidence suggests that some receptors (including several receptor variants created by site-directed mutagenesis — see Chapter 2) are constitutively active, i.e., they exhibit some activity even when no agonist is present. A possible explanation, in keeping with what has been learned from studies of single-channel function, is that such receptors can isomerize spontaneously to and from an active form:

$$R \rightleftharpoons R^*$$
$$\text{(inactive)} \quad \text{(active)}$$

In principle, both forms could combine with agonist, or indeed with any ligand, L, with affinity:

$$\text{(inactive)} \quad R \rightleftharpoons R^* \quad \text{(active)}$$
$$+ \qquad\qquad +$$
$$L \qquad\qquad L$$
$$K_{LR} \Big\updownarrow \qquad\qquad \Big\updownarrow K_{LR^*}$$
$$\text{(inactive)} \; LR \qquad\quad LR^* \; \text{(active)}$$

Suppose that L combines only with the inactive, R, form. Then the presence of L, by promoting the formation of LR at the expense of the other species, will *reduce* the proportion of receptors in the active, R*, state, and L is said to be an ***inverse agonist*** or ***negative antagonist.*** If, in contrast, L combines with the R* form alone, the outcome will be an increase in the proportion in the active state, and so L will behave as a conventional agonist. If, however, L has equal affinity for R and R*, its presence will not affect the fraction of receptors in the active state. It will, however, reduce the action of either a conventional or an inverse agonist, and so in effect is an antagonist.

As shown in Section 1.8 (see the solution to Problem 1.4), application of the law of mass action to this scheme provides the following expression for the proportion of receptors that are in the active state (i.e., $p_{R*} + p_{LR*}$) at equilibrium:

$$p_{\text{active}} = \cfrac{1}{1 + K\left(\cfrac{1 + \cfrac{[L]}{K_{LR}}}{1 + \cfrac{[L]}{K_{LR*}}}\right)} \tag{1.30}$$

Here the equilibrium constant K is defined by p_R/p_{R*}, K_{LR} by [L] p_R/p_{LR}, and K_{LR*} by [L] p_{R*}/p_{LR*}. Figure 1.10 plots this relationship for three hypothetical ligands which differ in their relative affinities for the active and the inactive states of the receptor. The term α has been used to express the ratio of K_{LR} to K_{LR*}. When $\alpha = 0.1$, the ligand is an inverse agonist, whereas when $\alpha = 100$ it is a conventional agonist. In the third example, with a ligand which shows no selectivity between the active and inactive forms of the receptor ($\alpha = 1$), the proportion of active receptors remains unchanged as [L] and therefore receptor occupancy is increased.

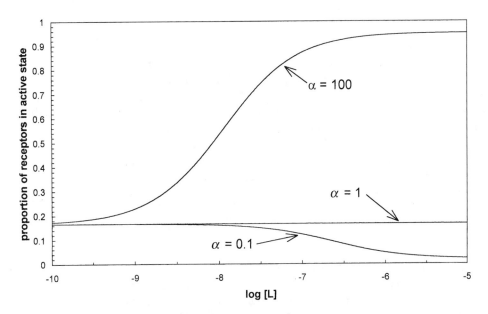

FIGURE 1.10 The relationship between the total fraction of receptors in the active state ($p_{R*} + p_{AR*}$) and ligand concentration ([L]) for a constitutively active receptor. The curve has been drawn according to Equation 1.30, using the following values: $K = 5$, $K_{LR} = 200$ nM, α (= K_{LR}/K_{LR*}) = 0.1, 1, and 100, as shown. Note that on this model some of the receptors (a fraction given by $1/(1+K) = 0.167$) are active in the absence of ligand.

1.4.6 Interpretation of Efficacy for Receptors Acting Through G-Proteins

Some of the most informative studies of partial agonism (including Stephenson's seminal work) have been done with tissues in which G-proteins (see Chapter 8) provide the link between receptor activation and the final response. In contrast to the situation with "fast" receptors with intrinsic ion channels (see above), it is not yet possible to observe the activity of individual G-protein-coupled receptors (with the potential exception of some that are linked to potassium channels). However, enough is known to show that the mechanisms involved are complex. The interpretation of differences in efficacy for agonists acting at such receptors is correspondingly less certain.

The simplest possible model for the action of such receptors is as follows:

$$A + R \underset{}{\overset{K_A}{\rightleftharpoons}} AR$$

$$AR + G \underset{}{\overset{K_{ARG}}{\rightleftharpoons}} ARG*$$

Here the agonist-receptor complex (AR) combines with a G-protein (G) to form a ternary complex (ARG*) which can initiate further events, such as the activation of adenylate cyclase.

Application of the law of mass action to the two equilibria, and the use of the "conservation rule" (see earlier, and the solution to Problem 1.3 in Section 1.8) leads to the following expression for p_{ARG*}:

$$p_{ARG*} = \frac{[G]_T [A]}{K_A K_{ARG} + \left([G]_T + K_{ARG}\right) [A]} \tag{1.31}$$

Here it has been assumed that the concentration of G does not fall as a consequence of the formation of ARG*. This would be so if the total concentration of G, $[G]_T$, greatly exceeds the concentration of receptors ($[R]_T$), so that the concentration of G could be regarded as a constant, approximately equal to $[G]_T$.

Note that Equation 1.31 is formally similar to the expression for p_{AR*} on the del Castillo-Katz scheme (see Equation 1.26) with K_1 replaced by K_A, and K_2 by $K_{ARG}/[G]_T$. If a very large concentration of A is applied, the value of p_{ARG*} asymptotes to $\frac{1}{1 + \frac{K_{ARG}}{[G]_T}}$ (cf. $\frac{1}{1 + K_2}$ on the del Castillo-Katz scheme). Thus the intrinsic efficacy of an agonist is influenced by both K_{ARG} and $[G]_T$.

However, can we really regard [G] as constant? Suppose instead that $[R]_T \gg [G]_T$, rather than the reverse. Then Equation 1.31 has to be replaced by

$$p_{ARG*} = \frac{[G]_T [A]}{K_A K_{ARG} + \left([R]_T + K_{ARG}\right)[A]} \tag{1.32}$$

Now the intrinsic efficacy of the agonist would be influenced by $[R]_T$ as well as by K_{ARG} and $[G]_T$.

Clearly, it would be best to avoid the need to have to make any assumptions about either the constancy of [G] or the relative magnitudes of $[R]_T$ and $[G]_T$. This can be done, and the outcome is a somewhat more complex expression for the concentration of ARG*, which is obtainable from the roots of the following quadratic equation:

$$[ARG*]^2 - \left(Q + [G]_T + [R]_T\right)[ARG*] + [R]_T [G]_T = 0 \tag{1.33}$$

where
$$Q = K_{ARG}\left(1 + \frac{K_A}{[A]}\right)$$

This predicts a nonhyperbolic relationship between [ARG] and [A], as well as between binding and [A]. Efficacy is determined in general by K_{ARG} and by both $[R]_T$ and $[G]_T$, with the relative importance of these concentrations depending on their respective magnitudes.

These expressions are easily extended* to include the possibility that the AR complex may have to isomerize to an active form (as in the del Castillo-Katz scheme) in order to become capable of activating the G-protein. Equations 1.31 and 1.32 then become, respectively,

$$p_{ARG^*} = \frac{[G]_T[A]}{K_A K_{AR} K_{ARG} + \left\{[G]_T + K_{ARG}\left(1 + K_{AR}\right)\right\}[A]} \tag{1.34}$$

and

$$p_{ARG^*} = \frac{[G]_T[A]}{K_A K_{AR} K_{ARG} + \left\{[R]_T + K_{ARG}\left(1 + K_{AR}\right)\right\}[A]} \tag{1.35}$$

Here K_{AR} is the isomerization constant (equivalent to K_2 in Equation 1.22). Equation 1.33 will still hold, but now with

$$Q = K_{ARG}\left\{1 + K_{AR}\left(1 + \frac{K_A}{[A]}\right)\right\}$$

Further analysis is outside the scope of this introductory account. However, it has to be mentioned that the schemes outlined, complex as they may seem, are in fact gross oversimplifications. Among factors which have been ignored are

1. The receptor combines with the G-protein in its G_{GDP} form, with the consequence that GTP can replace GDP.
2. The likelihood that some receptors are coupled to G-protein even in the absence of agonist.
3. The heterotrimeric nature of the G-protein: once activated as a consequence of combination with GTP, it dissociates into its α and $\beta\gamma$ subunits, each of which may be capable of eliciting cellular responses.
4. The dynamic nature of G-protein activation. The α-subunit can hydrolyze the GTP which is bound to it, thereby allowing the regeneration of G_{GDP}. The lifetime of individual α_{GTP} subunits will vary (cf. the lifetimes of open ion channels), adding a further complication. Moreover, some receptors are constitutively active (Section 1.4.5).
5. The possession by many cells of more than one type of G-protein, with characteristic cellular actions.

Efforts are now being made to incorporate at least some of these complexities into models of receptor activation. Such models by necessity have many disposable parameters, and require preknowledge of at least some of the rate and equilibrium constants if they are to be testable. One experimental approach is to alter the relative proportions of receptors and G-proteins, and then test whether the efficacy of agonists changes in the way to be expected on the basis of the models.

---

* For Equation 1.31 see the solution to the third problem in Section 1.8.

1.5 INHIBITORY ACTIONS AT RECEPTORS: SURMOUNTABLE ANTAGONISM

1.5.1 OVERVIEW OF DRUG ANTAGONISM

Many of the most useful drugs are antagonists, i.e., substances that reduce the action of another agent which is often an endogenous agonist (e.g., a hormone or neurotransmitter). Though the most common mechanism is simple competition, antagonism can occur in a variety of ways.

1.5.1.1 Mechanisms Not Involving the Receptor Macromolecule Through Which the Agonist Acts

1. Chemical antagonism. The antagonist combines directly with the substance being antagonized. Receptors are not involved.

   Example: the chelating agent EDTA is used to treat inorganic lead poisoning (a less toxic chelate is formed, and excreted).

2. Functional or physiological antagonism. The 'antagonist' is actually an agonist which produces an opposite biological effect to the substance being antagonized. Each substance acts through its own receptors. See also *indirect antagonism* (below)

   Example: adrenaline relaxes bronchial smooth muscle, and can thereby reduce the bronchoconstriction caused by histamine and the leukotrienes.

3. Pharmacokinetic antagonism. Here the 'antagonist' effectively reduces the concentration of the active drug at its site of action.

   Example: repeated administration of phenobarbitone induces an increase in the activity of hepatic enzymes that inactivate the anticoagulant drug warfarin. Hence if phenobarbitone and warfarin are given together, the plasma concentration of warfarin is reduced, so that it becomes less active.

4. Indirect antagonism. The antagonist acts at a second 'downstream' receptor which links the action of the agonist to the final response observed.

   Example 1. β-adrenoceptor blockers such as propranolol reduce the increase in heart rate caused by indirectly acting sympathomimetic amines such as tyramine. This is because tyramine acts by releasing noradrenaline from noradrenergic nerve endings, and the released noradrenaline acts on β-adrenoceptors to increase heart rate:

   tyramine → release of noradrenaline → β-receptor activation → response

   Another possibility is that the antagonist interferes with other postreceptor events which contribute to the tissue response.

   Example 2. Calcium channel blockers ("calcium antagonists") such as verapamil block the influx of calcium needed for smooth muscle contraction, and hence they reduce the contractile response to acetylcholine.

   Some pharmacologists prefer to describe this as a variant of functional antagonism (see above).

1.5.1.2   Mechanisms Involving the Agonist Receptor Macromolecule

The binding of agonist and antagonist is mutually exclusive. This may be because the agonist and antagonist compete for the same binding site, or combine with adjacent sites which overlap. A third possibility is that different sites are involved but that they influence the receptor macromolecule in such a way that agonist and antagonist molecules cannot be bound at the same time. This type of antagonism can take two forms:

1. The agonist and antagonist form only short-lasting combinations with the receptor, so that equilibrium between agonist, antagonist and receptors can be reached during the presence of the agonist. The interaction between the antagonist and the binding site is freely reversible. Hence the blocking action can always be surmounted by increasing the concentration of agonist which will then occupy a higher proportion of the binding sites. This is described as ***reversible competitive antagonism*** (see later).

    Example: atropine competitively blocks the action of acetylcholine on muscarinic receptors.

2. The antagonist combines irreversibly (or effectively so within the time scale of the agonist application) with the binding site for the agonist. When enough receptors have been irreversibly blocked in this way, the antagonism is ***insurmountable*** (i.e., no amount of agonist can produce a full response because too few unblocked receptors are left). Note that most pharmacologists now describe this as ***irreversible competitive antagonism***, which is the term used in this account: others have regarded it as *noncompetitive*.

    Example: phenoxybenzamine forms a covalent bond at or near the agonist binding sites on the α-adrenoceptor, resulting in insurmountable antagonism.

The agonist and the antagonist can be bound at the same time, to different regions of the receptor. This is **noncompetitive antagonism.** It is sometimes also referred to as **allotopic** antagonism (*allotopic* means "different place" in contrast to *syntopic,* meaning "same place"). In principle, noncompetitive antagonists can be either reversible or irreversible. Example: hexamethonium reversibly reduces the action of acetylcholine at the nicotinic receptor of sympathetic ganglion cells by blocking the ion channel which is intrinsic to the nicotinic receptor.

Note that the term noncompetitive is sometimes extended (quite understandably) to include forms of antagonism which do not involve the agonist receptor macromolecule (see, e.g., indirect antagonism in Section 1.5.1.1).

1.5.2 Reversible Competitive Antagonism

We start by examining how a reversible competitive antagonist (for example, atropine) alters the concentration-response relationship for the action of an agonist (for example, acetylcholine). It is found experimentally that the presence of the antagonist causes the agonist log concentration-response curve to be shifted to the right, without any change in slope or maximal response. The antagonism is *surmountable* over a wide range of concentrations. This is illustrated in Figure 1.11.

The extent of the shift is best expressed as a ***concentration ratio****. This is defined as the factor by which the agonist concentration must be increased to restore a given response in

---

* Or dose ratio — both terms are used.

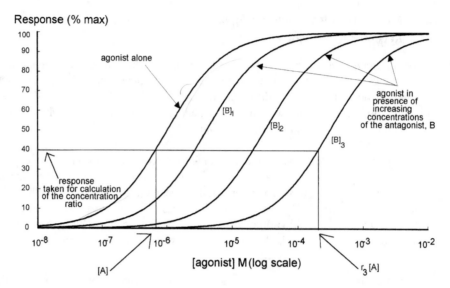

FIGURE 1.11   The predicted effect of three concentrations of a reversible competitive antagonist, B, on the response to an agonist. The calculation of the concentration ratio for the highest concentration of antagonist is also illustrated.

the presence of the antagonist. The calculation of the concentration ratio is done as follows. First, a certain magnitude of response is selected. This is often 50% of the maximum attainable, but in principle any value would do;* 40% has been taken in the illustration. In the absence of antagonist, this response is elicited by a concentration [A] of agonist. When the antagonist is present, the agonist concentration has to be increased by a factor r, i.e., to r[A]. Thus, for antagonist concentration $[B]_3$ in Figure 1.11, the concentration ratio is r_3 ($= r_3[A]/[A]$).

The negative logarithm of the concentration of antagonist which causes a concentration ratio of x is sometimes denoted by pA_x. This term was introduced by H. O. Schild as an empirical measure of the activity of an antagonist. The value most often quoted is pA_2, where

$$pA_2 = -\log [B]_{r=2}$$

To illustrate this notation we consider the ability of atropine to block the muscarinic receptors for acetylcholine. A concentration of only 1 nM makes it necessary to double the acetylcholine concentration needed to elicit a given submaximal response of a tissue. Hence $pA_2 = 9$ for this action of atropine ($-\log (10^{-9}) = 9$).

We next look at why there should be a parallel shift in the curves, and at the same time we will derive a simple but most important relationship between the amount of the shift, as expressed by the concentration ratio, and the concentration of the antagonist. We assume for simplicity that when the tissue is exposed to the agonist and the antagonist at the same time, the two drugs come into equilibrium with the binding sites on the receptor macromolecules. At a given moment an individual site may be occupied by either an agonist or an antagonist molecule, or it may be vacant. The relative proportions of the total population of binding sites occupied by agonist and antagonist are governed, just as Langley had surmised, by the concentrations of agonist and antagonist, and by the affinities of the sites for each. Because

---

* Though clearly it is sensible to avoid the extreme ends of the range. The concentration ratio can also be estimated by using a computer-aided least-squares procedure to fit the Hill equation, or some other suitable function, to each of the concentration-response curves. This also allows the parallelism of the curves to be assessed. A further possibility is to fit all the curves (i.e., with and without antagonist) simultaneously.

the agonist and the antagonist combine reversibly with the receptor, raising the agonist concentration will increase the proportion of sites occupied by the agonist at the expense of antagonist occupancy. Hence the response will increase.

We begin by assuming that both the agonist, A, and the antagonist, B, combine with their binding site according to the law of mass action, and in a way that can be represented by the two reactions below.

$$A + R \rightleftharpoons AR$$

$$B + R \rightleftharpoons BR$$

Our first task is to work out how the proportion of receptors occupied by the agonist varies with the concentrations of the agonist and the antagonist. Equilibrium is assumed. Applying the law of mass action gives

$$[A]\,[R] = K_A\,[AR]$$

$$[B]\,[R] = K_B\,[BR]$$

where K_A and K_B are the dissociation equilibrium constants for the combination of A and B, respectively, for the binding sites.

As in Section 1.2.1, these equations can be rewritten in terms of the proportions of binding sites that are free (p_R) or occupied by either A (p_{AR}) or B (p_{BR}):

$$[A]\; p_R = K_A \; p_{AR} \tag{1.36}$$

$$[B]\; p_R = K_B \; p_{BR} \tag{1.37}$$

An individual site is either vacant or occupied by an agonist or an antagonist molecule. Hence we can write

$$p_R + p_{AR} + p_{BR} = 1 \tag{1.38}$$

What we need to know is p_{AR}, so we use Equations 1.36 and 1.37 to substitute for p_R and p_{BR} in Equation 1.38:

$$\frac{K_A}{[A]} \cdot p_{AR} + p_{AR} + \frac{[B]}{K_B} \cdot \frac{K_A}{[A]} \cdot p_{AR} = 1$$

$$p_{AR} = \frac{[A]}{K_A \left(1 + \dfrac{[B]}{K_B}\right) + [A]} \tag{1.39}$$

This is the relationship we require and it embodies the "law" that Langley had inferred must exist for the action of a competitive antagonist (see Section 1.1). Termed the **Gaddum equation**, after J. H. Gaddum, it expresses how p_{AR} depends on the concentrations of A and B. If [B] is set to zero, we have the Hill-Langmuir equation (Section 1.2.1).

In order to apply this expression to the practical problem of how a competitive antagonist will affect the response to the agonist, we need to make an assumption about the relationship that exists between the response and the proportion of receptors occupied by agonist. Gaddum and Schild recognized that the best way to proceed was to assume that the same response (say 30% of the maximum attainable) corresponded to the same receptor occupancy by agonist, whether the agonist was acting alone or in the presence of the competitive antagonist. This assumption makes it unnecessary to know the exact form of the relationship between occupancy and response. This was a most important advance, however obvious it might seem in retrospect.

We can now consider an actual experiment in which a certain response, say 30% of the maximum, is elicited first by a concentration [A] of agonist acting alone, and then by a concentration r[A] when the agonist is applied in the presence of the antagonist. Here r is the concentration ratio, as already defined.

Since p_{AR} is assumed to be the same in the two situations, we can then write

$$\frac{[A]}{K_A + [A]} = \frac{r[A]}{K_A\left(1 + \dfrac{[B]}{K_B}\right) + r[A]}$$

$$= \frac{[A]}{K_A\left(\dfrac{1 + \dfrac{[B]}{K_B}}{r}\right) + [A]}$$

If the expressions on the right and the left are to take the same value, the following equality must hold:

$$\frac{1 + \dfrac{[B]}{K_B}}{r} = 1$$

Hence

$$r - 1 = \frac{[B]}{K_B} \tag{1.40}$$

This is the ***Schild equation*** which was first applied to the study of competitive antagonism by H. O. Schild in 1949. It is probably the most important single quantitative relationship in pharmacology, and has been shown to apply to the action of many competitive antagonists over a wide range of concentrations. Though originally derived (as here) on the basis of the simple scheme for receptor activation described in Section 1.2, it holds equally for the more realistic models considered in Sections 1.4.4, 1.4.5, and 1.4.6. Note also that the underlying assumption is that binding of agonists and antagonists is mutually exclusive (see Section 1.5.1.2).

One of the predictions of the Schild equation is that a reversible competitive antagonist should cause a parallel shift in the log agonist concentration response curve (as illustrated in Figure 1.11 — see also Figure 1.13). This is because for a given value of [B] and of K_B the concentration ratio, r, should also be constant, regardless of the concentration and even the identity of the agonist (provided that it acts through the same receptors as the antagonist). With a logarithmic scale, a constant value of r corresponds to a constant separation of the concentration-response curves, i.e., parallelism (because log (r[A]) – log [A] = log r + log [A] – log [A], = log r, regardless of the value of [A]).

Perhaps the most important application of the Schild equation is that it provides a way of estimating the dissociation equilibrium constant for the combination of an antagonist with its binding sites. A series of agonist concentration-response curves is established, first without and then with increasing concentrations of antagonist, and tested for parallelism. If this condition is met, the value of $(r - 1)$ is plotted against the antagonist concentration. This should give a straight line of slope equal to the reciprocal of K_B.

More usually, both $(r - 1)$ and [B] are plotted on logarithmic scales (the **Schild plot**). The outcome should be a straight line with a slope of unity, and the intercept on the x-axis provides an estimate of $\log K_B$. The basis for these statements can be seen by expressing the Schild equation in logarithmic form:

$$\log (r-1) = \log [B] - \log K_B \tag{1.41}$$

A Schild plot (based on the results of a student class practical on the effect of atropine on the contractile response of guinea-pig ileum to acetylcholine) is shown in Figure 1.12. Note that the line is straight, and its slope close to unity, as Equation 1.41 predicts.

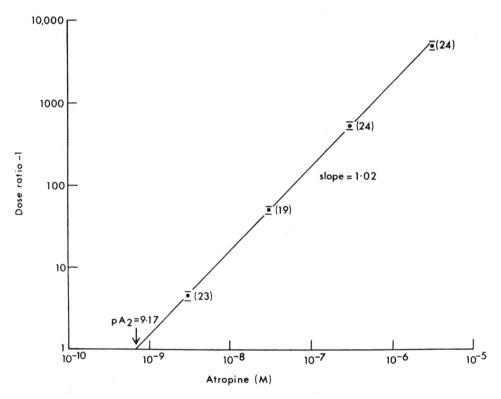

FIGURE 1.12   Schild plot for the action of atropine in antagonizing the action of acetylcholine on guinea-pig ileum. Each point gives the mean ± the standard error of the mean of the number of observations shown. From a student class experiment.

How might the value of pA_2 (see page 37) be interpreted in these terms? *If the Schild equation is obeyed,* pA_2 then gives an estimate of $-\log K_B$, because (from Equation 1.41)

$$\log (2-1) = \log (1) = 0 = \log[B]_{r=2} - \log K_B$$

$$\therefore -\log [B]_{r=2} = pA_2 = -\log K_B$$

The term pK_B is often used* to denote $-\log K_B$.

To summarize to this point, reversible competitive antagonism has the following characteristics:

1. *The action of the antagonist can be overcome by a sufficient increase in the concentration of agonist (i.e., the antagonism is surmountable).*
2. *In the presence of the antagonist, the curve relating the log of the agonist concentration to the size of the response is shifted to the right in a parallel fashion.*
3. *The quantitative relationship between the magnitude of the shift (as expressed by the concentration ratio) and the antagonist concentration obeys the Schild equation.*

1.5.3 APPLICATIONS OF THE STUDY OF COMPETITIVE ANTAGONISM

The quantitative study of competitive antagonism by the methods just described has important practical applications.

1. *The characterization and classification of receptors.* Measuring the value of K_B for the action of a well-characterized competitive antagonist can allow the identification of a particular type of receptor in a tissue or cell preparation. To illustrate, if a tissue is found to respond to acetylcholine, and if the response is antagonized by atropine with a pK_B value of about 9, then the receptor involved is likely to be muscarinic. Preferably more than one antagonist should be used, and this can then allow receptor subtypes to be identified. For example, if the response just mentioned is blocked by the muscarinic antagonist pirenzepine, with a pK_B of 7.9 to 8.5, whereas the corresponding value for the antagonist himbacine is found to be 7 to 7.2, then the receptor is very probably of the M_1 subtype.
2. *The assessment of new competitive antagonists.* The procedures developed by Gaddum and Schild have been invaluable for the development of new competitive antagonists. Examples include the H_2-receptor antagonists such as cimetidine which reduce gastric acid secretion (see below), and the $5HT_3$-receptor antagonists such as ondansetron, which can control the nausea and vomiting caused by cytotoxic drugs. These competitive antagonists, and others, were discovered by careful examination of the relationship between chemical structure and biological activity, as assessed by the methods of Gaddum and Schild. Having a reliable measure of the change in affinity (as assessed by the reciprocal of K_B) which results from modifying the chemical structure of a potential drug provides the medicinal chemist with a powerful tool with which to discover new compounds with greater activity and selectivity.
3. *The classification of agonists.* At first sight, this may seem a surprising application of a method developed primarily for the study of antagonists. However, recall that only the *ratio* of agonist concentrations appears in the Schild equation, not the actual values of the concentrations. It follows that for a given competitive antagonist acting at a fixed concentration, the concentration ratio should be the same for all agonists acting through the receptors at which the antagonist acts. So it is possible

---

* The distinction between pK_B and pA_2 is subtle but can be important. pA_2, *as Schild defined it,* is an empirical measure of the action of an antagonist, without reference to theory: it can be measured whether or not the predictions of the Schild equation have been met. Thus the intercept of a Schild plot on the abscissa gives an estimate of pA_2 even if the slope of the line is not unity. If, however, the line is adequately defined experimentally, and is straight (but has a slope which is not unity, though not differing significantly from it), it is common, and appropriate, to constrain the slope to unity. The intercept on the abscissa then provides an estimate not of pA_2 but of pK_B, as defined above. pK_B and pA_2 coincide only if the slope is exactly unity, and there are no complicating factors. If the slope of the Schild plot differs significantly from unity, so that the Schild equation does not hold, K_B cannot be estimated (unless the cause of the deviation is identified and analyzed — see later).

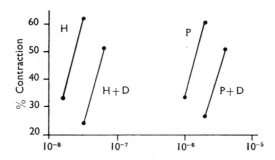

FIGURE 1.13   Responses of guinea-pig ileum to histamine (H) and pyridylethylamine (P) in the absence and presence of diphenhydramine (D, at 3.3 ng/ml). The equal shift in the lines (from H to H+D, and from P to P+D) suggests that the two agonists act on the same receptor. From O. Arunlakshana and H. O. Schild, *Br. J. Pharmacol.,* 14, 48-58, 1959. With permission.)

to test if a new agonist acts at a given receptor by examining whether the concentration ratio is the same for the agonist as it is for a well-characterized agonist known to act at that receptor. Figure 1.13, from the work of Arunlakshana and Schild, illustrates the approach. It can be seen that the competitive antagonist diphenhydramine, which acts at H_1-receptors, caused exactly the same shift (i.e., the same concentration ratio) of the log concentration-response curve for pyridylethylamine as for histamine. This strongly suggested that pyridylethylamine was acting through the same receptors as histamine, even though it is almost 100 times less active as an agonist.

The application of these principles is well illustrated by the classical work of J. W. Black and colleagues which led to the discovery of the first competitive antagonists acting at the H_2-receptors for histamine. Although the overall aim of the study was to develop compounds that would reduce gastric acid secretion in disease, much of the work was done not with secretory tissue, but with two isolated tissue preparations, guinea-pig atria and rat uterus. These could be used because they were first shown to possess histamine receptors of the same kind (H_2) as concerned in gastric acid secretion. Also, their responses to histamine (increased rate of contraction of the atria; relaxation of the rat uterus) were more easily measured than was gastric secretion. This allowed large numbers of compounds to be tested.

The successful outcome included the synthesis of burimamide, the first H_2-receptor antagonist to be tested in humans. Table 1.1 compares its ability to antagonize the actions of three agonists on guinea-pig atria: histamine, 4-methylhistamine, and 2-methylhistamine. The K_B values are almost the same, despite the varying potencies of the agonists. This suggested that all three agonists were acting through the same receptors (see 3 above).

TABLE 1.1

Comparison of the Antagonism by Burimamide of the Actions of Histamine and Two Related Agonists on Guinea-Pig Atria

Agonist	EC_{50} on guinea-pig atria	Dissociation equilibrium constant (K_B) for the blocking action of burimamide
Histamine	1.1 µM	7.8 µM
4-Methylhistamine	3.1 µM	7.2 µM
2-Methylhistamine	19.8 µM	6.9 µM

From Black, J. W. et al., *Nature,* 236, 385-390, 1972. With permission.

Table 1.2 shows that the value of K_B for blockade by burimamide of the action of histamine on the rat uterus is almost the same as for the guinea-pig atria, as would be expected were the receptors in the two tissues to be the same (see 1 above). In contrast, when burimamide was tested for its inhibitory action against the H_1-mediated contractile action of histamine on guinea-pig ileum, it was found to be approximately 40-fold less active (as judged by the apparent K_B value). Moreover, inhibition no longer conformed to the predictions of competitive antagonism. For example, the slope of the Schild plot, at 1.32, was significantly greater than unity. Further, when burimamide was tested against carbachol, which also contracts the guinea-pig ileum (though through muscarinic rather than H_1 receptors), the slope was similarly divergent, and the apparent K_B value was of the same order. This suggested that the inhibition by burimamide of the response of the ileum to both agonists was more likely to have resulted from a nonspecific depression of the tissue rather than from weak competitive antagonism at both H_1 and muscarinic receptors.

TABLE 1.2

Comparison of the Ability of Burimamide to Block the Actions of Histamine on Guinea-Pig (G.-P.) Ileum and Atrium, and on Rat Uterus

Tissue	Agonist	n_s (slope of Schild plot)	Apparent dissociation equilibrium constant (K_B) for the blocking action of burimamide
G.-P. atrium (H_2)	Histamine	0.98	7.8 μM
Rat uterus (H_2)	Histamine	0.96	6.6 μM
G.-P. ileum (H_1)	Histamine	1.32	288 μM
G.-P. ileum	Carbachol	1.44	174 μM

From Black, J. W. et al., *Nature*, 236, 385-390, 1972. With permission.

1.5.4 Complications in the Study of Competitive Antagonism

Though the predictions of competitive antagonism are often fulfilled over a wide range of agonist and antagonist concentrations, divergencies sometimes occur, and much can be learned from them. Two examples follow.

Example 1

Figure 1.14 shows two Schild plots, one of which (open circles) is far from the expected straight line of unit slope. Both sets of experiments were done with a smooth muscle preparation, the isolated nictitating membrane of the cat's eye. This tissue receives a dense noradrenergic innervation and contracts in response to noradrenaline, which was the agonist used. The adrenoceptors concerned are of the α-subtype and can be blocked by the reversible competitive antagonist phentolamine. In accounting for the nonlinear Schild plot, the key observation was that when the experiments were repeated, but with a nictitating membrane which had previously been denervated (i.e., the adrenergic nerve supply had been cut and allowed to degenerate), the concentration ratios became larger, and moreover, the Schild plot was now linear with a slope near to unity.

This suggested an explanation in terms of the presence in the normal but not the denervated muscle of the neuronal uptake mechanism (uptake$_1$) for noradrenaline. This uptake process can be so effective that when noradrenaline is added to the bathing fluid, the concentration attained in the interior of the preparation (especially if it is relatively thick) may be much less than that applied. As noradrenaline diffuses in, some of it is taken up by the adrenergic nerves, so that a large concentration gradient is maintained. In keeping with this, blockade of uptake$_1$ (for example, by cocaine) can greatly potentiate the action of noradrenaline.

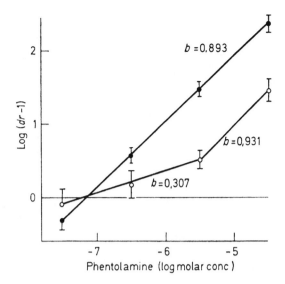

FIGURE 1.14   Schild plots for the antagonism of noradrenaline by phentolamine, studied in the isolated nictitating membrane of the cat. The values plotted are the means (± S.E. bars) for four to five experiments; (●), denervated nictitating membrane; O, normal membrane, b indicates the slope. The slope values for normal membrane were calculated for the three lowest concentrations and the two highest concentrations of phentolamine. (From R. F. Furchgott, *Handbk. Exp. Pharmacol.*, 23, 283-335, 1972, based on the results of S. Z. Langer and U. Trendelenburg, *J. Pharmacol. Exp. Ther.*, 167, 117-142, 1969. With permission.)

This is illustrated schematically in Figure 1.15. The left-most full line shows the control concentration-response curve for an adrenergically innervated tissue. The dotted line (extreme left) represents the consequence of blocking the uptake process: much lower concentrations of noradrenaline are now sufficient to elicit a given response*. The full line on the right shows the displacement of the control curve caused by the application of phentolamine, and the dotted line just to its left depicts the effect of blocking uptake when phentolamine is present. Note that this dotted line is closer to the full line than is seen with the pair of curves on the left. This is because the influence of uptake (which is a saturable process) on the local concentration of noradrenaline will be proportionately smaller when a large noradrenaline concentration is applied, as is required to restore the response in the presence of phentolamine. Hence the concentration ratio will be greater in the absence of uptake$_1$.

Example 2

Figure 1.16, like Figure 1.14, shows two Schild plots, one of which (open circles) departs greatly from the expected behavior. The deviation occurs when noradrenaline is the agonist, and again it can be accounted for in terms of the reduction in local concentration caused by the uptake$_1$ process (the tissue used, the atrium of the guinea-pig, has a dense adrenergic innervation). Isoprenaline is not subject to uptake$_1$. Accordingly, the Schild plot with this agonist is linear with a slope close to unity. In keeping with this explanation (and with the prediction that the concentration ratio should be the same for different agonists, provided that they act through the same receptors — see Section 1.5.3), blockade of uptake$_1$ by the inclusion of cocaine in the bathing fluid causes the concentration ratio for noradrenaline to increase to the same value as seen with isoprenaline as agonist.

Deviations from the expected behavior will also be seen when the antagonist has additional actions at the concentrations examined. An example is provided by the ability of the

---

* The curves in Figure 1.15 are stylized: the leftward shift which results from the blockade of noradrenaline uptake would not be expected to be exactly parallel.

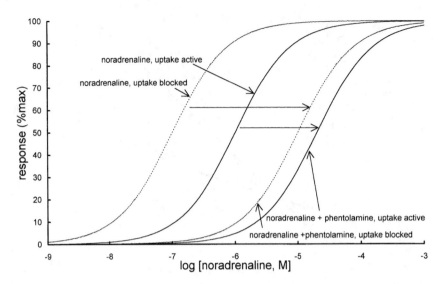

FIGURE 1.15 Hypothetical concentration-response curves to illustrate how the uptake$_1$ process can influence the study of the antagonism of noradrenaline by phentolamine. The two full lines show the response to noradrenaline, first in the absence and then in the presence of phentolamine. If the experiment is repeated, but with the uptake process blocked, the dotted lines would be obtained. Noradrenaline becomes more active, and phentolamine now causes a greater shift (compare the lengths of the two horizontal arrows) for reasons explained in the text.

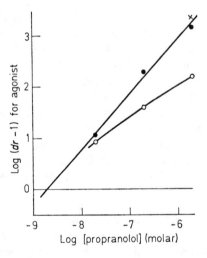

FIGURE 1.16 Schild plots for the antagonism by propranolol of the actions of noradrenaline (O) and isoprenaline (●) on the contractile force of the isolated atrium of the guinea pig; x shows the value obtained with noradrenaline as agonist, but in the presence of cocaine (20 μM). (From R. F. Furchgott, *Handbk. Exp. Pharmacol.*, 23, 283-335, 1972, based on the results of J. R. Blinks, *Ann. N.Y. Acad. Sci.*, 139, 673-685, 1967. With permission.)

reversible competitive antagonist tubocurarine to block the ion channels which open when nicotinic receptors are activated. This is described in Chapter 7, as are the complications introduced by the possession by such receptors of two agonist binding sites which may or may not have equal affinities for the antagonist. Nonlinear Schild plots can arise in many other ways. One cause is failure to allow sufficient time for the antagonist to reach equilibrium with the receptors. As discussed in Section 1.3.2, the rate of combination of a ligand with its binding sites becomes slower at lower concentrations (see Figure 1.3). Hence, if the exposure is too short, the concentration ratio will be disproportionately low at such concentrations, and the Schild plot will be steeper in this region than predicted. Nonlinear Schild plots can also result when the response of a tissue is mediated by more than one receptor with different affinities for the antagonist. These complications, and several others, have been described in the book by T. P. Kenakin whose detailed account of the analysis of competitive antagonism is recommended (see Further Reading, Section 1.9).

1.6 INHIBITORY ACTIONS AT RECEPTORS INSURMOUNTABLE ANTAGONISM

1.6.1. IRREVERSIBLE COMPETITIVE ANTAGONISM

In this form of drug antagonism, the antagonist forms a long-lasting or even irreversible combination with either the agonist binding site or a region related to it in such a way that agonist and antagonist molecules cannot be bound at the same time. *Irreversible* in this context means that the dissociation of the antagonist from its binding site is very slow (sometimes taking hours or even days) in relation to the duration of the agonist application.*

An example of an irreversible antagonist is ***phenoxybenzamine,*** which blocks α-adrenoceptors and also (though less potently) H_1-histamine receptors as well as muscarinic receptors. Its structure is shown below. Also illustrated is ***benzilylcholine mustard,*** which is an effective and selective irreversible blocker of muscarinic receptors.

phenoxybenzamine   benzilylcholine mustard

Both compounds are β-*haloalkylamines*, i.e., they contain the group

where X is a halogen atom. Once in aqueous solution, such compounds cyclize to form an unstable ethyleneiminium** ion. This is likely to have a greater affinity for the binding site

---

* Under physiological conditions, a naturally occurring agonist (e.g., a neurotransmitter) may be present for a very brief time indeed — only a millisecond or so for acetylcholine released from motor nerve endings. This is unlikely to be long enough to allow an appreciable fall in receptor occupancy by a competitive antagonist such as the neuromuscular blocking agent tubocurarine, which would therefore be effectively irreversible *on this time scale*. If, however, the interaction between acetylcholine and tubocurarine is studied in the classical pharmacological manner, in which both agents are applied for long enough for equilibrium to be reached, the antagonism then shows all the characteristics of reversible competitive antagonism (albeit with the additional feature that tubocurarine also blocks open ion channels — see Chapter 7).

** Or *ethyleneimmonium*, or *aziridinium* ion — all these terms are used.

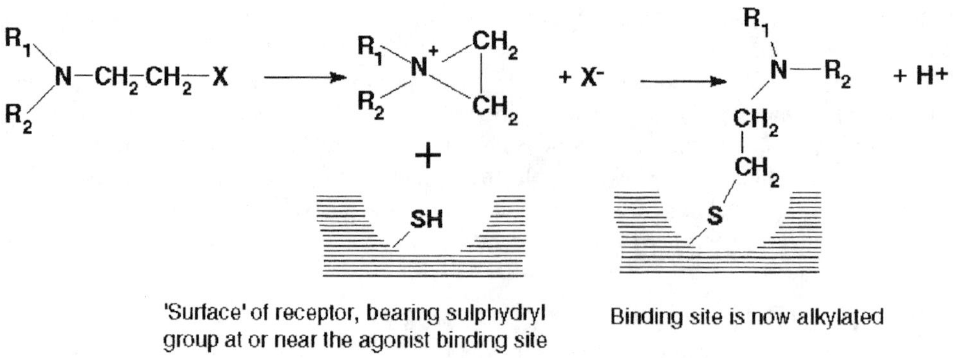

'Surface' of receptor, bearing sulphydryl   Binding site is now alkylated
group at or near the agonist binding site

FIGURE 1.17   Alkylation of a receptor by a β-haloalkylamine.

on the receptor than does the parent molecule, because an ionic bond can now be formed. When the ethyleneiminium ion first docks with the binding site, there are two possible outcomes. One is merely that after a short interval it dissociates from the site. The other is that the ethyleneiminium ring opens to create a reactive intermediate, with the consequence that a covalent bond between the drug molecule and the binding site can be formed. In effect, the receptor becomes alkylated* as illustrated in Figure 1.17.

Groups that can be alkylated in this way include –SH, –OH, = NH, and –COOH. However, not all irreversible antagonists act by forming a covalent bond. Some may 'fit' the receptor so well that the combined strength of the other kinds of intermolecular interaction (ionic, hydrophobic, Van der Waals, hydrogen bonds) that come into play approaches that of a covalent link.

1.6.2. Practical Applications of Irreversible Antagonists

1.6.2.1   Labeling Receptors

Alkylation of the kind illustrated in Figure 1.17, but using a radiolabeled ligand, provides a means of labeling the binding site(s) of receptor macromolecules.** The tissue is exposed to the labeled antagonist for long enough to allow combination with most of the receptors. It is then washed with ligand-free solution so that unbound or loosely bound antagonist can diffuse away, leaving (under ideal circumstances) only the receptors covalently labeled. A related approach is to use a photoaffinity label. This is a substance which has affinity for the receptor, and also has the property of breaking down to form a reactive intermediate following absorption of light energy of the appropriate wavelength. Light sensitivity of this kind can often be achieved by attaching an azido group ($-N_3$) to a drug molecule. The resulting photoaffinity label is allowed to equilibrate with a tissue or membrane preparation, which is then exposed to intense light. The outcome (for an azide) is the formation of a highly reactive nitrene which combines with immediately adjacent structures (including, hopefully, the binding regions of the receptor) to form covalent bonds, so 'tagging' the binding site(s).*** This can provide a first step towards receptor isolation.

---

* Possibly via the formation of a reactive carbonium ion: $R_1R_2NCH_2CH_2^+$.
** As well as β-haloalkylamines, substances with haloalkyl groups attached to carbons bonded to oxygen can be used. An interesting example is bromoacetylcholine, which acts as a "tethered agonist" acting on nicotinic receptors.
*** Some drugs are intrinsically photolabile. Examples include tubocurarine and chlorpromazine, each of which has been used to label the binding regions of receptors.

1.6.2.2   Counting Receptors

The same general procedure can be used to estimate the number of receptors in an intact tissue, provided that the specific activity (i.e., the radioactivity expressed in terms of the quantity of material) of the ligand is known. An example is the application of ^{125}I- or ^{131}I-labeled α-bungarotoxin to the determination of the number of nicotinic receptors at the endplate region of skeletal muscle. This revealed that the muscular weakness which characterizes myasthenia gravis, a disease affecting the transmission of impulses from motor nerves to skeletal muscle, results from a reduction in the number of nicotinic receptors. A variant of the technique, using α-bungarotoxin labeled with a fluorescent group, allows the nicotinic receptors to be visualized by light microscopy.

1.6.2.3   Receptor Protection Experiments

The rate at which an irreversible antagonist inactivates receptors can be slowed by the simultaneous presence of a reversible agonist or competitive antagonist which acts at the same binding site (for a quantitative account, see Chapter 5). The reversible agent, by occluding the sites, reduces the number that are irreversibly blocked within a given period: the receptors are said to be 'protected'. This can be a useful tool for the characterization of drugs as well as of receptors. For example, R. F. Furchgott (who introduced the method) tested the ability of three agonists (noradrenaline, adrenaline, and isoprenaline) to protect against the alkylating agent dibenamine (a phenoxybenzamine-like compound) applied to rabbit aortic strips. Each agonist protected the response to the other two. Thus after the tissue had been exposed to dibenamine in the presence of a large concentration of noradrenaline, followed by a drug-free washing period, adrenaline and isoprenaline as well as noradrenaline were still able to cause contraction. The same exposure to dibenamine on its own abolished the response to the subsequent application of each of the same agonists. This provided evidence that all three agonists caused contraction by acting at a common receptor (now well established to be the α-adrenoceptor subtype) which was uncertain at the time.

Another example of receptor protection, but using a competitive antagonist rather than an agonist, is provided by the ability of tubocurarine to slow the rate of binding of α-bungarotoxin at the neuromuscular junction (see Chapter 5). Note that the degree of receptor protection will depend not only on the relative concentrations of the reversible and irreversible antagonists, but also on the period allowed for their interaction with the receptors. Given enough time, a completely irreversible antagonist will eventually occupy all the receptors even in the presence of a reversible ligand.

1.6.3   Effect of an Irreversible Competitive Antagonist on the Response to an Agonist

An adequate exposure of a tissue to an irreversible antagonist results in *insurmountable antagonism* — the response cannot be fully restored by increasing the concentration of agonist, applied for the usual period. This is because an individual binding site, once firmly occupied by antagonist, is 'out of play', in contrast to the dynamic equilibrium between agonist and antagonist that is characteristic of reversible competitive antagonism. Hence it is usual in work with irreversible antagonists which form covalent bonds to apply the compound for just long enough for it to occupy the required fraction of the receptors, and then to wash the tissue with drug-free solution so that unbound antagonist can diffuse away. The change in the response to the agonist can then be studied. The results of experiments of this kind are illustrated in Figures 1.18 and 1.19.

The family of concentration-response curves in Figure 1.18 shows the effect of an alkylating agent on the contractile response of rabbit aorta to adrenaline. Note the reduction in

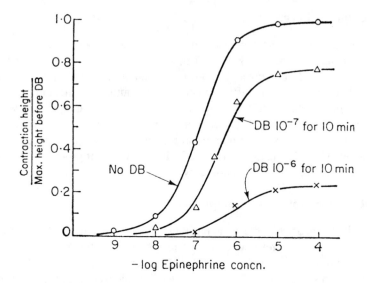

FIGURE 1.18   Effect of a 10-min exposure to different concentrations of a phenoxybenzamine-like compound, dibenamine (DB), on the contractile response of a strip of rabbit aorta to adrenaline (epinephrine in the U.S.). (From R. F. Furchgott, *Adv. Drug Res.*, 3, 21-55, 1966. With permission.)

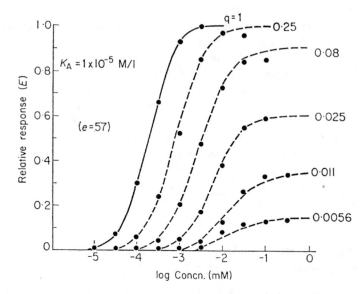

FIGURE 1.19   The effect of progressive blockade by dibenamine on the response of guinea-pig ileum to histamine. Five successive exposures to 1 μM dibenamine each for 10 min, were used, and the response to histamine was tested after each exposure. The results were analyzed as described in Section 1.6.4, and the value of q listed for each curve gives an estimate of the fraction of receptors remaining unblocked. The dashed curves were constructed from the original pre-dibenamine curve by inserting these estimates of q and also the value of K_A shown, into the equations set out in Section 1.6.4 (which see). (From R. F. Furchgott, *Adv. Drug Res.*, 3, 21-55, 1966, based on data obtained by E. J. Ariens et al., *Arch. Int. Pharmacodynamie*, 127, 459-478, 1960. With permission.)

the maximal response, the departure from parallelism, and also the fact that the exposure times as well as the concentration of the antagonist have been given for each curve.

Figure 1.19 shows the influence of the same irreversible antagonist on the contractile response of the guinea-pig ileum to histamine. The full line is the control concentration-response curve, and the dotted lines show the consequences of five successive exposures to 1 μM dibenamine, with testing of histamine after each exposure. A striking feature is that the first application of the antagonist caused an almost parallel shift of the curve. Only after further applications of dibenamine did the maximal response become smaller in the expected way (compare Figure 1.18). The most likely explanation is as follows. Although the first application of dibenamine blocked many receptors, enough remained to allow histamine (albeit at a higher concentration) to produce a full response. Only when the number of receptors had been reduced even further by the subsequent applications of dibenamine was there an appreciable fall in the maximal response attainable. The implication is that in this tissue not all the receptors have to be occupied by histamine in order to elicit a maximal response. There are, in effect, *spare receptors*. This does not of course mean that there are two kinds, 'spare' and 'used' — the receptors do not differ. However, only a few need to be activated to cause a large or even maximal response. This can occur when the response of the tissue is limited not by the receptors but by some subsequent event. For example, a piece of smooth muscle may not be able to shorten further. This maximal shortening may occur in response to a rise in cytosolic calcium that is much less than can be elicited by activating all the receptors.

The situation is different with a partial agonist (see Section 1.4.1). Inactivation of any of the receptors by, e.g., dibenamine or phenoxybenzamine will then reduce the maximal response to the partial agonist, without the initial parallel shift in the log concentration-response curve which would be seen (e.g., Figure 1.19) with a full agonist if the tissue has a substantial receptor reserve.

1.6.4 USING AN IRREVERSIBLE COMPETITIVE ANTAGONIST TO FIND THE DISSOCIATION EQUILIBRIUM CONSTANT FOR AN AGONIST

The availability of irreversible antagonists suggested a possible way to estimate the equilibrium constant for the combination of an agonist with its receptors. It was first described by R. F. Furchgott. The experimental procedure is to compare the concentrations of agonist needed to produce a selected response (say 40% of the maximum) before and after the tissue has been exposed to an irreversible antagonist. In the fresh tissue, the response is elicited by a concentration [A]; after the antagonist has acted, this has to be increased to $[A]'$. The fraction of receptors left free after the application of antagonist is denoted by q. (If only 10% of the receptors remained unblocked, q would be 0.1.)

First we recall the definition of p_{AR}, the proportion of receptors occupied by A:

$$p_{AR} = \frac{[AR]}{[R]_T}$$

where [AR] is the nominal "concentration" (number per unit membrane area) of receptors occupied by A, and $[R]_T$ refers to the total "concentration" of receptors. Hence:

$$[AR] = [R]_T \frac{[A]}{K_A + [A]}$$

from the Hill-Langmuir equation.

After the irreversible antagonist has acted, $[R]_T$ is reduced to $q[R]_T$, and a greater concentration of agonist, $[A]'$, must now be applied in order to achieve the same value of [AR] as before:

$$[AR] = q[R]_T \frac{[A]'}{K_A + [A]'}$$

Furchgott then went on to assume that the same (submaximal) response of the tissue before and after antagonist corresponds to the same receptor occupancy by the agonist.* Hence he equated

$$[R]_T \frac{[A]}{K_A + [A]} = q[R]_T \frac{[A]'}{K_A + [A]'}$$

Canceling $[R]_T$, and inverting, gives

$$\frac{K_A}{[A]} + 1 = \frac{1}{q} \frac{K_A}{[A]'} + \frac{1}{q}$$

$$\frac{1}{[A]} = \frac{1}{q} \frac{1}{[A]'} + \frac{1}{K_A} \left(\frac{1}{q} - 1 \right)$$

Hence a plot of $1/[A]$ against $1/[A]'$ should give a straight line with a slope of $1/q$ and an intercept of $(1 - q)/q.K_A$. The value of q is obtained from the reciprocal of the slope, and that of K_A from (slope − 1)/intercept.

Applying this method to the results of Figure 1.19, Furchgott estimated K_A to be 10 μM for the combination of histamine with its receptors. He used this figure, and the values of q obtained as just described, to construct the dashed curves in the illustration. These lie close to the experimental points, which is certainly in keeping with the validity of the treatment which has been outlined, though equally certainly not providing decisive proof that it is correct. A key assumption, and one that is difficult to test, is that the irreversible antagonist has had no action other than to inactivate the receptors under study. Were it, for example, to have interfered with one or more of the steps that link receptor activation to the observed response, the approach would be invalid.

Furchgott therefore sought further evidence, and devised the ingenious experiment illustrated in Figure 1.20. He began by using the method just described to determine the dissociation equilibrium constant for the combination of a partial agonist, pilocarpine, with the muscarinic receptor subserving contraction in smooth muscle. He then exposed the tissue to the irreversible antagonist (dibenamine) for a second time, to a point at which there was no longer an appreciable response to pilocarpine. However, the muscarinic agonist carbachol (carbamoylcholine), which has a much higher efficacy than pilocarpine, was still able to elicit a small response. This allowed him to use pilocarpine again, but this time as a competitive antagonist of carbachol. Hence he could obtain a second estimate of the dissociation equilibrium constant for the combination of pilocarpine with the receptors. This should of course agree with the first one, and in fact the agreement was satisfactory, as can be seen from the similarity between the values for K_A and K_B given in Figure 1.20. However, the method is limited to partial agonists.

We can now return to the experiment of Figure 1.19. In the fresh tissue, the concentration of histamine needed to produce a half-maximal contraction was about 180 nM. The value of K_A was estimated to be 10 μM, as we have seen. We can substitute these figures in the Hill-Langmuir equation to obtain a value for the receptor occupancy needed to elicit half the maximal response. This comes to only 0.0177: there is a large receptor reserve. Furchgott went one step further and used this value to obtain an estimate of the efficacy of histamine, in the sense used by Stephenson. Since the response is half maximal, the "stimulus" as defined

---

* Note that this assumption was made in relation to the classical model (Hill, Clark, Gaddum) of receptor action, which does not distinguish clearly between receptor *occupation* and *activation* by an agonist. This is considered further at the end of the section.

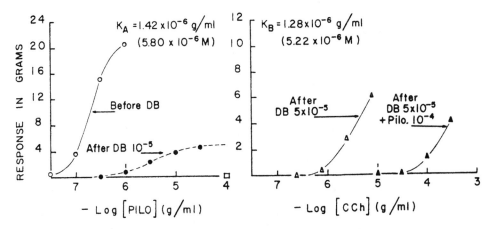

FIGURE 1.20 Comparison of the dissociation equilibrium constant of pilocarpine (pilo) as agonist (K_A) with that of the same drug as an antagonist (K_B) for parasympathetic receptors of stomach muscle. Paired strips from the fundus of same stomach were used. Concentration-response data for pilocarpine were obtained before and after incubation with 1×10^{-5} dibenamine (DB) for 20 min. In the graph on the left, concentration-response data for the first strip are plotted. From these data a q value of 0.0078 and the K_A value shown were calculated. The dashed curve is the theoretically predicted curve for this q value. Both strips were then incubated with 5×10^{-5} g/ml dibenamine for 20 min, after which there was no detectable response to pilocarpine, (indicated by □ in graph on left). Concentration-response data were then obtained for carbamoylcholine (CCh) on both strips. After washout, pilocarpine (1×10^{-4} g/ml) was added only to the second strip for 15 min and concentration-response data were again obtained for CCh on both strips. The graph on the right shows log concentration-response curves of the second strip to CCh in absence and in presence of pilocarpine. (The position of the first curve has been corrected for a small shift to the right exhibited by the curves of the first strip which had no pilocarpine and served as a control.) The dissociation equilibrium constant of pilocarpine as an antagonist (K_B) was calculated from the dose ratio corresponding to the displacement of the two curves shown. (From R. F. Furchgott and P. Bursztyn, *Ann. N.Y. Acad. Sci.,* 139, 882, 1967. With permission.)

by Stephenson is unity, so that the efficacy is $1/0.0177 = 57$, the value given in Figure 1.19 (see also Method 3 in Section 1.4.3).

As already mentioned, Furchgott's procedure as it was originally described is based on the classical model of Hill, Clark, and Gaddum. If instead we assume that receptor activation requires two steps (first occupation and then activation of the receptor — see Equation 1.22 in Section 1.4.4), and then follow Furchgotts's arguments, as set out above, we find that a plot of $1/[A]$ against $1/[A]'$ should give a straight line, as before. However, as shown in the second of the worked examples in Section 1.8, the value of (slope – 1)/intercept of the line now gives, not K_A as in the classical model, but

$$K_{\text{eff}} = \frac{K_1 K_2}{1 + K_2}$$

Only if K_2 is very large in relation to unity (i.e., were A to be a very weak partial agonist) does K_{eff} approximate to K_1.

Note that a direct radioligand measurement (in the absence of desensitization and other complicating factors) would also yield an estimate of K_{eff}, and not K_1 (see also Chapter 5).

1.6.5 REVERSIBLE NONCOMPETITIVE ANTAGONISM

In this variant of insurmountable antagonism, the antagonist acts by combining with a separate inhibitory site on the receptor macromolecule. Agonist and antagonist molecules can be bound

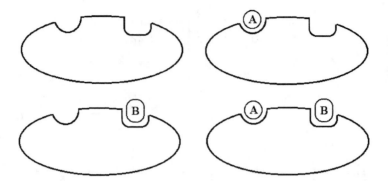

FIGURE 1.21 Noncompetitive antagonism. A stylized receptor carries two sites, one of which can combine with agonist (A) and the other with antagonist (B). There are four possible states, only one of which (agonist site occupied, antagonist site empty — see upper right) is active.

at the same time, though the receptor becomes active only when the agonist site alone is occupied (Figure 1.21).

In the presence of a large enough concentration of an antagonist of this kind, the antagonism will become insurmountable: not enough activatable receptors will remain to give a full response, even if all the agonist sites are occupied. The point at which this occurs in a particular tissue will depend on the numbers of spare receptors, just as with an irreversible competitive antagonist (see Section 1.6.3). If a full agonist is used, and the tissue has a large receptor reserve, the first effect of a reversible noncompetitive antagonist will be to shift the log concentration-response curve to the right. Eventually, when no spare receptors remain, the maximum will be reduced. In contrast, if there is no receptor reserve, the antagonist will depress the maximum from the outset.

If we apply the law of mass action to this form of antagonism, the proportion of the inhibitory sites occupied by the antagonist will be given by the Hill-Langmuir equation:

$$p_{BR} = \frac{[B]}{K_B + [B]}$$

Hence the proportion free of antagonist will be

$$1 - p_{BR} = \frac{K_B}{K_B + [B]}$$

If we assume for simplicity that each receptor macromolecule carries one agonist and one antagonist (inhibitory) site, the proportion of the receptors in which the agonist site is occupied is also given by the Hill-Langmuir equation. However, only a fraction of these agonist-combined receptor macromolecules are free of antagonist, and so able to initiate a response. To obtain the proportion in this state we simply multiply the fraction that is occupied by agonist by the fraction free of antagonist:

$$p_{active} = \frac{[A]}{K_A + [A]} \cdot \frac{K_B}{K_B + [B]} \tag{1.42}$$

Figure 1.22 shows log concentration-response curves drawn according to this equation. In A, the response has been assumed to be directly proportional to the fraction of receptors which are active (p_{active}): there are no spare receptors. In B, spare receptors have been assumed to

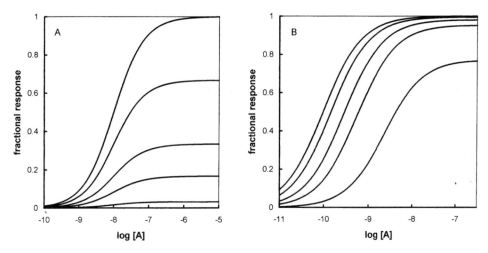

FIGURE 1.22 The effect of a reversible noncompetitive antagonist. Each of the sets of curves has been constructed using Equation 1.42, and shows the effect of four concentrations of the antagonist (5, 20, 50, and 300 µM). K_A has been taken to be 10 nM, and K_B to be 10 µM. For A, the response has been assumed to be directly proportional to the proportion of receptors in the active state. B has been drawn using the same values, but now assuming the presence of spare receptors. This has been modeled by supposing that the relationship between the response, y, and the proportion of active receptors is given by $y = \frac{1.01 \times p_{active}}{0.01 \times p_{active}}$, so that a half-maximal response occurs when just under 1% of the receptors are activated.

be present, and accordingly the presence of a relatively low concentration of the antagonist causes an almost parallel shift before the maximum is reduced.

The initial near-parallel displacement of the curves in Figure 1.22B raises the question of whether the Schild equation would be obeyed under these conditions. If we consider the two concentrations of agonist ([A] and r[A], respectively, where r is the concentration ratio) that give equal responses before and during the action of the antagonist, and repeat the derivation set out in Section 1.5.2 (though using Equation 1.42 rather than 1.39) we find that the expression equivalent to the Schild equation is

$$r - 1 = \frac{[B]}{K_B}\left(1 + \frac{r[A]}{K_A}\right)$$

If $r[A]/K_A \ll 1$ (i.e., if the proportion of receptors occupied by the agonist remains small even when the agonist concentration has been increased to overcome the effect of the reversible noncompetitive antagonist) this expression approximates to

$$r - 1 = \frac{[B]}{K_B}$$

Hence the Schild equation *would* apply, albeit over a limited range of concentrations which is determined by the receptor reserve. Moreover, the value of K_B obtained under such conditions will provide an estimate of the dissociation equilibrium constant for the combination of the antagonist with its binding sites.

A corollary is that a demonstration that the Schild equation holds over a small range of concentrations must not be taken as proof that the action of the antagonist under study is competitive. Clearly, as wide as practicable a range of antagonist concentrations should be tested, especially if there is evidence for the presence of spare receptors.

Open channel block. Studies of the action of ligand-gated ion channels have brought to light an interesting and important variant of reversible noncompetitive antagonism. It has been found that some antagonists block only those channels that are open, by entering and occluding the channel itself. In effect, the antagonist combines only with activated receptors. Examples include the block of neuronal nicotinic receptors by hexamethonium, and of *N*-methyl-D-aspartate receptors by dizocilpine (MK801).

Such antagonists cause a characteristic change in the log concentration-response curve for an agonist. In contrast to what is observed with the other kinds of antagonism so far considered, the value of $[A]_{50}$ will become *smaller* rather than larger in the presence of the antagonist. This is illustrated in Figure 1.23, and is best understood in terms of the del Castillo-Katz model of receptor action (Section 1.4.4). Incorporating the possibility that an antagonist, C, is present which combines specifically with active receptors, we have

$$A + R \rightleftharpoons AR \rightleftharpoons AR^* + C \rightleftharpoons AR^*C$$
$$\text{(inactive)} \quad \text{(inactive)} \quad \text{(active)} \quad \text{(inactive)}$$

Hence there are four states of the receptor, R, AR, AR*, and AR*C, of which only AR* is active. This scheme predicts that at equilibrium* the proportion of active receptors is given by

$$p_{AR^*} = \frac{[A]}{K_1 K_2 + \left(1 + K_2 + \dfrac{[C]}{K_C}\right)[A]} \tag{1.43}$$

where K_c is the dissociation equilibrium constant for the combination of C with the activated receptor, AR*. This equation has been used to draw the curves shown in Figure 1.23. Note how $[A]_{50}$ decreases as the antagonist concentration is increased. In effect, the combination of the antagonist with AR* causes a rightward shift in the positions of the other equilibria expressed in Equation 1.43.

Note, too, the convergence of the curves plotted in Figure 1.23 at low agonist concentrations. The antagonist becomes less active, because there are fewer receptors in the AR* form available to combine with C. Again, in contrast to the other kinds of antagonism that have been described, there is no initial parallel displacement of the curves (even if there are many spare receptors) and the Schild equation is never obeyed.

Some antagonists combine the ability to block open ion channels with a competitive action at or near the agonist binding site. A well-characterized example is the nicotinic blocker tubocurarine, as described in Chapter 7. Agonists may also be open channel blockers, so limiting the maximal response that they can elicit. Such agents (e.g., decamethonium) may therefore behave as partial agonists when tested on an intact tissue.**

The scheme illustrated in Figure 1.21 assumes that the accessory site is inhibitory. It is now known that some agonists (e.g., glutamate) may only be effective in the presence of another ligand (e.g., glycine in the case of glutamate receptors) which binds to its own site on the receptor macromolecule. Under this circumstance, glutamate is referred to as the ***primary agonist***, and glycine as a ***co-agonist***. In principle, an antagonist could act by competing with either the primary agonist or the co-agonist. These interactions can be analyzed by the methods already outlined but are beyond the scope of the present chapter.

---

* See Chapter 7 for an account of the kinetics of open channel block.
** As noted in Section 1.4.4, the characterization of a substance as a partial agonist does not presuppose a particular mechanism for its failure to elicit a maximal effect.

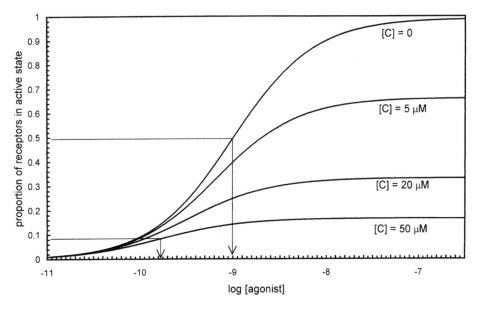

FIGURE 1.23 Curves drawn using Equation 1.43 to illustrate the effect of three concentrations of an open channel blocker, C, on the response to an agonist acting on a ligand-gated ion channel. Values of 0.1, 0.01, and 10 μM were taken for K_1, K_2, and K_C, respectively. The vertical arrows show the concentrations of agonist causing a half-maximal response in the absence and presence of C at 50 μM.

1.7 CONCLUDING REMARKS

Modeling the action of receptors in the ways outlined in this chapter has been, and is likely to remain, a powerful tool. In particular, it has allowed the actions of drugs to be better described, quantified, and analyzed. Nevertheless, it should not be overlooked that each of the key advances in the understanding of receptor action has come not from modeling and equation-writing (informative as this can be) but rather from new experimental techniques such as the radioligand binding method, single-channel recording, and most recently, the procedures of molecular biology which allow the structure of receptors not only to be established but also modified in precise ways by site-directed mutagenesis. These and other advances are the subjects of the chapters that follow.

1.8 PROBLEMS

PROBLEM 1.1

A competitive antagonist (B) is applied to a tissue and produces a concentration ratio r_B. A second competitive antagonist (C) acting at the same receptors produces a concentration ratio r_C, under identical conditions. The tissue is now exposed to both antagonists together, at the same concentrations as in the separate applications.

What will the new concentration ratio, r_{B+C}, be in terms of r_B and r_C?

PROBLEM 1.2

Show that on the following scheme for receptor action (see Section 1.4.4), Furchgott's

$$A + R \xrightleftharpoons{K_1} AR \xrightleftharpoons{K_2} AR^* \quad \text{(active)}$$

irreversible antagonist method (Section 1.6.4) for measuring the dissociation equilibrium constant for the combination of an agonist with its binding sites will estimate

$$K_{eff} = \frac{K_1 K_2}{1 + K_2}$$

PROBLEM 1.3

What quantity would Furchgott's method (Section 1.6.4 and Problem 1.2 above) estimate if the occupied receptor, AR, has first to isomerize to a second form, AR* which then attaches to another entity, such as a G-protein, in order to elicit a response? Assume that the G-protein is present in great excess in relation to the "concentration" of receptors.

PROBLEM 1.4

Derive Equation 1.30 (Section 1.4.5), which expresses how the proportion of receptors in the active form varies with the concentration of a ligand for a receptor with constitutive activity.

1.9 FURTHER READING

General

More detailed accounts of much of the material in this chapter can be found in three excellent books:

Kenakin, T.P., *Pharmacologic Analysis of Drug-Receptor Interaction,* 2nd ed., Raven Press, New York, 1993.

Limbird, L.E., *Cell Surface Receptors: A Short Course on Theory and Methods,* 2nd ed., Martinus Nijhoff, Boston, 1996.

Pratt, W.B. and Taylor, P., *Principles of Drug Action,* Churchill Livingstone, New York, 1990 (see in particular Chapters 1 and 2).

Early work, now of mainly historical interest

The application of the law of mass action to the kinetics of drug-receptor interaction.

Hill, A.V., The mode of action of nicotine and curari, determined by the form of the contraction curve and the method of temperature coefficients, *J. Physiol.,* 39, 361-373, 1909.

The Hill equation

Hill, A.V., The possible effects of the aggregation of the molecules of haemoglobin on its dissociation curve, *J. Physiol.,* 40, iv-vii, 1910.

A.J. Clark's modeling of the concentration-response relationship.

Clark, A.J., The reaction between acetylcholine and muscle cells, *J. Physiol.,* 61, 530-547, 1926.

The Gaddum equation

Gaddum, J.H., The quantitative effect of antagonistic drugs, *J. Physiol.,* 89, 7-9P, 1937.
Gaddum, J.H., The antagonism of drugs, *Trans. Faraday Soc.,* 39, 323-332, 1943.

The pA scale

Schild, H.O., pA — a new scale for the measurement of drug antagonism, *Br. J. Pharmacol.,* 2, 189-206, 1947.

The Schild equation

Schild, H.O., pA$_x$ and competitive drug antagonism, *Br. J. Pharmacol.,* 4, 277-280, 1949.
Schild, H.O., Drug antagonism and pA$_x$, *Pharmacol. Rev.,* 9, 242-246, 1957.

Efficacy

Stephenson, R.P., A modification of receptor theory, *Br. J. Pharmacol.,* 11, 379-393, 1956.
Colquhoun, D., Affinity, efficacy and receptor classification: is the classical theory still useful?, in *Perspectives on Receptor Classification*, Black, J.W., Jenkinson, D.H., and Gerskowitch, V.P., Eds., Alan R. Liss, New York, 1987, chap. 11.
Samama, P., Cotecchia, S., Costa, T., and Lefkowitz, R.J., A mutation-induced activated state of the β$_2$-adrenergic receptor: extending the ternary complex model, *J. Biol. Chem.,* 268, 4625-4636, 1993.

Examples of the practical application of Schild's approach

Arunlakshana, O. and Schild, H.O., Some quantitative uses of drug antagonists, *Br. J. Pharmacol.,* 14, 48-58, 1959.
Black, J.W., Duncan, W.A.M., Durant, C.J., Ganellin, C.R., and Parsons, E.M., Definition and antagonism of histamine H$_2$-receptors, *Nature,* 236, 385-390, 1972.

Additional example of analysis of deviations from the Schild equation

Black, J.W., Leff, P., and Shankley, N.P., Further analysis of anomalous pK$_B$ values for histamine H$_2$-receptor antagonists on the mouse isolated stomach assay, *Br. J. Pharmacol.,* 86, 581-587, 1985.

Application of irreversible antagonists (determination of K_A for agonists, receptor protection experiments)

Furchgott, R.F., The use of β-haloalkylamines in the differentiation of receptors and in the determination of dissociation constants of receptor-agonist complexes, *Adv. Drug Res.,* 3, 21-55, 1966.

Recent example of use of receptor protection technique

Eglen, R.M. and Harris, G.C., Selective inactivation of muscarinic M$_2$ and M$_3$ receptors in guinea-pig ileum and atria *in vitro, Br. J. Pharmacol.,* 109, 946-952, 1993.

1.10 SOLUTIONS TO PROBLEMS

PROBLEM 1.1

We have three experimental situations to consider:

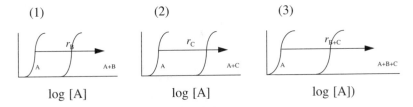

(1) and (2) are straightforward (see Section 1.5.2) whereas (3) breaks new ground.

When B and C are applied together, as in (3) above, and the agonist A is also present, there will be three simultaneous equilibria (at least in principle):

$$A + R \rightleftharpoons AR$$

$$B + R \rightleftharpoons BR$$

$$C + R \rightleftharpoons CR$$

Applying the law of mass action:

$$[A]p_R = K_A p_{AR}$$

$$[B]p_R = K_B p_{BR}$$

$$[C]p_R = K_C p_{CR}$$

Also (see Section 1.5.2), $p_R + p_{AR} + p_{BR} + p_{CR} = 1$
From these equations,

$$p_{AR} = \frac{[A]}{K_A\left(1 + \dfrac{[B]}{K_B} + \dfrac{[C]}{K_C}\right) + [A]}$$

Hence, equating equal receptor occupancies by the agonist (at which it is assumed that the responses would also be equal), first in the absence of any antagonist and then in the simultaneous presence of B and C:

$$\frac{[A]}{K_A + [A]} = \frac{r_{B+C}[A]}{K_A\left(1 + \dfrac{[B]}{K_B} + \dfrac{[C]}{K_C}\right) + r_{B+C}[A]}$$

$$\frac{[A]}{K_A + [A]} = \frac{[A]}{K_A\left(\dfrac{1 + \dfrac{[B]}{K_B} + \dfrac{[C]}{K_C}}{r_{B+C}}\right) + [A]}$$

$$\frac{1 + \dfrac{[B]}{K_B} + \dfrac{[C]}{K_C}}{r_{B+C}} = 1$$

$$r_{B+C} - 1 = \frac{[B]}{K_B} + \frac{[C]}{K_C}$$

$$r_{B+C} - 1 = \left(r_B - 1\right) + \left(r_C - 1\right)$$

$$\therefore\ r_{B+C} = r_B + r_C - 1$$

This relationship has been used to obtain evidence that two antagonists act at the same site.

PROBLEM 1.2

It was shown in Section 1.4.4 that on this model the proportion of activated receptors is given by

$$p_{AR*} = \frac{[A]}{K_1 K_2 + (1 + K_2)[A]}$$

Recalling that p_{AR*} is defined as $[AR*]/[R]_T$, we can rewrite this as

$$[AR*] = \frac{[R]_T [A]}{K_1 K_2 + (1 + K_2)[A]}$$

If the tissue is now exposed for a fixed period to an irreversible antagonist, so that the "concentration" of receptors is reduced, it will afterwards become necessary to increase the agonist concentration in order to restore a previous value of $[AR*]$. Hence if we consider the agonist concentrations, $[A]$ and $[A]'$, (respectively, that elicit the same response before and after the inactivation of some of the receptors, and if we assume that this response corresponds to equal concentrations of activated receptors, we can write

$$\frac{[R]_T [A]}{K_1 K_2 + (1 + K_2)[A]} = \frac{q[R]_T [A]'}{K_1 K_2 + (1 + K_2)[A]'}$$

where q is the fraction of receptors remaining after the action of the irreversible antagonist.

Canceling $[R]_T$, and inverting (as in Section 1.6.4), we have

$$\frac{1}{[A]} = \frac{1}{q} \frac{1}{[A]'} + \left(\frac{1 + K_2}{K_1 K_2}\right)\left(\frac{1}{q} - 1\right)$$

Hence the slope of a plot of $1/[A]$ against $1/[A]'$ (will be $1/q$, and the quantity estimated by (slope $-$ 1)/intercept will be

$$\frac{K_1 K_2}{1 + K_2}$$

PROBLEM 1.3

Here the scheme for receptor activation is

$$A + R \underset{}{\overset{K_A}{\rightleftarrows}} AR \underset{}{\overset{K_{AR}}{\rightleftarrows}} AR* + G \underset{}{\overset{K_{ARG}}{\rightleftarrows}} AR*G* \qquad (1.44)$$

(inactive)   (inactive)   (active but uncoupled)   (active and coupled)

There are three equilibria, and applying the law of mass action to each gives

$$[A]p_R = K_A p_{AR}$$

$$p_{AR} = K_{AR} p_{AR*}$$

$$[G]p_{AR*} = K_{ARG} p_{AR*G*}$$

Also,

$$p_R + p_{AR} + p_{AR*} + p_{AR*G*} = 1 \tag{1.45}$$

Using the three mass law equilibrium equations to substitute for p_R, p_{AR}, and p_{AR*} in this expression, we obtain

$$p_{AR*G*} = \frac{[G]_T[A]}{K_A K_{AR} K_{ARG} + \left\{[G]_T + K_{ARG}\left(1 + K_{AR}\right)\right\}[AR]} \tag{1.46}$$

It has been assumed here that G is present in such excess that its total concentration $[G]_T$ does not fall appreciably when AR*G* is formed. [G] in the mass law equation can therefore be replaced by $[G]_T$.

If we now consider Furchgott's experiment, and make the same assumptions as in the answer to Problem 1.2, we can write

$$\frac{[R]_T[G]_T[A]}{K_A K_{AR} K_{ARG} + \left\{[G]_T + K_{ARG}\left(1 + K_{AR}\right)\right\}[A]} = \frac{q[R]_T[G]_T[A]'}{K_A K_{AR} K_{ARG} + \left\{[G]_T + K_{ARG}\left(1 + K_{AR}\right)\right\}[A]'}$$

Here, just as before, [A] and [A]′ are the concentrations of the agonist A that produce the same response (assumed to correspond to the same concentrations of receptors in the active, AR*G*, form) before and after reducing the total "concentration" of receptors from $[R]_T$ to $q[R]_T$.

Canceling $[R]_T$, and inverting, we obtain

$$\frac{1}{[A]} = \frac{1}{q}\frac{1}{[A]'} + \left(\frac{[G]_T + K_{ARG}\left(1 + K_{AR}\right)}{K_A K_{AR} K_{ARG}}\right)\left(\frac{1}{q} - 1\right)$$

Hence a plot of 1/[A] against 1/[A]′ should again give a straight line of slope 1/q, and the quantity estimated by (slope −1)/intercept would be

$$\frac{K_A K_{AR} K_{ARG}}{[G]_T + K_{ARG}\left(1 + K_{AR}\right)}$$

This is just what would be estimated by a direct ligand binding experiment were this scheme for receptor occupation and activation to apply.

PROBLEM 1.4

The model is

$$\text{(inactive)} \quad R \overset{K}{\rightleftharpoons} R* \quad \text{(active)}$$

$$+ \qquad +$$

$$L \qquad L$$

$$K_{LR} \big\Updownarrow \qquad \big\Updownarrow K_{LR*}$$

$$\text{(inactive) LR} \qquad \text{LR* (active)}$$

from which we see that there are three equilibria to consider. Applying the law of mass action to each, we have

$$p_R = K \; p_{R*}$$

$$[L]p_R = K_{LR} \; p_{LR}$$

$$[L]p_{R*} = K_{LR*} \; p_{LR*}$$

where the equilibrium constants K, K_{LR}, and K_{LR*} are as defined in Section 1.4.5. Also,

$$p_R + p_{R*} + p_{LR} + p_{LR*} = 1$$

By using the mass law equilibrium expressions to substitute for p_R, p_{R*}, and p_{LR} in the last equation, we obtain

$$p_{LR*} = \frac{[L]}{[L] + K_{LR*} + K \cdot K_{LR*}\left(1 + \dfrac{[L]}{K_{LR}}\right)} .$$

From this, and using the third of the equilibrium expressions, we also have

$$p_{R*} = \frac{K_{LR*}}{[L] + K_{LR*} + K \cdot K_{LR*}\left(1 + \dfrac{[L]}{K_{LR}}\right)}$$

What we wish to know is the total fraction of receptors in the active state,

$$p_{active} = p_{R*} + p_{LR*}$$

$$= \frac{[L] + K_{LR*}}{[L] + K_{LR*} + K \cdot K_{LR*}\left(1 + \dfrac{[L]}{K_{LR}}\right)}$$

$$= \frac{1}{1 + K\left(\dfrac{1 + \dfrac{[L]}{K_{LR}}}{1 + \dfrac{[L]}{K_{LR*}}}\right)}$$

This derivation has followed the same general procedure applied throughout this chapter. Another route is instructive:

$$p_{active} = p_{R*} + p_{LR*}$$

$$= \frac{[R^*] + [LR^*]}{[R^*] + [LR^*] + [R] + [LR]}$$

$$= \frac{1}{1 + \left(\dfrac{[R] + [LR]}{[R^*] + [LR^*]}\right)}$$

Considering just the term in brackets, and making use of the three equilibrium equations, we have

$$\frac{[R] + [LR]}{[R^*] + [LR^*]} = \frac{[R]}{[R^*]} \left(\frac{1 + \dfrac{[LR]}{[R]}}{1 + \dfrac{[LR^*]}{[R^*]}} \right) = K \left(\frac{1 + \dfrac{[L]}{K_{LR}}}{1 + \dfrac{[L]}{k_{LR^*}}} \right)$$

Hence Equation 1.30 has been derived.

Section II

Molecular Structure of Receptors

2 Molecular Structure of G-Protein-Coupled Receptors

Thue W. Schwartz

CONTENTS

0-8493-9227-6/96/$0.00+$.50
© 1996 by CRC Press, Inc.

2.1. G-PROTEIN-COUPLED RECEPTORS CONSTITUTE A UNIFYING SIGNAL TRANSDUCTION MECHANISM

2.1.1 GTP BINDING PROTEINS ACT AS TRANSDUCERS BETWEEN RECEPTORS AND EFFECTOR SYSTEMS

In 1969 it was suggested by Martin Rodbell and co-workers that a series of hormones, all of which stimulated adenylate cyclase, acted by binding to specific receptors, "discriminators", which were linked to intracellular adenylate cyclase, the "amplifier", through a so-called "transducer" system. The common transducer for all of these hormones was subsequently characterized as being one of several heterotrimeric guanine nucleotide binding proteins, G-proteins. In the signal transduction mechanism, receptor activation leads to an exchange of GDP with GTP in the G-protein, which becomes active and can stimulate various intracellular effector systems until its GTPase activity hydrolyzes GTP to GDP and turns the system off again (see Chapter 8). Besides adenylate cyclase, a number of amplifiers or effector systems like phospholipases and phosphodiesterase, as well as ion channels, are regulated by the G-protein subunits in a sophisticated signal-processing system. The number of hormone receptors as well as receptors for other chemical messengers acting through G-proteins is now known to be very large. It is clear that G-protein-coupled receptors constitute one of the major signal transduction systems in eukaryotic cells.

2.1.2 A LARGE SUPERFAMILY OF PROTEINS WITH SEVEN-TRANSMEMBRANE (7TM) SEGMENTS

Rhodopsin, the light-sensing molecule which binds the chromophore retinal was the first G-protein-coupled molecule to be cloned. The most conspicuous structural feature of this photoreceptor was the seven hydrophobic segments believed to constitute seven-transmembrane helices — in analogy to the seven-transmembrane helices of the proton pump, bacteriorhodopsin. When the β-adrenoreceptor, the first neurotransmitter/hormone receptor, was subsequently cloned, this protein turned out to be surprisingly homologous with rhodopsin and to have a similar overall structure, with seven-transmembrane segments. The subsequent characterization of a multitude of different receptors has demonstrated that, independent of the chemical nature of the natural ligand, all G-protein-coupled receptors are members of a gigantic superfamily of 7TM proteins. Although most of the receptors have turned out to be homologous with rhodopsin, several distantly related families of receptors were discovered with the only apparent common structural feature being the seven hydrophobic segments.

2.1.3 A MULTITUDE OF VERY DIFFERENT CHEMICAL COMPOUNDS ACT THROUGH 7TM RECEPTORS

The number of cloned and characterized G-protein-coupled receptors are counted in hundreds and the number of different types of 7TM receptors which are expressed, for example, in humans is presumably several hundred. The spectrum of hormones, neurotransmitters, paracrine mediators, etc. which act through G-protein-coupled receptors includes all kinds of chemical messengers: **ions** (calcium ions acting on the parathyroid and kidney chemosensor; plus possibly other chemical sensors), **amino acids** (glutamate and γ-amino butyric acid — GABA), **monoamines** (catecholamines, acetylcholine, serotonin, etc.), **lipid messengers** (prostaglandins, thromboxane, anandamide [endogenous cannabinoid], platelet activating factor, etc.), **purines** (adenosine and ATP), **neuropeptides** (tachykinins, neuropeptide Y, endogenous opiates, cholecystokinin, vasoactive intestinal polypeptide [VIP], plus 30 to 40 others), **peptide hormones** (angiotensin, bradykinin, glucagon, calcitonin, parathyroid hormone, etc.),

chemokines (interleukin-8, fMFL [formyl-Met-Phe-Leu], RANTES, etc.), **glycoprotein hormones** (TSH, LH/FSH, choriongonadotropin, etc.), as well as **proteases** (thrombin). In sensory systems, G-protein-coupled receptors are involved both as the light-sensing molecule in the eye, **rhodopsin,** and as several hundred distinct **odorant receptors** in the olfactory system and in sperm cells.

2.2   G-PROTEIN-COUPLED RECEPTORS ARE SEVEN-HELICAL-BUNDLE PROTEINS EMBEDDED IN THE CELL MEMBRANE

The problem of characterizing the three-dimensional structure of G-protein-coupled receptors by X-ray crystallography or NMR has been particularly difficult to solve. The receptors are complicated membrane proteins which are hard to produce in sufficiently large quantities; and when they have been available it has been impossible to make them form useful crystals. However, through cryoelectron microscopic analysis of two-dimensional membrane crystals, it has been possible to construct electron density maps of both bacteriorhodopsin and of bovine rhodopsin — a real G-protein-coupled protein. The two structures exhibit some similarities, but are also significantly different. It should be noted that bacteriorhodopsin is a proton pump and not a G-protein-coupled receptor, and that there is no real sequence similarity between bacteriorhodopsin and rhodopsins. However, both protein structures are folded as seven helical bundles. The electron density map of rhodopsin is shown in Figure 2.1 along with a helical wheel diagram interpretation. Since side chains are not yet obvious in the cryoelectron microscopic pictures of rhodopsin, we cannot assign the individual helices to the individual electron densities. In fact, we do not even know whether the helices are oriented in a clockwise or an anticlockwise fashion. Nevertheless, there is evidence to support the notion that transmembrane segment III is the central helix in the bundle and that the helices are placed in an anticlockwise fashion as viewed from outside the cell (Figure 2.1). This basic principle of helix packing is employed in many molecular models which are currently used to try to understand the structure and functional aspects of 7TM receptors.

It should also be noted that even though these characterizations will become more detailed in the coming years, at present we still only have static pictures. In the future, the dynamic interchange between different conformations of these proteins needs to be understood. This question is starting to be addressed through different biophysical means, for example, experiments using spin-labels, fluorescent probes, etc.

2.3   THERE ARE SEVERAL FAMILIES OF G-PROTEIN-COUPLED RECEPTORS

Most of the G-protein-coupled receptors are homologous with rhodopsin. However, other quantitatively minor families, as well as some individual receptors, do not share any of the structural features common to the rhodopsin family; for example, the glucagon/VIP/calcitonin receptor family, the metabotropic glutamate receptor family, yeast pheromone receptors, or the Dictyostelium cAMP receptor (Figure 2.2).

Thus, the only structural feature that all G-protein-coupled receptors have in common is the seven-transmembrane helical bundle. Nevertheless, most non-rhodopsin-like receptors have certain minor structural features in common with the rhodopsin-like receptors; for example, a disulfide bridge between the top of TM-III and the middle of extracellular loop 3, and a cluster of basic residues located just below TM-VI.

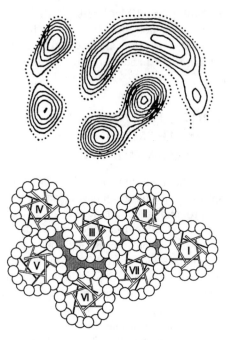

FIGURE 2.1 Electron density map of bovine rhodopsin obtained through cryoelectron microscopy analysis of two-dimensional membrane crystals. The lower figure shows a helical-wheel diagram. TM-III is believed to be the main, middle helix and the rest of the seven-helical bundle arranged anticlockwise as viewed from outside the cell. The helices are rotated relative to each other and shifted vertically in order to optimize interactions, as deduced from structure-function studies in various receptor systems. (Redrawn from Schertler, G.F., Villa, C., and Henderson, R., *Nature,* 362, 770, 1993; and Baldwin, J.M., *EMBO J.,* 12, 1693, 1993. With permission.)

2.3.1 G-Protein-Coupled Receptors Have Evolved Through Divergent and Convergent Evolution

The evolutionary tree for rhodopsin-like receptors indicates that they have evolved both as a consequence of selection for coupling to different G-proteins and selection for reaction with different ligands. However, these two developments would appear to have occurred independently and through different mechanisms. Subtypes of receptors which bind the same ligand generally have evolved within a given branch of the tree through ordinary **divergent evolution** (see, for example, D2, D3, and D4 dopamine receptors and the muscarinic receptors in Figure 2.3). However, subtypes of receptors are also frequently found in separate branches of the tree. Aminergic (i.e., binding monoamines) receptors are examples of how receptors that couple to a particular G-protein, but bind different ligands, can be more homologous to each other than receptor subtypes which bind the same transmitter. Thus, it appears that the ability to bind, for example, dopamine, has evolved in different evolutionary branches of G-protein-coupled receptors, which through divergent evolution had already segregated from each other (see D1 and D5 vs. D2, D3, and D4 in Figure 2.3). Similarly, histamine H_1 and H_2 receptors are only approximately 20% identical in their transmembrane segments and are, in fact, more similar to receptors that bind acetylcholine and adrenergic ligands, respectively. Apparently, receptors have picked up the same ligand in different evolutionary branches — **convergent evolution**.

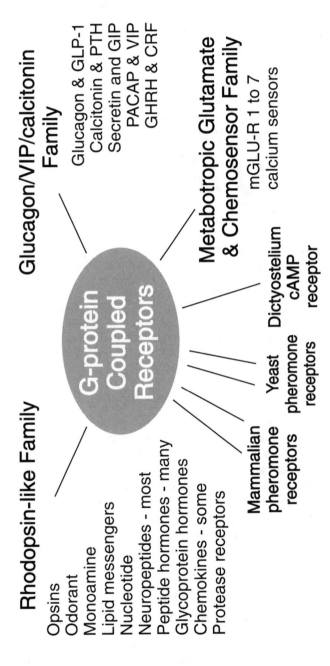

FIGURE 2.2 The three main families of mammalian G-protein-coupled receptors in mammals. No obvious sequence identity is found between the rhodopsin-like family, the glucagon/VIP/calcitonin family, and the metabotropic glutamate/chemosensor family of G-protein-coupled receptors, with the exception of a presumed disulfide bridge between the top of TM-III and the middle of extracellular loop 2 (see Figures 2.4 and 2.5). Similarly, there is no sequence identity between members of these three families and, for example, the yeast alpha- and a-factor receptors and the Dictyostelium cAMP receptor. Bacteriorhodopsins, which are not G-protein-coupled proteins but proton pumps, are totally different in respect to amino acid sequence but have a seven-helical bundle arranged rather similarly to the G-protein-coupled receptors.

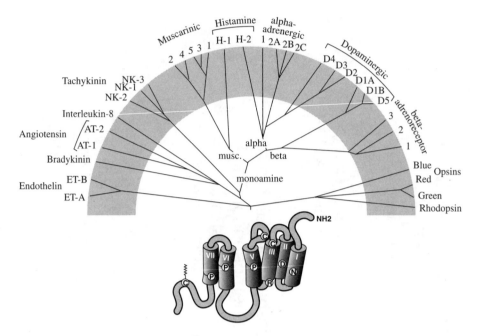

FIGURE 2.3 Part of an evolutionary tree for rhodopsin-like 7TM receptors. Only a few branches of the tree are shown to highlight certain principles. The sequence similarity scale starting at the center of the tree is not linear and does not start at zero. All rhodopsin-like receptors are at least 15 to 20% homologous; for example, rhodopsin compared with the monoamine receptors or rhodopsin compared with peptide receptors. The shaded area indicates more than 70% sequence identity which covers most receptor subtypes. Note that certain receptor subtypes appear to originate from different branches (here: histamine, dopamine, and angiotensin), indicating a possible convergent evolution during which receptors may have picked up ligands. (From Donally, D., Findlay, J.B.C., and Blundell, T.L., *Receptors and Channels,* 2, 61, 1994, and supplementary material from D. Donally.)

2.3.2 Subtypes of Receptors Have Evolved For Several Reasons

For many hormones and transmitters there are several subtypes of receptors. As discussed above, structurally these subtypes of receptors may or may not be very similar. However, the different subtypes usually all bind the natural ligand with high affinity, and originally they were identified mainly by means of their different reactions with synthetic agonists and antagonists. In some cases the functional significance of receptor subtypes is rather obvious; for example, receptor subtypes frequently give the transmitter or hormone the opportunity to couple through different G-proteins and thereby activate different effector systems. However, in many cases the functional significance of receptor subclasses is more subtle — for example, where subtypes only display slight differences in desensitization properties or differences in their ability to be constitutively active (see below).

2.4 RHODOPSIN-LIKE 7TM RECEPTORS — THE QUANTITATIVELY DOMINATING FAMILY

The archetype of G-protein-coupled receptors is the rhodopsin-like receptor. A series of 'fingerprint' residues, most of which are located within the transmembrane segments, have been conserved among the rhodopsin-like receptors, as indicated in Figure 2.4. These fingerprint residues are conserved in 95 to 98% of the receptors and any given receptor will contain most of them. Nevertheless, among all rhodopsin-like G-protein-coupled receptors only one single residue is totally conserved: ArgIII:26 at the intracellular pole of TM-III. This residue is believed to be involved in signaling to the G-protein (see below).

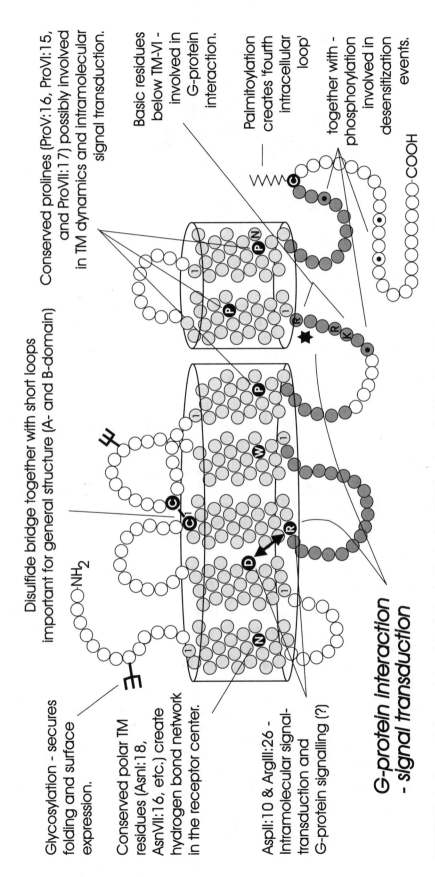

FIGURE 2.4 Structural characteristics of the rhodopsin-like family of 7TM receptors. Residues located in the transmembrane helices are shaded light gray. The subunits of the G-proteins are believed to interact mainly with residues located in the segments which are shaded dark gray. The precise delineation of the transmembrane segments (TM) is obviously unclear, however in each of the segments several residues are conserved among the family members. The key fingerprint residues of each helix are highlighted: AsnI:18, AspII:10, CysIII:01, ArgIII:26, TrpIV:06, ProV:16, ProVI:15, and ProVII:17.

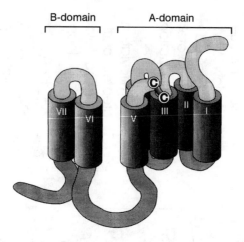

FIGURE 2.5 The possible structural and functional division of rhodopsin-like 7TM receptors into an A- and a B-domain. The A-domain is defined by a series of short loops conserved in absolute length, yet not conserved in amino acid sequence. An obligatory disulfide bridge between the top of the central TM-III column and the middle of extracellular loop 2 creates two extra loops which presumably ensure a close interaction between TM-IV and especially TM-V and TM-III. The loop between TM-VI and -VII in the B-domain is also short, whereas the loop between the two putative domains, connecting TM-V and -VI, is not conserved in length and can in fact be very long, for example, in certain monoamine receptors.

2.4.1 A Conserved Disulfide Bridge Creates Two Extra Loops From the Top of TM-III

One of the most highly conserved features among 7TM receptors is the disulfide bridge between the Cys at the top of TM-III and a Cys situated somewhere in the middle of the second extracellular loop. This loop is thereby transformed into two loops connecting the top of TM-III with the top of both TM-VI and -V. These two "extra" loops tie up TM-IV and -V close to TM-III, which generally is considered to be the central column in the seven-helical bundle. In the ACTH and MSH receptors, this disulfide bridge is absent. However, in these cases only two hydrophilic residues separate TM-IV and -V, which is just another way of holding TM-V closely together with the rest of the A-domain (see Figure 2.5).

2.4.2 A Network of Relatively Short and Well-Conserved Loops Define Two Domains

Despite the fact that the amino acid sequence of 7TM receptors is rather poorly conserved, especially outside the transmembrane segments, the *length* of most of the loops is surprisingly well conserved. The loops connecting TM-I and -II and TM-II and -III are short and of almost the same length in all rhodopsin-like receptors, despite great variance in the actual amino acid sequences. As discussed above, the conserved disulfide bridge creates two short loops which tether TM-IV, and especially TM-V, close together with the first three transmembrane segments. The two C-terminal transmembrane segments, TM-VI and -VII, are also connected by a shorth intracellular loop of approximately ten residues. However, the loop connecting TM-V and TM-VI is remarkably poorly conserved in respect of both sequence and length, and is often relatively long — sometimes up to several hundred residues. Thus, it appears that the rhodopsin-like receptors are structurally composed of two intramolecular domains, held together by a network of relatively short loops — an A-domain consisting of TM-I through TM-V and a B-domain consisting of TM-VI and -VII (Figure 2.5). In fact, the two hypothetical domains can form a fully functional split-receptor upon coexpression of two plasmids, which each codes for one of the domains.

2.4.3 SOME RECEPTORS HAVE DISULFIDE-RICH, LIGAND-BINDING N-TERMINAL DOMAINS

The N-terminal extracellular segment is very variable both in length and sequence. In the subfamily of receptors which binds the glycoprotein hormones TSH, FSH/LH, and chorion-gonadotropin, this segment is very long and contains a set of conserved cysteines which are expected to form a network of disulfide bridges, thus creating a well-defined, globular domain. In this subfamily of receptors, the glycoprotein hormones obtain most of their binding energy by interaction with the large N-terminal domain which, in some cases even in a truncated soluble form, is capable of binding the hormone.

2.4.4 GLYCOSYLATION IS IMPORTANT FOR PROTEIN FOLDING AND INTRACELLULAR TRANSPORT

Nearly all 7TM receptors are glycosylated. Usually several Asn-X-Thr/Ser recognition sequences for N-linked glycosylation are found in the amino-terminal segment, but occasionally also elsewhere. The glycosylation is not directly important for ligand binding. However, as is the case for most other membrane proteins expressed at the cell surface, the glycosylation appears to be a posttranslational modification which, through recognition by specific proteins in the endoplasmic reticulum, ensures that the protein is retained in the cellular export machinery until it is correctly folded.

2.4.5 CONSERVED PROLINE IN THE TM SEGMENTS MAY BE OF FUNCTIONAL IMPORTANCE

Due to the fact that the pyrrolidine ring of the imino acid proline involves the backbone nitrogen, it prevents the formation of one of the stabilizing hydrogen bonds in the α-helix backbone. Thus, prolines rarely occur in α-helices in globular proteins. Nevertheless, proline residues are among the well-conserved fingerprint residues in several of the transmembrane helices. In the static 2D crystal structure of bacteriorhodopsin, prolines in several but not all cases cause a kink in the transmembrane helix. The conserved prolines in TM-V, -VI, and -VII of the 7TM receptors will create weak points in these helices. Thus, it may be speculated that the proline residues serve an important role in the dynamic function of the receptors, possibly by facilitating the interchange between different conformations or by allowing the otherwise very stable transmembrane helices to wobble in order for ligands and G-protein subunits to associate and dissociate.

2.4.6 G-PROTEINS BIND TO SEVERAL INTRACELLULAR LOOPS IN AN AS YET ILL-DEFINED WAY

There is no real consensus sequence for G-protein binding to the receptors. However, based on competition experiments with synthetic peptides corresponding to the intracellular parts of receptors and mutational mapping experiments, it is thought that intracellular loops 2 and 3 and the first part of the C-terminal tail are especially important for G-protein interaction. It is mainly the part of the loops closest to the membrane that are involved. It has been possible to differentiate between segments which are important only for high affinity binding, and segments which convey specificity in the G-protein association. Rather few details are yet known, but in certain receptor systems it is clear that the segment just below TM-V in intracellular loop 3 determines the selective binding of a particular type of G-protein. Another important epitope in the same loop is the segment just below TM-VI which is particularly rich in positively charged amino acid residues — through which the G-protein may induce the high affinity conformation of the receptor. In several systems, mutations in this area of the receptor lead to a phenotype which includes increased constitutive activity (see below) and high affinity for agonists. One hypothesis suggests that this part of intracellular loop 3 in the resting state is held in a conformationally constrained state which is released upon ligand binding, and that it is the loose, unfolded conformation of the loop which is recognized by the G-protein.

2.4.7 AN ARG SWITCH BELOW TM-III MAY CONVEY THE SIGNAL TO THE G-PROTEIN

The totally conserved Arg residue located just below TM-III is probably, in some crucial way, involved in the signal transduction process. In one model, the signal is believed to be conveyed by a conformational interchange of the guanidino function of this Arg between an *internal position* in the receptor structure (conceivably up towards the highly conserved acidic residue in TM-II and the surrounding hydrogen bond network) and an *external position*, in which it would interact with the G-protein.

2.4.8 IONS CAN ALLOSTERICALLY INFLUENCE THE LIGAND AFFINITY

A series of relatively well-conserved polar residues, for example Asn in TM-I and TM-VII and Asp in TM-II, are believed to form a hydrogen-bond network in the center of the receptors facing towards the intracellular surface of the membrane. In several receptors, cations (especially Na^+) will modulate the binding affinity of the agonist, presumably through an interaction with the hydrogen-bond network relatively deep in the middle of the receptor. Most ligands are believed to bind either to the exterior part of the receptor or between the outer parts of the transmembrane segments, depending on the size and chemical structure of the ligand (see below). The effect of the cations is, therefore, considered to be allosteric in nature.

2.4.9 PHOSPHORYLATION IS INVOLVED IN DESENSITIZATION EVENTS

Stimulation of the receptor will, in many cases, lead to phosphorylation of Thr and Ser residues in the intracellular loop 3 and in the C-terminal tail. At least two types of kinases are involved in this process, PKA (protein kinase A) which is regulated by cAMP, and βARK-like enzymes (β-adrenergic receptor kinases) which are relatively specific for 7TM receptors and especially modify residues in the C-terminal tail. The recognized consequence of phosphorylation is desensitization or downregulation of the receptor (see below). However, it should be noted that the functional consequences of the phosphorylation vary considerably among the receptors and, for example, can be dependent upon which type of G-protein is involved in the coupling process.

2.4.10 PALMITOYLATION IN THE C-TERMINAL TAIL CREATES AN EXTRA INTRACELLULAR LOOP

In many 7TM receptors a single or a couple of Cys residues are located 15 to 20 residues C-terminally to TM-VII. In several cases it has been demonstrated that palmitoylation occurs at this position. The covalently coupled fatty acid will associate this point of the tail closely with the membrane and thereby create a fourth intracellular loop. Like the phosphorylation event, the palmitoylation process appears to be dynamically regulated by receptor occupancy and is also involved in the desensitization phenomenon. The two posttranslational modifications can influence each other. For example, the conformational constraint induced by palmitoylation may alter the accessibility of certain phosphorylation sites. Like the phosphorylation process, the functional consequences of palmitoylation also appear to vary from receptor to receptor.

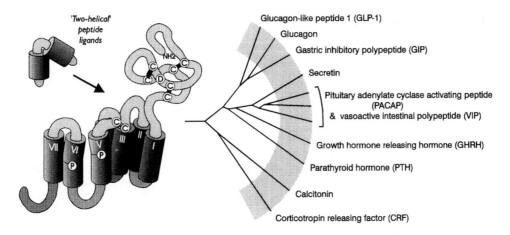

FIGURE 2.6   The glucagon/VIP/calcitonin family of 7TM receptors. On the right is an evolutionary tree for the receptors of this family. The shaded area indicates 70% sequence identity. Most of the peptides appear to have a common secondary structure and will fold into a characteristic two-helical conformation at low water activity, as determined by NMR experiments. Only a few of the common fingerprint residues of this family are indicated in the serpentine model. Note that members of this family do not share any of the TM fingerprint residues of the rhodopsin-like family. However, they do have the potential to form a disulfide bridge from the top of TM-III and the middle of extracellular loop 2. Also, they have some conserved prolines in the TM segments but not at positions corresponding to the prolines of the rhodopsin-like family.

2.5   A DISTINCT FAMILY OF GLUCAGON/VIP/CALCITONIN 7TM RECEPTORS

Receptors for a series of peptide hormones and neuropeptides constitute a separate family of G-protein-coupled receptors devoid of the classical fingerprint residues of rhodopsin-like receptors, as shown in Figure 2.6. This family includes receptors for hormones involved in calcium metabolism (calcitonin and parathyroid hormone — PTH), glucose metabolism (glucagon; glucagon-like peptide I — GLP-I), gastrointestinal tract function (secretin; gastric inhibitory polypeptide — GIP) as well as neurohormones involved in pituitary function (growth hormone releasing factor — GHRH; ACTH releasing factor — CRF) and important neuropeptides (vasoactive intestinal polypeptide — VIP; pituitary adenylate cyclase stimulatory peptide — PACAP). In view of the physiological importance of these peptides, it is likely that receptors of this family will become major targets for the development of non-peptide drugs in the years to come.

Besides their seven-transmembrane segments, the most conspicuous common feature among these receptors is their large extracellular N-terminal domain. This segment contains a set of six conserved Cys residues, conceivably interconnected by a number of disulfide bridges, thus forming a globular domain supposedly involved in ligand binding (Figure 2.6). Two more Cys residues, at the top of TM-III and in the middle of extracellular loop 2, are also conserved and could form a disulfide bridge similar to the one found in the rhodopsin-like receptors. The first extracellular loop is variable in length and can be up to 30 residues long. As in the large rhodopsin-like family, a number of proline residues are conserved in the transmembrane segments of the glucagon/VIP/calcitonin-like receptors (Figure 2.6). However, in this family the prolines are located in TM-IV, -V, and -VI and not in TM-VII. In TM-V and -VI the prolines are located at different positions from the conserved prolines of the rhodopsin-like receptors. All receptors from this family stimulate adenylate cyclase and, therefore, couple through a Gs protein. The coupling mechanism including the Gs molecule appears to be shared with rhodopsin-like receptors, despite the lack of sequence homology. In addition, some of these receptors may also activate other effector systems.

2.6 A THIRD FAMILY OF METABOTROPIC GLUTAMATE RECEPTORS AND CHEMOSENSORS

Members of another family of G-protein-coupled receptors, which are not homologous to rhodopsin, either bind glutamate or they act as chemical sensors for calcium ions. Glutamate is an important excitatory amino acid in the nervous system, reacting both with a family of ligand-gated ion channels (see Chapter 3) and also with a series of G-protein-coupled receptors called metabotropic glutamate receptors. Among the chemical sensors known to couple through G-proteins, the calcium sensors of the parathyroid and the kidney are homologous to the metabotropic glutamate receptors.

Structurally, these receptors are characterized by an unusually large (500 to 600 residues) N-terminal extracellular segment and frequently also by a similarly large intracellular C-terminal domain separated by a domain of 7TM segments. The transmembrane segments are connected by short loops and differ totally in sequence from the other families presented above. Interestingly, the large extracellular domains bear some resemblance to a family of bacterial binding proteins that function as transporters for amino acids and other small molecules across the periplasmic space. X-ray structures of several of these proteins are known. Molecular models and mutational analysis support the notion that glutamate binds between two large subdomains in the extracellular N-terminal segment of the metabotropic receptor, analogous to the binding of amino acids in the bacterial transport proteins.

2.7 THERE ARE MULTIPLE *AGONIST* BINDING MODES IN 7TM RECEPTORS

It was initially believed that there would be a common "lock" on all the receptors into which all agonists in some way would fit. It was envisioned that in the different 7TM receptors this lock had, during evolution been specifically equipped to recognize the specific agonists. However, as shown in Figure 2.7, mutational analysis of the receptors has demonstrated that the chemically very different ligands apparently bind in rather different fashions. Unfortunately, most of our knowledge on ligand-receptor interactions is based on loss-of-function experiments, i.e., mutations or substitutions which impair binding or coupling. In fact, very few of these presumed points of interaction have been studied in greater detail using alternative, supplementary methods.

2.7.1 MONOAMINES AND OTHER SMALL MESSENGERS BIND BETWEEN THE TRANSMEMBRANE SEGMENTS

Retinal is known to attach to the ε-amino group of a lysine residue located in the middle of transmembrane segment VII and to make a Schiff-base interaction with a glutamate residue located at the top of TM-III in rhodopsin (GluIII:04). In the adrenergic system, the specific and direct interaction of the amine group of the ligand with the carboxylic group of a totally conserved aspartic acid residue in transmembrane segment III (AspIII:08) has been substantiated in great detail through the combined use of molecular biology and medicinal chemistry. The interaction was first probed both by destroying the binding and activation of the receptor by mutating the Asp to a Ser (converting the carboxylic acid to a hydroxyl group) and by destroying the binding of the ligand by changing the amine to a ketone or an ester. However, in contrast to the wild-type receptor, the receptor which had a serine residue in place of the aspartate in TM-III bound ligands with ketones or esters in place of the amine with high

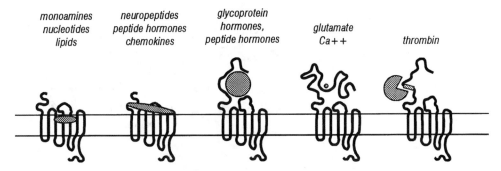

monoamines   neuropeptides   glycoprotein
nucleotides   peptide hormones   hormones,   glutamate
lipids   chemokines   peptide hormones   Ca++   thrombin

FIGURE 2.7   Overview of different patterns of ligand binding to 7TM receptors shown schematically in two-dimensional serpentine models. There appear to be multiple different ways for ligands to bind and activate 7TM receptors, conceivably because these agonists primarily serve only to stabilize an active conformation which the receptor can fold into by itself. In the thrombin receptor, shown on the right, the enzyme cleaves the N-terminal segment and discloses an oligopeptide (gray box), which then activates the receptor while it is still covalently tethered to the transmembrane domain.

affinity. In other words, the specific interaction between the amine and the carboxylic acid group of the receptor could be reintroduced by an intelligent, complementary modification of both the ligand and the receptor: a double revertant experiment. Unfortunately, it has not yet been possible to substantiate other interactions in 7TM receptors by similar deliberate knowledge-based experiments of the gain-of-function type. Thus, most points of interaction and molecular models are based mainly on more or less indirect evidence.

However, the currently favored picture of the binding of adrenalin to the β-adrenoreceptor is that the ligand binds in a pocket between TM-III, -V, and -VI. The amine of the ligand interacts with the carboxylic acid group of the conserved Asp in TM-III, whereas the catechol ring is oriented through hydrogen-bond interactions with two serine residues at the top of TM-V, while the ring itself makes an aromatic-aromatic interaction with a phenylalanine residue in TM-VI (Figure 2.8). Acetylcholine, histamine, dopamine, serotonin, and the other amines are believed to bind in a similar fashion by making interactions with residues located at corresponding or neighboring positions in their target receptors.

2.7.2   PEPTIDES BIND IN SEVERAL MODES WITH MAJOR INTERACTION SITES IN THE EXTERIOR PARTS

The large glycoprotein hormones achieve most of their binding energy by interaction with the large N-terminal segment of their receptors. Medium and small neuropeptides and peptide hormones usually have major points of interaction located in the N-terminal segment of their receptors. However, additional contact points have been identified in the loops and around the outer portion of the transmembrane segments. In some cases, such as the angiotensin AT–1 receptor, a picture is emerging where the contact points, which are scattered in the primary structure, appear to be located in close spatial proximity in a folded molecular model of the receptor (Figure 2.9). For smaller peptides like TRH and the chemoattractant formyl peptide, it appears that most of the interaction points are located deeper in the receptor, relatively close to where the contact points for the monoamines are found.

An interesting case is the thrombin receptor, where the ligand is part of the N-terminal segment of the receptor as such. Thrombin will bind and cleave off most of this segment and thereby disclose or reveal the free N-terminus of a small pentapeptide which is still covalently bound to the rest of the receptor. This peptide will interact with other parts of the exterior of the receptor and thereby activate it (Figure 2.7). Thus, this receptor has a shielded or caged peptide ligand already covalently tethered to the N-terminal segment. It could be imagined that several other peptides act as pseudotethered ligands, which by initial interaction with

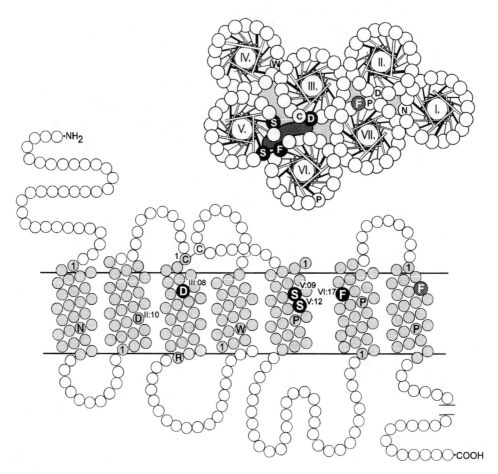

FIGURE 2.8 Binding site for catecholamines in the adrenergic receptors. The main contact residues for norepinephrine are indicated in white on black. The monoamine *agonist*, indicated as a dark gray oval in the helical wheel diagram, is believed to interact with: AspIII:08, SerV:09, SerV:12, and PheVI:17. The chemical interaction between the amine group of the monoamine ligand and the carboxylic acid group of AspIII:08 has convincingly been demonstrated by combined modifications of the receptor by mutagenesis and complementary modifications of the ligand performed by medicinal chemistry. In white on darker gray is indicated an important interaction point for monoamine *antagonists* in TM-VII, i.e., residue VII:06, which in the beta-adrenoreceptor is a Phe.

the N-terminal segment of their target receptors become pseudotethered and then, through secondary interactions with the main domain of the receptor, complete the activation process.

2.8 *ANTAGONIST* MAY BIND LIKE THE AGONISTS OR THEY MAY BIND VERY DIFFERENTLY

Originally it was suggested that competitive antagonists would bind to the same site as the agonists and function simply by hindering the agonist from binding to the receptor. During the last couple of years it has become clear that antagonists, whether or not they behave in a classical competitive manner, may act independent of the agonist. In other words, antagonism is a property in itself. Most if not all antagonists are **inverse agonists** that inhibit the constitutive activity of the receptor and, therefore, do not just hinder the access of the agonist to the receptor. In agreement with this, it is not surprising that antagonists have binding sites of their own, which may or may not coincide with those of the corresponding agonists.

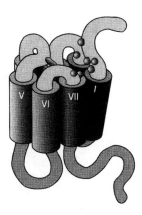

FIGURE 2.9 Clustering of putative contact residues for a peptide ligand in a model of the three-dimensional, folded structure of the receptor. The contact residues for angiotensin in the AT–1 receptor are shown as small spheres in the N-terminal extension, in extracellular loop 1, and around the top of TM-VII. In other peptide receptors similar interaction points have been identified together with interaction points around the top of TM-III and in some cases also around the top of, for example, TM-V and -VI. Although the structure of the loops is very ill-defined, it is clear that these residues which are scattered in the primary structure of the receptor may form a pocket between the outer portions of the TM segments. It is unclear to what degree the different peptide ligands may also reach down between the TM segments.

2.8.1 MONOAMINE ANTAGONISTS OFTEN BIND CLOSE TO WHERE THE AGONISTS BIND

Many antagonists for monoamine receptors are chemically similar to the corresponding agonists, i.e., an agonist can, through relatively small chemical modifications, be converted into an antagonist. In most of these systems, it has been demonstrated or it is assumed that the antagonists, like the agonists, are interacting with the conserved Asp in TM-III and that they occupy much of the same space that the agonists normally occupy in the pocket between TM-III, -V, and -VI. However, several antagonists have been shown to have interaction points, for example at the top of TM-VII, which are not shared with the agonists. Thus, antagonists for monoamines, which in many cases are classical competitive antagonists, to a large extent bind to the same site as the corresponding agonists, i.e., they function as *isosteric competitive antagonists*.

2.8.2 NONPEPTIDE ANTAGONISTS MAY BIND RATHER DIFFERENTLY FROM THE AGONISTS

For many years, analogues of peptides have been known that act as antagonists or partial agonists. The antagonistic property was obtained, for example, by substitutions with D-amino acids, introduction of reduced peptide bonds, or substitution with conformationally constrained amino acid analogues. Such peptide antagonists share much of their binding site with the natural peptide agonists and, in general, are therefore also isosteric competitive antagonists. However, nonpeptide compounds have recently been developed in many peptide receptor systems. These compounds, which are discovered through chemical file screenings, do not chemically resemble the corresponding peptide ligands. Nevertheless, they act as specific competitive antagonists on the peptide receptor. Mapping of binding sites for nonpeptide antagonists has revealed that they often bind rather differently from the peptide agonists. The nonpeptide compounds typically have interaction points located relatively deep in the pocket between TM-III, -V, -VI, and -VII, corresponding to where agonists and antagonists for the monoamine receptors bind (Figure 2.10). As discussed above, many of

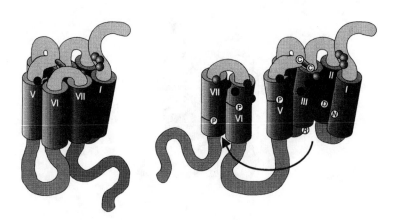

FIGURE 2.10   Different binding site for peptide agonist and nonpeptide antagonist in the NK-1 (substance P) receptor. The presumed contact points for the natural *agonist,* substance P, are indicated as light gray spheres and the presumed contact residues for the quinuclidine, nonpeptide antagonist CP96,345 are indicated as dark gray spheres. To the left a model of the folded NK-1 receptor is shown, and to the right the receptor model is opened up to display the location of the presumed contact points more clearly. Mutational analysis of these interactions have not pointed to any clear common point of interaction on the receptor for these two competitive ligands. Conceivably the ligands act as allosteric competitive ligands, competing for binding to the receptor by binding to different sites displayed in different conformations of the receptor: an active conformation and one of the many inactive conformations, respectively. In this way, binding of one ligand excludes the binding of the other type.

the peptide agonists do not reach into the lower part of this pocket. Thus, in some cases nonpeptide antagonists for peptide receptors can act as *allosteric competitive antagonists,* i.e., they bind to a different epitope from the agonist, but the two ligands still compete for occupancy of the receptor as such. The competitive kinetics is a result of the phenomenon that the binding of one ligand excludes the binding of the other ligand through a very large degree of negative cooperativity. The mutually exclusive binding pattern is probably a result of the fact that the agonist and antagonist preferentially bind to different conformational states of the receptor, i.e., an active and an inactive conformation, respectively (see Chapter 1). In the substance P receptor, the binding site for a nonpeptide antagonist has even been exchanged by a metal ion binding site (through systematic introduction of His residues) without any effect on the binding of the agonist. In the mutant receptor, zinc ions have replaced the nonpeptide antagonist in antagonizing both the binding and the function of substance P. It is believed that the nonpeptide compound and the zinc ions act as antagonists by selecting and stabilizing an inactive conformation that prevents the binding and action of the agonist.

Thus, for both monoamine receptors and peptide receptors a picture is emerging where presumed interaction points for ligands are clustering in molecular models in what appears to be "binding pockets". However, only in very few cases is there any hard evidence identifying the actual chemical interaction between a particular chemical moiety on the ligand and a particular side chain of the receptor. As discussed above, the mapping of such interactions should be based on real gain-of-function experiments. Thus, we are still surprisingly far away from knowing the actual orientation of the natural messengers and drugs within their binding pockets.

2.9   7TM RECEPTORS ARE IN AN EQUILIBRIUM BETWEEN ACTIVE AND INACTIVE CONFORMATIONS

As presented above, 7TM receptors are activated by ligands of very wide chemical variance. On the other hand, all the receptors are homologous or at least belong to a few families of

7TM proteins which all couple through a relatively small family of homologous G-proteins. It would, therefore, be expected that the molecular signal transduction process from the receptor to the G-protein would be similar, and that the conformational change in the receptor occurring upon activation would be similar among the many different receptors. Nevertheless, there is no evidence that all the different ligands recognize or activate a common structural "lock" in their respective receptors. In contrast, there appear to be many different 'locks'. The mechanism by which this variety of chemical ligands all can act as agonists on 7TM receptors appears to be one whereby the active conformation of the receptors is not *induced* by the ligand as such. Rather, the receptor folds into the active conformation by itself. The receptor is a dynamic membrane protein which exists naturally in an equilibrium between inactive and active conformations.

The currently accepted model for G-protein-coupled receptor function is the **allosteric ternary complex** model of Lefkowitch and Costa. The principal signaling form of the receptor is the one which occurs in the so-called ternary complex, consisting of the agonist, the receptor, and the G-protein (Figure 2.11). From this point in the signal transduction process, the G-protein will continue the mission (as presented in Chapter 8). Importantly, however, a certain fraction of the receptors — for example, 5 to 20% depending on the receptor type — will be able to bind the G-protein without any agonist present and they will together form an active, constitutively signaling binary complex. Both agonist and G-protein will have high affinity for a so-called "isomerized" form of the receptor (placed in the center of Figure 2.11). Agonists will have a significantly lower affinity for the G-protein-uncoupled form of the receptor; whereas antagonists will rather bind G-protein independently. However, it is becoming more and more clear that, in fact, many antagonists have the highest affinity for the G-protein-uncoupled conformation of the receptor. In other words, from this point of view agonists and antagonists bind preferentially to distinct and complementary conformational populations of their common receptor target.

2.9.1 Agonists and Antagonists Act by Stabilizing Active and Inactive Receptor Conformations

The **agonist** thus stimulates the receptor merely by stabilizing an active conformation. This can be achieved in many different ways depending on the chemical nature of the ligand and on the structure of the receptor. A small monoamine will, for example, be most efficient in stabilizing the active conformation by binding between the transmembrane segments. In contrast, large peptides and proteins can achieve a similar stabilizing function through multiple interactions at the exterior parts of their target receptors. In addition, such ligands may or may not reach relatively deep into the receptor structure.

An **antagonist** is a compound which stabilizes one of probably many different inactive conformations of the receptor, and thereby prevents the receptor from going into the active, signaling conformation. Thus, like ligand-gated ion channels, 7TM receptors are allosteric proteins which obey the basic principle of the concerted type of allostery of Monod, Wyman and Changeux, i.e., they interchange between different conformations which are stabilized by ligands. It is likely that when the details of ligand-receptor interactions are studied, some degree of induced fit will also be found to be taking place. However, the important issue is the concept that both agonists and antagonists become "active" or "passive" compounds, by stabilizing active and passive conformations, respectively, of a dynamic membrane protein.

2.9.2 Constitutively Elevated Levels of Second Messengers Are Normalized by Inverse Agonists

If a fraction of the receptor population at a given time will be in the active conformation, without any ligand present, then 7TM receptors should display some degree of constitutive

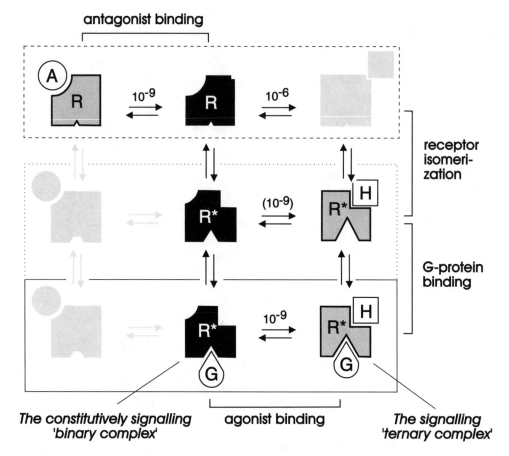

FIGURE 2.11 A schematic model for ligand interactions in different conformational states of 7TM receptors. This model is an extended version of the so-called "allosteric ternary complex model" of Lefkowitz and Costa. The agonist or hormone is indicated as the square H and the antagonists as the circle A. The G-protein is shown as the droplet-shape 'G'. A series of different putative conformations of the receptor R and R* are shown as squares with indentations indicating the binding sites and the "affinities" for the different ligands. A few affinities are indicated to underline the fact that the agonists have low affinity (10^{-7} mol/l) for the G-protein-uncoupled receptor (black R at the top in the middle) but have high affinity (10^{-9} mol/l) for the G-protein-coupled form of the receptor. The antagonists bind relatively G-protein-independently, but with a somewhat higher affinity for the uncoupled form. The *hatched square* indicates the G-protein-uncoupled part of the scheme which the antagonist will preferentially be involved in, and the *solid square* indicates the complementary G-protein-coupled part of the scheme, which the agonist will prefer. (Redrawn from: Rosenkilde, M.M., Cahir, M., Gether, U., et al., *J. Biol. Chem.*, 269, 28160, 1994. With permission.)

activity. That is, in fact, the case in many systems. In cells transfected with 7TM receptors the level of the intracellular second messenger is increased — without any agonist being present. Furthermore, the higher the expression level the higher is the intracellular level of second messengers. This is most clearly observed in receptor systems that couple through stimulation of cAMP production. This phenomenon of **constitutive activity** of the receptors is clearly demonstrated by the effect of antagonists, which inhibit the "unstimulated" function of the receptor and thus normalize the increased second messenger level to that found in untransfected cells (Figure 2.12). These antagonists are called "inverse agonists", which underlines the fact that they have a property of their own independent of the agonist, i.e., the

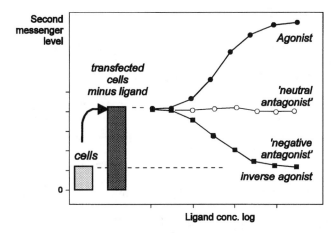

FIGURE 2.12 Opposite but functionally equipotent effects of agonists and inverse agonists (negative antagonists). The second messenger level is higher in transfected cells than in untransfected control cells although no agonist is present, and the second messenger level is dependent on the number of receptors expressed on the cells (most clearly seen with cAMP). Agonists will increase the second messenger level further, whereas antagonists (inverse agonists) will decrease the spontaneously increased level back to the level of the untransfected cells. Thus inverse agonists have a property of their own, being antagonistic, independent of the presence of the agonists.

ability to inhibit the constitutive activity of the receptors. Importantly, the constitutive activity of 7TM receptors can also be observed in untransfected primary cell cultures.

2.9.3 POINT MUTATIONS CAN SHIFT THE EQUILIBRIUM TOWARDS THE ACTIVE CONFORMATION

Alterations in the normal conformational equilibrium of receptors have been demonstrated to be the genetic basis of diseases. For example, mutations which shift the equilibrium totally towards the constitutively active form of the TSH or the LH receptors are responsible for the development of certain thyroid adenomas and the development of puberty in small children. In the case of the thyroid adenomas, a normal TSH receptor is expressed in the surrounding normal thyroid tissue. Mutations that cause increased constitutive activity of 7TM receptors are frequently located in the lower part of TM-VI. However, other locations for such mutations have also been reported.

2.10 DESENSITIZATION MECHANISMS TURN SIGNALING OFF DURING PROLONGED STIMULATION

During prolonged stimulation of G-protein-coupled receptors the signal is attenuated by one of several different processes, which allows the cell to adapt to the increased stimulatory situation. Within just a few minutes, the ligand-occupied receptors are sequestered into intracellular vesicles where the low pH leads to dissociation of the ligand, which in most cases is subsequently degraded. In contrast, the receptor is shunted back to the surface membrane. A more prolonged desensitization is achieved through interaction of the receptor with an intracellular protein, arrestin, which preferentially will bind to the phosphorylated form of the receptor. A family of arrestin molecules occurs with more or less specificity for certain receptors and with a variable preference for phosphorylated forms of these receptors. An even slower and more prolonged downregulation results from the decreased synthesis of new receptor molecules.

2.11 FURTHER READING

Baldwin, J.M., The probable arrangement of the helices in G protein-coupled receptors, *EMBO J.,* 1993, 12:1693-1703.

Coughlin, S.R., Expanding horizons for receptors coupled to G proteins: diversity and disease, *Curr. Opinion Cell Biol.,* 1994, 6:191-197.

Dohlman, H.G., Thorner, J., Caron, M.G., and Lefkowitz, R.J., Model systems for the study of seven-transmembrane segment receptors, *Annu. Rev. Biochem.,* 1991, 60:653-688.

Donelley, D., Findlay, J.B.C., and Blundell, T.L., The evolution and structure of aminergic G protein-coupled receptors, *Receptors Channels,* 1994, 2:61-78.

Elling, C.E., Nielsen, S.M., and Schwartz, T.W., Conversion of antagonist-binding site to metal-ion site in the tachykinin NK-1 receptor, *Nature,* 1995, 374:74-77.

Findlay, J. and Eliopoulos, E., Three-dimensional modeling of G protein-linked receptors, *TIPS,* 1990, 11:492-499.

Hargrave, P.A., Seven-helix receptors, *Struct. Biol.,* 1991, 1:575–581.

Kobilka, B., Adrenergic receptors as models for G protein-coupled receptors, *Annu. Rev. Neurosci.,* 1992, 15:87-114.

Lefkowitz, R.J., Cotecchia, S., Samama, P., and Costa, T., Constitutive activity of receptors coupled to guanine nucleotide regulatory proteins, *Trends Pharmacol. Sci.,* 1993, 14:303-307.

Rosenkilde, M.M., Cahir, M., Gether, U., Hjorth, S.A., and Schwartz, T.W., Mutations along transmembrane segment II of the NK-1 receptor affect substance P competition with non-peptide antagonists but not substance P binding, *J. Biol. Chem.,* 1994 269:28160-28164.

Savarese, T.M. and Fraser, C.M., In vitro mutagenesis and the search for structure-function relationships among G protein-coupled receptors, *Biochem. J.,* 1992, 283:1-19.

Schertler, G.F., Villa, C., and Henderson, R., Projection structure of rhodopsin, *Nature,* 1993, 362:770-772.

Schwartz, T.W., Locating ligand-binding sites in 7TM receptors by protein engineering, *Curr. Opinion Biotechnol.,* 1994, 5:434-444.

Strader, C.D., Sigal, I.S., and Dixon, R.A.F., Structural basis of β-adrenergic receptor function, *FASEB J.,* 1989, 3:1825-1832.

Strader, C.D., Gaffney, T., Sugg, E.E., Candelore, M.R., Keys, R., Patchett, A.A., and Dixon, R.A.F., Allele-specific activation of genetically engineered receptors, *J. Biol. Chem.,* 1991, 266:5-8.

Strosberg, A.D., Structure, function and regulation of adrenergic receptors, *Protein Sci.,* 1993, 2:1198-1209.

3 Molecular Structure of Ligand-Gated Ion Channels

Jan Egebjerg

CONTENTS

3.1 INTRODUCTION

Ligand-gated ion channel receptors are integral glycoproteins that transverse the cell membrane. All molecularly characterized ligand-gated ion channel receptors are multisubunit complexes. The receptors generally exist in one of three functional states: resting (or closed), open, or desensitized. Each functional state may reflect many discrete conformational states with different pharmacological properties. The receptors in the resting state will, in the presence of agonist, undergo a fast transition to the open state, called gating, and for most agonists also a transition to the desensitized state. Because the desensitized state often exhibits higher agonist affinity than the open state, most of the receptors will be in the desensitized state after prolonged agonist exposure.

    The receptors or channels have three important properties: (1) they are activated in response to specific ligands, (2) they conduct ions through the otherwise impermeable cell membrane, and (3) they select among different ions.

0-8493-9227-6/96/$0.00+$.50
© 1996 by CRC Press, Inc.

Molecular cloning combined with a variety of different techniques have revealed the existence of at least three structurally different families of receptors. These families can be classified as the four-transmembrane domain (4-TM) receptors, the excitatory amino acid receptors (3-TM), and the ATP receptors (2-TM).

3.2 4-TM RECEPTORS

The 4-TM family of receptors consists of the nicotinic acetylcholine receptors (nAChR), serotonin receptors ($5HT_3$), glycine receptors, and γ-aminobutyric acid receptors ($GABA_A$).

nAChRs are the primary excitatory receptors in the skeletal muscle and the peripheral nervous system of vertebrates. In the central nervous system nAChRs are present in much smaller numbers than the excitatory amino acid receptors. $5HT_3$ receptors are also cation-selective receptors but are located exclusively on neurones.

Glycine and GABA are the major inhibitory neurotransmitters. GABA predominates in cortex and cerebellum, whereas glycine is most abundant in the spinal cord and brainstem. Both ligands activate a chloride current.

3.2.1 MOLECULAR CLONING

The 4-TM receptors are pentameric complexes composed of subunits of 420 to 550 amino acids (Table 3.1). The subunits exhibit sequence identities from 25 to 75%, with a similar distribution of hydrophobic and hydrophilic domains. The hydrophilic 210- to 230-amino acid N-terminal domain is followed by three closely spaced hydrophobic and putative trans-membrane domains, then by a variable-length intracellular loop, and finally by a fourth putative transmembrane region shortly before the C-terminus (Figure 3.1). Of the four candidate transmembrane regions there is evidence for one α-helix. The structures of the other hydrophobic regions have not been resolved.

TABLE 3.1

	nAChR					$5HT_3$	Glycine receptors		$GABA_A$				
$\uparrow$	$\alpha 1$	$\beta 1$	γ	δ	ϵ	A	$\alpha 1$	β	$\alpha 1$	$\beta 1$	$\gamma 1$	δ	ρ
60–70%	$\alpha 2$	$\beta 2$					$\alpha 2$		$\alpha 2$	$\beta 2$	$\gamma 2$		
$\downarrow$	$\alpha 3$	$\beta 3$					$\alpha 3$		$\alpha 3$	$\beta 3$	$\gamma 3$		
	$\alpha 4$	$\beta 4$							$\alpha 4$				
	$\alpha 5$								$\alpha 5$				
	$\alpha 6$								$\alpha 6$				
	$\alpha 7$												
	$\alpha 8$												
	$\alpha 9$												
	$\longleftarrow$ 40% $\longrightarrow$								$\longleftarrow$ 40% $\longrightarrow$				

Molecular cloning has resulted in the identification of the muscle nAChR subunits $\alpha 1$, $\beta 1$, γ, δ, and ϵ, and the structurally related neuronal subunits $\alpha 2$ to $\alpha 9$ and $\beta 2$ to $\beta 4$. The agonist binding site is mainly located on the α-subunit. The neuronal nAChR subunits $\alpha 2$ to $\alpha 4$ can assemble with $\beta 2$ or $\beta 4$ and generate functional heteromeric receptors, while the $\alpha 7$ to $\alpha 9$ subunits can generate functional homomeric receptors. The heteromeric nAChR assembles according to the general stoichiometry $(\alpha)_2(\beta)_3$ with a β-subunit between the α-subunits (Figure 3.2). Obviously, the properties of the receptor depend on the subunit composition. If the assembly process was not controlled in cells that express more than two

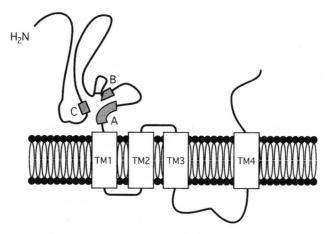

FIGURE 3.1 Schematic representation of the transmembrane topology of the 4-TM receptor family. A, B, and C indicate regions involved in agonist binding. Both the N-terminus (indicated by H_2N) and the C-terminus are located extracellularly. The cytoplasmic loop between TM3 and TM4 is variable in size and contains putative phosphorylation sites.

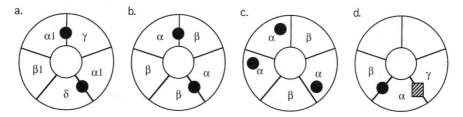

FIGURE 3.2 Schematic representation of the subunit organization in the most abundant heteromeric receptor complex: **a.** embryonic muscle nicotinic acetylcholine receptor (nAChR), **b.** neuronal nAChR, **c.** glycine receptors, and **d.** GABA$_A$ receptors. The circles indicates the location of the agonist binding site at the interface between the subunits in nAChR and GABA$_A$ receptors. The square indicates the location of the benzodiazepine binding site. The depicted GABA$_A$ receptor model is the general model with at least one GABA and one benzodiazepine binding site. The number of different binding sites on the GABA$_A$ receptor depends on the final stoichiometry of the pentameric complex. Adult muscle nAChR has the stoichiometry $(\alpha 1)_2\beta\varepsilon\delta$.

different subunits, it would result in a very large number of different receptor types. At least in muscle cells, where four different subunits are expressed at the same time, the subunits must be assembled in an ordered sequence to achieve the correct stoichiometry and neighborhood relationship.

Four glycine receptor subunits have been identified: three α-subunits and one β-subunit. When expressed in heterologous systems, homomeric receptors generate functional channels and the current is inhibited by strychnine and picrotoxin. A more detailed analysis revealed that the β-subunit, probably in the stoichiometry $\alpha_3\beta_2$, is necessary to generate channel properties similar to the channels studied in adult spinal cord neurones, while the embryonic glycine receptor is homomeric with no β-subunit.

The diversity of the GABA$_A$ subunits (Figure 3.2d and Table 3.1) is reflected in very complex pharmacology. The receptor can be modulated by a number of agents that either enhance the channel current (benzodiazepines, barbiturates) or reduce the channel current (bicuculline, β-carbolines, picrotoxin). The GABA binding site is located on the β-subunit, but coexpression with an α-subunit is necessary for significant functional expression. The complexity of the benzodiazepine pharmacology is illustrated by the observation that heteromeric α/β receptors are modulated by barbiturates and blocked by picrotoxin, but not potentiated by benzodiazepine. This was surprising, since cross-linking experiments assigned the benzodiazepine binding site to the α-subunit. Only coexpression of the α- and β-subunits with a γ-subunit generates receptors that are potentiated by benzodiazepine. Thus benzodiazepine pharmacology depends on the α-subunit, but in order to have any functional implications, the receptor complex must also contain a γ-subunit. The basic unit in the GABA receptor is believed to be an α-, β-, and γ-subunit with a GABA and benzodiazepine binding site at the α-β and β-γ interfaces, respectively. The pharmacology of the receptor will not only depend on these three subunits but also on the remaining two subunits.

3.2.2 THE 3-D STRUCTURE

The nAChRs of skeletal muscles and the fish electric organ are the best-characterized ligand-gated ion channels. The receptor is a 290-kDa complex, composed of four distinct subunits assembled into a heterologous $(\alpha1)_2\beta1\gamma\delta$ pentameric complex. In muscle, the γ-subunit present in the embryo is replaced by an ε-subunit in the adult. The receptor complex in the resting state, in electron micrographs from the synaptic site viewed perpendicular to the plane of the membrane, appears as a ring-like particle with an outer diameter of 80 Å and an inner tube of 20 to 25 Å. Viewed from the side (Figure 3.3), the receptor looks like a 125-Å-long cylinder, protruding 60 Å into the synaptic cleft and 20 Å into the cytoplasm. The cation-conducting pathway consist of three parts. In the synaptic portion, it forms a water-filled tube 20 Å in diameter and 60 Å long. The next part, across the membrane, forms a more constricted region about 30 Å long (the pore). Near the middle of the membrane, the pathway becomes constricted in a region where the pathway is blocked when the channel is closed (the gate). In the cytoplasmic part the pathway forms a cylinder 20 Å in diameter and 20 Å long. A close inspection of the electron micrographs revealed that each subunit has an α-helical-like segment lining the pore. This segment consist of two α-helices separated by a kink around the midpoint, pointing inwards (in the resting state), giving the pore an "hourglass" shape with the kink located at the most constricted point. When the receptor is activated by ACh, each of the helical segments rotates, opening up the gate. In the open state the pore narrows from the outer side to the cytoplasmic side, where the diameter is roughly 11 Å. Thus the flexure between the two α-helices provides an effective way of altering the shape and size of the pore (Figure 3.4).

3.2.3 THE RECEPTOR PORE

The ability of a receptor channel to conduct ions, which is measured as the conductance (the reciprocal of resistance) of the channel, depends on TM2. The experiments which showed this were based on the observation that receptors made of *Torpedo* α-, β-, γ- and δ-subunits had a different conductance from receptors made of *Torpedo* α-, β-, γ- and calf δ-subunits. When chimeric δ-subunits, in which parts of the *Torpedo* sequences were replaced by the corresponding calf sequences, were coexpressed with the *Torpedo* α-, β- and γ-subunits, it was demonstrated that the entire difference in conductance could be attributed to the TM2 region.

The structure of the TM2 regions is obviously not a perfect α-helix. However, assuming a symmetric, pentameric distribution of α-helices gives us a useful structural model to describe the molecular environment an ion has to pass through when permeating the receptor channel. Amino acids assigned to the same position in the sequence alignments will, because of the symmetric distribution around the pore, form a ring in the three-dimensional model (Figure 3.5).

Important clues to how the pore is structurally organized were obtained by examining the distribution of the charged and uncharged residues in the *Torpedo* nAChR subunits. As

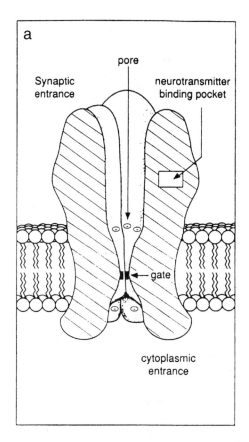
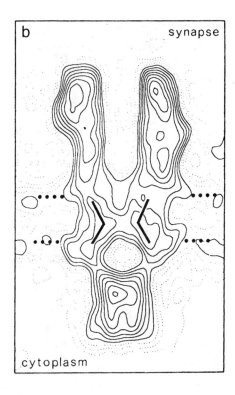

FIGURE 3.3   a. Model of the 4-TM receptors based on data obtained from the nAChR. The model shows the ligand binding site, the membrane bilayer, and the position of the channel gate. **b.** Electron density map of the nAChR in profile with the membrane indicated by dots. The bend α-helical segment, believed to be TM2, is depicted as solid lines. The square-like density in the cytoplasmic region arises from an associated 43-kDa protein (Courtesy of N. Unwin).

expected for a hydrophobic segment, the TM2 bears no charged residues. However, a number of charged and polar residues were located at both ends of TM2 (Figure 3.5). According to the 4-TM model, the charged residues in the TM1-TM2 loop will be located at the entrance to the pore from the cytoplasmatic side while the charged residues in the TM2-TM3 loop will be located at the pore entrance from the extracellular side. Since nAChR conducts cations, the negatively charged rings are expected to line the channel and also attract permeant cations to the pore. Indeed, when the number of charged amino acids in the intermediate ring was reduced from the four negative charges in the native *Torpedo* receptor, there was a clear reduction in the conductance of the channel. Mutations which altered the charge of the inner and the outer rings also changed the conductance, but to a much lesser extent. Thus, these residues must be exposed to the lumen of the pore, although additional experiments suggest that the inner and outer rings are more involved in regulating the access of the cations to the channel than being in direct contact with the permeating ions. The optimal effect of the negatively charged rings on the current is a subtle balance between attracting monovalent ions and boosting the current on one hand, and on the other hand attracting divalent ions which bind to the residues in the charged rings with high affinity, thus reducing the current. These counteracting effects might explain why some functional nACh receptor subunits encode positively charged amino acids at the ring positions.

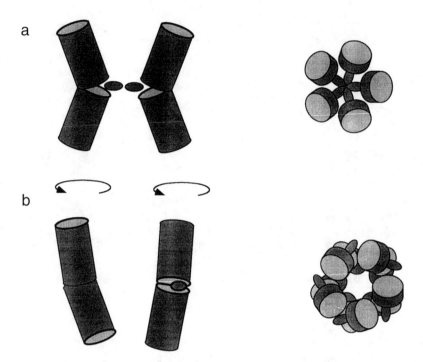

FIGURE 3.4   The orientation of the TM2 helical segment in (**a**) the closed and (**b**) the open state of the channel. On the left: a view of two of the five helices from the side where the helical segment is illustrated as two rods separated by a kink and where the leucine (ellipse) is located. On the right: the five helices viewed from the synaptic side where the leucines will block the pore. The binding of an agonist causes the helical segments to rotate and the narrowest region is then in the open state at the cytoplasmic part of the pore.

```
              Inner ring  Intermediate ring  Serine ring  Threonine ring  Leucine ring  Valine ring  Outer leucine ring  Outer ring        Selectivity

Torpedo α     DSG  EKMTLSISVLLSLTVFLLVIVELIP
Torpedo β     DAG  EKMSLSISVLLSLTVFLLVIVELIP
Torpedo γ     QAGGQKCTLSISVLLAQTIFLFLIAQKVP
Torpedo δ     ESG  EKMSTAISVLLAQAVFLLLTSQRLP

Rat α7        DSG  EKISLGITVLLSLTVFMLLVAEIMP         +

GlyR α1       DAAPARVGLGITTVLTMTTQSSGSRASLP        –
GABA α1       ESVPARTVFGVTTVLTMTTLSISARNSLP        –
                   **                  *

Mut 1         DSG  AKISLGITVLLSLTTFMLLVAEIMP        +
Mut 2         DSGPAKISLGITVLLSLTTFMLLVAEIMP        –
```

FIGURE 3.5   Alignment of the TM2 amino acid sequences. Residues in the rings line the pore. The nomenclature of the rings are based on the α7 sequence. 'Selectivity' indicates the charge of the permeant ions. Mut1 and Mut2 are site-directed mutants (indicated by asterisks) of the α7 subunit (see text).

In the GABA and glycine receptors, where the permeant ion is negatively charged, the inner ring remains negatively charged and the outer is either negative or neutral. The question is then: What determines the ion selectivity of the channel? An alignment of the TM2 region between the nAChR subunit α7, which generates functional homomeric receptors, and glycine and GABA subunits revealed amino acid differences at five of the rings which line the pore, and in addition an extra amino acid was present at the N-terminal end of the TM2 segment in the anion-selective channels (Figure 3.5b). Two mutations generated by site-directed mutagenesis are of particular interest. In the first mutation, Mut1 (Figure 3.5), the glutamate in the intermediate ring, is substituted by an alanine, and a valine which also faces the lumen of the pore is substituted by a threonine. In this mutant, the channel remains cation selective, although both mutations make the channel more like the pore of the anion-selective channel. In the second mutant, Mut2 (Figure 3.5), an additional proline was inserted in Mut1 at the N-terminus of the TM2 (i.e., between TM1 and TM2) and the channel was then converted to an anion-selective channel. Thus, the pore can be permeable to both cations and anions, consequently ion selectivity is not directly related to the amino acid sequence within the pore. However, slight changes in the position of the TM2 or in the surrounding amino acids apparently determines the ion selectivity.

It is important that conclusions based on mutagenesis studies are confirmed by other experiments, since mutations involving residues in key positions for structure or for function may cause their effect not only as a result of changes at the site of substitution, but also as a result of nonlocalized structural perturbations created to accommodate that change. In fact, most of the residues facing the lumen of the pore were also identified in labeling experiments using noncompetitive antagonists known to bind in the pore. When the noncompetitive antagonist [³H]chlorpromazine was photolabeled to the receptor, the cross-linked amino acids were located in the serine, threonine, and leucine rings (Figure 3.5). Evidence for structural changes in the pore was obtained by using the antagonist trifluoromethyl-iodophenyldiazirine, which in the absence of agonist cross-links amino acids present in the valine and the leucine ring. However, in the presence of agonist the labeling pattern extends down to the threonine and serine rings, indicating that the central valine, leucine, and threonine rings may correspond to the constricted region of the pore observed in the electron micrographs. The leucine is thought to be the gate-forming residue, pointing out from the kink in TM2. This is supported by mutagenesis studies which demonstrated that a substitution of the leucine with a smaller amino acid affected the ability of the receptor to close when in the desensitized state.

3.2.4 THE LIGAND BINDING SITE

To study the properties of the binding site, it is important to keep in mind that receptors exist in a number of conformations which may exhibit different binding properties. As mentioned, the affinity for the ligand of the open state is usually much lower (10- to 1000-fold) than the affinity in the desensitized state. Thus, in biochemical experiments where the receptor is exposed to a ligand for prolonged time periods, agonists-receptor interactions will reflect receptor conformation of the desensitized state while antagonist interaction may reflect conformations of either the resting state or the desensitized states. In contrast, electrophysiological studies of agonist interactions reflect the low affinity binding of the open state, except for certain mutants (see below). A second consideration is how ligands induce the activation of the receptor. At least two models can be proposed for the activation. First, an "induced fit" model where the agonist, by interacting with the receptor, induces a new agonist-dependent conformation. Second, the allosteric model, which proposes that the receptor, in the absence of agonist, already exists in a number of conformations with specific binding properties. The binding of an agonist will not affect the structure of the binding site or the physiological properties of the conformation, but will modify the equilibrium between the conformational states. A ligand will then stabilize the conformation it binds preferentially. Consequently, agonists will stabilize the open state (e.g., kainate on AMPA receptors [Figure 3.8] and also the desensitized state (ACh on nAChR receptors, AMPA on AMPA receptors [Figure 3.8]), while competitive antagonists stabilize the resting state (α-bungarotoxin on nAChR receptors, CNQX on glutamate receptors) and some, termed metaphilic, antagonists will stabilize the desensitized state.

Studies of the mutant α7-receptor, where the leucine ring is changed (see above), have been put forward as an example supporting the allosteric model. The mutant is characterized by (1) a decrease in the onset of desensitization; (2) an apparent affinity for ACh, estimated from dose-response relationships 150-fold higher than the wild type; and (3) activation by antagonists such as (+)-tubocurarine. The single-channel conductance induced by (+)-tubocurarine was different from the normal open state conductance, but similar to the conductance elicited by low concentrations of ACh. This was interpreted in favor of the allosteric model by assuming that (+)-tubocurarine and low concentrations of ACh bind to one of the high affinity, desensitized conformations which, because the mutation cannot close, exhibits a conductance different from the normal open state.

The ligand binding site has been studied by biochemical and molecular biological approaches. Affinity labeling of the *Torpedo* nAChR using photoactivated cholinergic agonists and competitive antagonists identified a number of aromatic residues and cysteines located in one of three regions (A, B, and C) in the amino-terminal part of the receptor α-subunit (Figure 3.6). In addition, (+)-tubocurarine was found to cross-link to aromatic residues in the γ- and δ-subunits. There are caveats to affinity labeling experiments. First, the photoreactive group may be added as a substituent to ligands without affecting the binding affinity of the ligands, implying that the photoreactive group is not located right in the binding site. Naturally occurring photoreactive antagonists generally are large molecules, so the same restrictions may apply to them. Second, photoreactive groups may preferentially react with aromatic residues. However, we can conclude that the agonist binding cavity is mainly generated by amino acids located distantly in the sequence. The binding site is located at the interface between different subunits, and there are a number of accessible aromatic residues lining the cavity, although other residues may be important for the agonist binding. The importance of region A, B, and C is emphasized when the nAChR sequences are aligned with the equivalent regions from other members of the receptor family (Figure 3.6). The presence of amino acids conserved between all subunits suggests that the folding of the regions (i.e., the peptide backbone) are similar, and the different binding properties result from changes in the amino acid side chains. This was demonstrated when the exchange of a single hydroxyl group (Tyr to Phe) in the glycine α1 subunit rendered the mutant receptor responsive to GABA. This observation also implies that the aromatic residues interact with the agonists, which is surprising since aromatic residues in most proteins are buried in the interior of the protein and are inaccessible to charged molecules such as the agonists. Thus, interactions with small, charged molecules in a hydrophobic pocket may cause large structural changes because the hydrophobic core in most proteins contributes significantly to their stabilization. Such an interpretation would favor an induced fit model for activation of the receptors. Currently there is not enough evidence to discriminate between the different models for activation.

Different biophysical data, including electron micrographs, show that the ACh binding cavities are located 30 Å above the membrane. It is not clear how the structural perturbations around the agonist binding site are transmitted to the pore region. However, the changes might be conserved in the family. When chimeric receptor subunits were constructed between the N-terminal part of the 5HT$_3$ subunit, including the binding regions, and the C-terminal pore region from the α7 ACh receptor, the chimeras were functional receptors with the 5HT$_3$ pharmacology at the agonist binding site and the pore properties of the α7 nACh receptor. This supports the notion that the overall structure and the conformational change during activation of the different members of the 4-TM family is highly conserved. Furthermore, the receptor subunits can be envisioned as at least a two-domain protein, with a binding domain and a membrane-spanning domain.

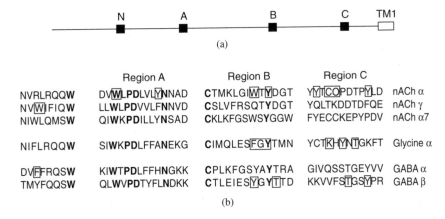

	Region A	Region B	Region C	
NVRLRQQW	DVWLPDLVLYNNAD	CTMKLGIWTYDGT	YYTCOPDTPYLD	nACh α
NVWIFIQW	LLWLPDVVLFNNVD	CSLVFRSQTYDGT	YQLTKDDTDFQE	nACh γ
NIWLQMSW	QIWKPDILLYNSAD	CKLKFGSWSYGGW	FYECCKEPYPDV	nACh α7
NIFLRQQW	SIWKPDLFFANEKG	CIMQLESFGYTMN	YCTKHYNTGKFT	Glycine α
DVFFRQSW	KIWTPDLFFHNGKK	CPLKFGSYAYTRA	GIVQSSTGEYVV	GABA α
TMYFQQSW	QLWVPDTYFLNDKK	CTLEIESYGYTTD	KKVVFSTGSYPR	GABA β

(b)

FIGURE 3.6 Regions involved in agonist binding: **a.** schematic model of the localization of the N, A, B, and C regions in the N-terminal domain of the nAChR α-subunit. A, B, and C are located on the same subunit, while the N-terminal region (N) is located on a different subunit. **b.** amino acid alignment of the four regions. Residues shown by affinity labeling or mutagenesis studies to be involved in agonist or antagonist binding are indicated by a box. Universally conserved residues are shown with bold type.

3.3 EXCITATORY AMINO ACID RECEPTORS

L-glutamate acts as an excitatory neurotransmitter at many synapses in the mammalian central nervous system. Electrophysiological measurements and the use of different selective agonists and antagonists indicate that different glutamate receptors coexist on many neurones.

The exogenous agonist *N*-methyl-D-aspartate (NMDA) activates receptors which are characterized by slow kinetics and a high Ca^{2+} permeability (Figure 3.8). These receptors require, in addition to glutamate (or NMDA), glycine as a coagonist. The current conducted by NMDA receptors is blocked by extracellular Mg^{2+} in a voltage-dependent manner (Figure 3.7). At the resting membrane potential (–70 mV), activation of the channel will only result in a low current because entry of Mg^{2+} ions into the channel will block the current. The affinity of the channel for the Mg^{2+} ions will decrease at smaller negative membrane potentials as the electrical driving force for Mg^{2+} is reduced and the block becomes ineffective (Figure 3.7). Another class of ionotropic glutamate receptors exhibits fast kinetics and, in most neurones, a low Ca^{2+} permeability when activated by glutamate. The selective agonist α-amino-3-hydroxy-5-methyl-4-isoxazole propionate (AMPA) activates a fast desensitizing current, as does glutamate, in a subset of these receptors. Consequently, this subtype is referred to as the AMPA receptor. Kainate activates a nondesensitizing current when applied to the AMPA receptor but it binds with high affinity to another receptor type, the kainate receptor. Kainate activates a slowly desensitizing current on the kainate receptor (Figure 3.8).

In addition to the three distinct ionotropic receptors, glutamate also activates the metabotropic G-protein-coupled glutamate receptors.

AMPA receptors mediate most of the fast excitatory neurotransmission in the mammalian brain. Their rapid kinetics and low Ca permeability make these receptors ideal for fast neurotransmission without creating sufficient changes in the intracellular calcium concentration to activate Ca^{2+}-dependent processes. The NMDA receptors are colocalized with the AMPA receptors on many synapses, but the slow kinetics of the NMDA receptor minimizes the NMDA receptor current because, after a single presynaptic glutamate release, the neurone quickly repolarizes, resulting in Mg^{2+} block. However, the NMDA receptor will be fully activated after extensive stimulation of the synapse where activation of the AMPA receptors will evoke sufficient depolarization of the postsynaptic membrane to relieve the NMDA

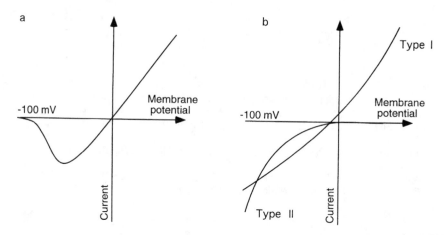

FIGURE 3.7   Current-voltage relationships for the NMDA and the non-NMDA glutamate receptors. **a.** Current-voltage relationship of the NMDA receptor subunit NR1 recorded in the presence of Mg^{2+}. The current through the channel becomes progressively smaller at negative membrane potentials due to the Mg^{2+} block. **b.** Expression of the AMPA and kainate receptor subunits generate either a linear (Type I) or a inwardly rectifying (Type II) current-voltage relationship, depending on the subunit composition of the receptor. If the receptor contains subunits edited at the Q/R site (i.e., GluR2 for the AMPA receptor, GluR5R or GluR6R for the kainate receptor) the current-voltage relationship is linear. Receptors made of unedited subunits alone or in combination with each other exhibit inwardly rectifying current-voltage relationships.

receptors of the Mg^{2+} block. This use-dependent Ca^{2+} influx has been interpreted as the underlying mechanism for many different processes including learning and memory.

3.3.1   MOLECULAR CLONING

The first glutamate receptor subunit was cloned by expression cloning in 1989. Currently, cDNAs encoding 16 subunits have been characterized. These subunits are based on sequence identities and are grouped into six different classes (Table 3.2). All the subunits have similar profiles in hydrophobicity plots and presumably have the same topology: a 400- to 500-amino acid extracellular N-terminal part followed by a 400-amino acid region encoding the trans-membrane domains (Figure 3.9). The C-terminus is intracellular and varies in size from 50 to 750 amino acids. The glutamate receptor subunits exhibit, in contrast to the 4-TM receptors, the highest sequence variability between the subunits at the N-terminal region, while the transmembrane domain is highly conserved.

3.3.1.1   AMPA Receptors

The GluR1–GluR4 subunits (also named GluRA–GluRD) coassemble into pentameric recep-tors with one another but not with subunits from the other classes. The functional profile of these cloned receptors demonstrated a desensitizing response to AMPA and a persistent response to kainate at high concentrations ($EC_{50} > 30\ \mu M$, Figure 3.8): features similar to AMPA receptors from the brain. The affinity for AMPA in binding experiments also resembles the affinities observed in brain tissue.

3.3.1.2   Kainate Receptors

The kainate receptors can be composed of subunits from the GluR5–GluR7 class and the KA1–KA2 class of subunits. Homomeric receptors of the former class (GluR5 and GluR6) generate functional receptors and bind kainate with an affinity of 50 to 100 nM. KA1 and

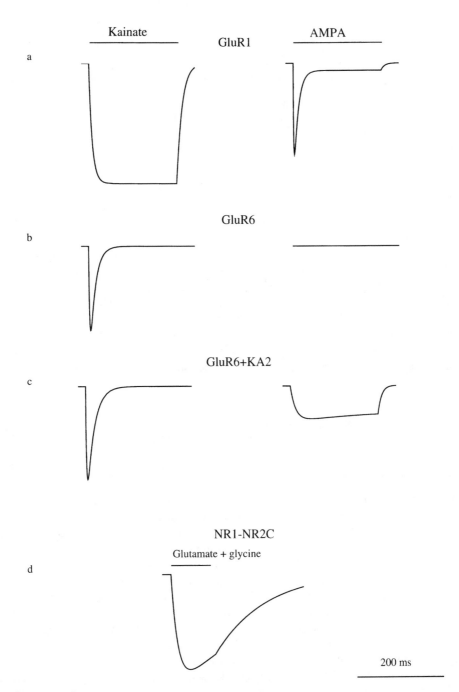

FIGURE 3.8 AMPA and kainate activate different current responses in the different classes of non-NMDA receptors: **a,** the AMPA receptor; **b, c,** the kainate receptors; **d,** glutamate + glycine activation of the NMDA receptor. The current response is characterized by a slow onset and offset compared to the non-NMDA receptors.

KA2 do not generate functional channels, but the receptors bind kainate with an affinity of 5 to 10 nM. Homomeric GluR6 and KA2 receptors are neither activated by AMPA nor bind AMPA. Interestingly, when they are coexpressed, heteromeric receptors respond to AMPA (Figure 3.8).

TABLE 3.2

AMPA receptors	Kainate receptors		NMDA receptors		Orphan subunits
GluR1 (A)	GluR5	KA1	NR1	NR2A	δ1
GluR2 (B)	GluR6	KA2		NR2B	δ2
GluR3 (C)	GluR7			NR2C	
GluR4 (D)				NR2D	

3.3.1.3 NMDA Receptors

The NMDA receptor can be reconstituted by subunits from two classes: the NR1 and the NR2 class (NR2A–NR2D). The NR2 subunits have the same basic structure as the other glutamate subunits, except for a large 400- to 630-amino acid C-terminal domain. Homomeric channels generated from NR1 display all the physiological and pharmacological character-istics of the NMDA channels expressed in neurones (see above). The NR2 class of subunits does not assemble into functional channels, but when coexpressed with the NR1 subunit, the heteromeric receptors conduct whole-cell currents a hundredfold larger than the currents recorded from homomeric NR1 receptors. This modulatory effect of the NR2 subunit, and other effects such as Mg^{2+} block, glycine sensitivity, deactivation kinetics, and the single-channel conductance, differ depending on which NR2 subunit coassembles with NR1.

3.3.1.4 Orphan Subunits

Two subunits, δ1 and δ2, have been identified that, based on sequence similarities, belong to the glutamate receptor family, although the function of the subunits is currently unknown.

3.3.2 TOPOLOGY

The hydrophobicity profile of the glutamate receptor subunits are similar, suggesting a similar membrane topology. However, the assignment of transmembrane regions is difficult because the hydrophobicity profile is ambiguous compared to the profile obtained for the 4-TM subunits. Recent studies using antibodies raised against the N-terminal part of the receptor subunits support the extracellular location predicted from the putative signal peptide, while the C-terminal part of the receptor subunit is located on the intracellular site of the membrane. Thus, there must be an odd number of transmembrane-spanning regions.

A more detailed understanding of the topology was obtained by studies of the extracel-lularly located Asn-glycosylation sites (N-type). Site-directed mutagenesis of all the consen-sus N-type glycosylation sites revealed that the receptor subunits are glycosylated at a number of sites in the N-terminal part and at the loop between TM3 and TM4.

So far, there is not sufficient experimental evidence to exclude one of the two incompatible models proposed to explain the glycosylation pattern. One model proposes a 5-TM topology as a modified version of the 4-TM receptors, where an extra TM (TM3a) region is introduced between TM3 and TM4. This model was proposed to account for a protein kinase A phos-phorylated site succeeding TM3 in GluR6. Recently the 5-TM model has been challenged by an increasing number of experiments favoring a 3-TM model (Figure 3.9).

N-type glycosylation sites, introduced by site-directed mutagenesis at different sites in the loop between TM3 and TM4 are all glycosylated, suggesting that the whole loop is extracellular. Deleting the putative TM1, TM2, or TM3 one by one, showed that deletion of TM1 and TM3 reverted the orientation of the receptor C-terminal while deletion of TM2 did not change the topology of the receptor, suggesting that TM1 and TM3 transverse the

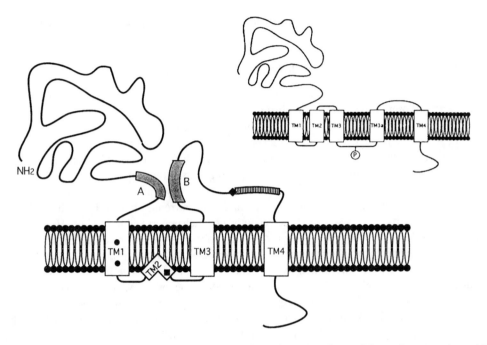

FIGURE 3.9 Schematic representation of the transmembrane topology of the excitatory amino acid receptors. The numbering of the TM regions follows, for historical reasons, the 4-TM numbering. The segments A and B represent the two lobes in the agonist binding site. The cross-hatched segment represents the alternatively spliced element (flip/flop) in the AMPA class of receptors. The edited sites are indicated by circles for the edited sites in TM1 of GluR6; square for the Q/R site; diamond for the G/R site. **Insert:** alternative model proposed to explain phosphorylation sites (marked by P) in GluR6.

membrane while TM2 does not. The 3-TM model has received further support from studies on the agonist binding site.

3.3.3 AGONIST BINDING SITE

The combination of comparative sequence analysis together with the use of standard cloning techniques to generate chimeric receptor subunits and site-directed mutants have been employed to explore the agonist binding site. Comparative sequence analysis revealed homology between a segment preceding TM1 (A) and the N-terminal part of the loop between TM3 and TM4 (B) of the glutamate receptor (Figure 3.9) with two segments in the bacterial periplasmic amino acid binding proteins. When the A and the B segments are exchanged between the kainate and the AMPA receptors the binding characteristics of the chimeric receptor subunit are specified by the A and B segments; that is, kainate receptors with AMPA A and B segments exhibit binding properties similar to AMPA receptors. A detailed analysis of the glycine binding site on the NR1 subunit identified two distinct sites in the A segment and one site in the B segment crucial for glycine binding. By analogy with the agonist binding pocket in the 4-TM receptors, aromatic residues were found to be very critical for the binding site in segment A.

The three-dimensional structure of a periplasmic amino acid binding protein shows that the protein is made of two globular lobes, where one lobe has homology with segment A and the other with segment B. The lobes are separated by a hinge region which corresponds to the channel-forming domain TM1–TM3 in the glutamate receptor. The ligand binding pocket is formed between the two lobes which can be positioned in either an open or a closed conformation where the opening-closing movement of the two lobes allow binding and dissociation of the ligand. Thus, changes in the relative position of the A and B segments after binding of an agonist might induce changes in the pore region that cause the channel to open.

3.3.4 POSTTRANSCRIPTIONAL MODIFICATIONS

One important form of regulation is achieved by splice variants exhibiting functional differences and differential regulation. For instance, a 38-amino acid segment preceding TM4 is present in one of two alternative spliced forms, called "flip or flop", in GluR1–GluR4. The current amplitude is smaller at the flop receptors compared with the flip receptors. This might be a mechanism that could enable the neurones to switch from a low-gain flop version to a high-gain flip receptor simply by alternative splicing of the transcripts.

Another form of regulation is editing of the RNA transcript. When GluR1, GluR3, or GluR4 are expressed individually or in combination, the current-voltage relationship exhibits an inwardly rectifying response and the receptor channel is permeable to Ca^{2+}. However, if the GluR2 subunit is part of the receptor the current-voltage relationship is linear and the channel is impermeable to Ca^{2+} (Figure 3.7). Site-directed mutagenesis demonstrated that the channel properties were determined by a single amino acid difference in the putative TM2. GluR2 encodes an arginine (R) at that position while the other AMPA receptor subunits encode a glutamine (Q); hence the name Q/R site. Analysis of the genomic sequences revealed that GluR2, as in other AMPA receptor subunits, encodes a glutamine (codon GAC) but the cDNA encodes an arginine (GGC) at that position. The A to G transition is catalyzed by an enzyme that recognizes an RNA structural element in the GluR2 transcript and then specifically deaminates the adenosine to an inosine (which is equivalent to a G). GluR6 is, in addition to the editing at the Q/R site in TM2, also edited at two sites in TM1 which influence the Ca^{2+} permeability. This suggests that TM1 might contribute to the pore in the glutamate receptors.

Another A to G editing, designated the R/G site, can occur immediately preceding the "flip-flop" segment in GluR2–GluR4. The "flip-flop" segment influences the rate of desensitization while the rate of recovery from the desensitized state depends on the R/G site where the edited form (G) recovers faster than the unedited R form.

3.3.5 THE SELECTIVITY FILTER

The interplay between the glutamate receptor subtypes depends in part on the ability of the different receptors to conduct Ca^{2+} ions vs. monovalent ions. For channels to be selective for different ions, the pore must be narrow enough to force the ions to interact with the pore. At this selective filter, water molecules binding the ion (or some of them) will be replaced by polar amino acids residues that line the wall of the pore. Consequently, the selectivity will depend on many parameters such as the size and charge of the ion, the hydration energy, and the size and geometry of the pore at the selectivity filter. The Q/R site defines an important part of the selectivity filter in the glutamate receptors. For instance, for the AMPA and kainate receptors, the presence of a subunit encoding an R at the Q/R site completely abolishes divalent ion flux but not the monovalent current. However, if all the subunits encode a Q at the Q/R site the divalent ion permeability is higher than the monovalent ion permeability.

3.4 ATP RECEPTORS

Extracellular ATP has been demonstrated to activate depolarizing currents in different neuronal and nonneuronal cells. Recently, two homologous subunits were cloned by an expression cloning strategy. The clones encoded proteins of 399 and 427 amino acids, respectively. Neither of the subunits expressed a signal sequence, indicating an intracellular location of the N-terminus. Considering the distribution of potential N-linked glycosylation sites, a region

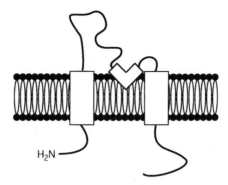

FIGURE 3.10   Schematic representation of the transmembrane topology of the ATP receptor.

that shows sequence similarity to an ATP binding site and the hydrophobicity profile, a 2-TM model was proposed with most of the protein in the extracellular domain and both the N and C termini located intracellularly. Some sequence similarity was observed between a hydrophobic segment preceding TM2 and the sequence which forms the lining of the pore in a number of potassium channels. Thus, the pore may by analogy with the potassium channels be formed by TM2 and this hydrophobic segment (Figure 3.10).

3.5 PROBLEMS

PROBLEM 3.1

The agonist binding site is located at the subunit interface in the 4-TM family. Argue for a similar location in the glutamate receptor family.

PROBLEM 3.2

Assume the assembly of nicotine acetylcholine receptor subunits is completely permissive. How many different receptors can be assembled in a cell expressing $\alpha 3$, $\beta 2$, and $\beta 4$? Group the receptors according to which are likely to have similar single-channel conductance and/or activation kinetics.

3.6 FURTHER READING

4-TM Receptors

Betz, H., Structure and function of inhibitory glycine receptors, *Q. Rev. Biophys.,* 25, 381-394, 1992.

Galzi, J.-L., Devillers-Thiéry, A., Hussy, N., Bertrand, S., Changeux, J.-P., and Bertrand, D., Mutations in the channel domain of a neuronal nicotinic receptor convert ion selectivity from cationic to anionic, *Nature*, 359, 500–505, 1992.

Karlin, A., Structure of nicotinic acetylcholine receptors, *Curr. Opin. Neurobiol.,* 3, 299-309, 1993.

Maricq, A. V., Peterson, A. S., Brake, A. J., Myers, R. M., and Julius, D., Primary structure and functional expression of the 5-HT3 receptor, a serotonin-gated ion channel, *Sceince,* 254, 432-437, 1991.

McDonald, R. L. and Olsen, R., GABA-A receptor channels, *Annu. Rev. Neurosci.,* 17, 569-602, 1994.

Sargent, P. B., The diversity of neuronal nicotinic acetylcholine receptors, *Annu. Rev. Neurosci.,* 16, 403-443, 1993.

Schmieden, V., Kuhse, J., and Betz, H., Mutation of glycine receptor subunit creates beta-alanine receptor responsive to GABA, *Science*, 262, 256-258, 1993.

Unwin, N., Nicotinic acetylcholine receptor at 9 Å resolution, *J. Mol. Biol.,* 229, 1101-1124, 1993.

Unwin, N., Acetylcholine receptor channel imaged in the open state, *Nature,* 373, 37-43, 1995.

Glutamate

Hollmann, M. and Heinemann, S., Cloned glutamate receptors, *Annu. Rev. Neurosci.,* 17, 31-108, 1994.

Hollmann, M., Maron, C., and Heinemann, S. F., N-glycosylation site tagging suggests a three trans-membrane domain topology for the glutamate receptor GluR1, *Neuron*, 13, 1331-1343, 1994.

Kuryatov, A., Laube, B., Betz, H., and Kuhse, J., Mutational analysis of the glycine-binding site of the NMDA receptor: structural similarity with bacterial amino-acid-binding proteins, *Neuron*, 12, 1291-1300, 1994.

Seeburg, P. H., The molecular biology of mammalian glutamate receptor channels, *Trends Neurosci.,* 16, 359-365, 1993.

Stern-Bach, Y., Bettler, B., Hartley, M., Sheppard, P. O., O'Hara, P. J., and Heinemann, S. F., Agonist selectivity of glutamate receptors is specified by two domains structurally related to bacterial amino acid binding proteins, *Neuron,* 13, 1345-1357, 1994.

Wo, Z. G. and Oswald, R. E., Transmembrane topology of two kainate receptor subunits revealed by N-glycosylation, *Proc. Natl. Acad. Sci. U.S.A.,* 91, 7154-7158, 1994.

ATP

Bean, B., Pharmacology and electrophysiology of ATP-activated ion channels, *Trends Pharmacol. Sci.,* 13, 87-90, 1992.

Brake, A. J., Wagenbach, M. J., and Julius, D., New structural motif for ligand-gated ion channels defined by an ionotropic ATP receptor, *Nature*, 371, 519-523, 1994.

Valera, S., Hussy, N., Evans, R. J., Adami, N., North, R., Surprenant, A., and Buell, G., A new class of ligand-gated ion channel defined by P2x receptor for extracellular ATP, *Nature*, 371, 516-519, 1994.

3.7 SOLUTIONS TO PROBLEMS

PROBLEM 3.1

Neither homomeric GluR6 nor homomeric KA2 receptors can bind AMPA, but the hetero-meric GluR6-KA2 receptor can. This suggests a location of the binding site where segment A from one subunit and segment B from the other might generate the binding site. In fact, mutant GluR6 can accommodate AMPA binding when the A segment is substituted with the corresponding segment from the AMPA receptors.

PROBLEM 3.2

Eight. In linear representation (1) α_3-β_2-α_3-β_2-β_2,(2) α_3-β_2-α_3-β_2-β_4, (3) α_3-β_2-α_3-β_4-β_2, (4) α_3-β_4-α_3-β_2-β_2, (5) α_3-β_2-α_3-β_4-β_4, (6) α_3-β_4-α_3-β_2-β_4, (7) α_3-β_4-α_3-β_4-β_2, (8) α_3-β_4-α_3-β_4-β_4. Combinations with similar stoichiometry would be likely to have similar conductances, i.e., four groups, 1, 2–4, 5–7, and 8. The subunit arrangement may be more important for the receptor kinetics since the agonist binding site is located between an α- and a β-subunit. If the binding site is assumed to be between the α-subunit and the β-subunit on the right (in this linear representation) there are three groups: 1–2, $2x(\alpha_3$-$\beta_2)$; 3–6, $(\alpha_3$-$\beta_2)(\alpha_3$-$\beta_4)$; and 7–8, $2x(\alpha_3$-$\beta_4)$.

4 Molecular Structure of Tyrosine Kinase-Linked Receptors

Steen Gammeltoft and C. Ronald Kahn

CONTENTS

4.1 INTRODUCTION

Membrane receptors can be classified structurally and functionally into three superfamilies that differ in the number and arrangement of membrane-spanning segments and signal transduction: (1) seven-transmembrane segment receptors coupled to G-proteins, (2) single-transmembrane segment receptors directly or indirectly coupled to intracellular enzymes, and (3) four-transmembrane segment receptors that form ligand-gated ion channels. Receptors for hormones, growth factors, and neurotransmitters are represented in all three groups, indicating that the ligand binding and signal transduction involved in their biological actions show significant variation. This chapter focuses on the superfamily of single-transmembrane segment receptors. Emphasis will be on structure and function of tyrosine kinase-linked receptors that mediate the action of a large number of polypeptide hormones, growth factors, and cytokines. The basic structural design of tyrosine kinase receptors is remarkably simple and constant. Each receptor polypeptide contains a single extracellular region that includes one or more ligand-binding domains, a single linear hydrophobic peptide region that makes one pass through the membrane bilayer, and a single peptide sequence that resides in the cytoplasm. The ligand-binding domain has only been grossly mapped in a limited number of receptors, and a detailed analysis awaits the resolution of the three-dimensional structure of the receptor by X-ray crystallography. The transmembrane domain is composed of 21 to

0-8493-9227-6/96/$0.00+$.50
© 1996 by CRC Press, Inc.

23 predominantly hydrophobic amino acids that forms an α-helix with 7 turns: a length (approximately 30 nm) sufficient to span the lipid membrane bilayer. Apart from the hydrophobic nature of the amino acids, no consensus sequence has been described. The cytoplasmic domain of the receptor contains the tyrosine kinase in a single linear sequence or two sequences bisected by an inserted domain. The activation of the receptor tyrosine kinase represents the initial cellular response to cell surface binding of growth factors, hormones, or cytokines.

Tyrosine kinase receptors belong to a superfamily including membrane-bound, cytoplasmic and nuclear tyrosine kinases that are involved in regulation of normal cell growth and differentiation. Several tyrosine kinases have been identified as protooncogenes that are capable of inducing a transformed, cellular phenotype after overexpression or after activating mutations. Viral oncogenes have developed the potential of cell transformation by virtue of acquiring a protooncogene and changing it into a viral oncogene by various mutations of the gene, resulting in amino acid substitutions and deletions in the oncogene protein that increase its transforming activity. Retroviral oncogenes have been identified as a cause of cancer in a variety of animal species, but not in humans. In human cancer, somatic mutations of protooncogenes that lead to gene amplification, overexpression, aberrant expression, or constitutive activation of oncogene proteins have been detected. The increased activity of these oncogene products may contribute to the development and maintenance of the tumor. In spite of the existence of multiple receptors and oncogene products with tyrosine kinase activity, phosphorylation of cellular proteins on tyrosine residues is a much less common event than serine phosphorylation, comprising about 0.1% of all protein phosphorylation in the resting cell and about 1% in dividing cells. Oncogene-transformed cells may contain up to 10% phosphotyrosine of the total phosphorylated proteins, implicating tyrosine kinases in the growth of cancer cells.

4.2 STRUCTURE OF TYROSINE KINASE-LINKED RECEPTORS

4.2.1 CLONING OF RECEPTORS

Receptor structures have been determined from the full-length nucleotide sequences of mRNA molecules encoding membrane receptors for hormones, growth factors, and neurotransmitters. One of the first membrane receptors to be sequenced was the epidermal growth factor (EGF) receptor. Because transmembrane receptors are not abundant molecules, their characterization involved a combination of biochemical and molecular biological techniques. Thus, the receptor proteins were first purified in small amounts, and short stretches of the amino acid sequence were determined. Oligonucleotide probes corresponding to the amino acid sequence were synthesized for screening of a cDNA library derived from a tissue or cell expressing mRNA for the receptor. Positive clones were selected by hybridization under stringent conditions, the cDNA insert of the phage was sequenced, and the amino acid sequence was deduced.

Following this basic approach, other techniques for cloning and sequencing of membrane receptors have been applied. Receptors with similar sequences were detected by screening the cDNA library with a known receptor cDNA probe under low stringency conditions. One example is the human EGF receptor homologue, HER-2, which was cloned and sequenced by screening with a cDNA probe for the viral oncogene v-erbB. The ligand was initially unknown and the receptor was designated an "orphan receptor". The ligand was later identified and termed either *Neu* differentiation factor, heregulin, or neuregulin. The polymerase chain reaction (PRC) technique has been used for amplification of an unknown receptor cDNA with synthetic oligonucleotide primers that are directed towards conserved domains based on a presumed sequence similarity with a known receptor. This cDNA fragment is then used as a specific probe for screening cDNA libraries under stringent conditions. Many of the G-protein-coupled receptors, including the thyroid-stimulating hormone receptor, have been cloned using this technique. Finally, expression-cloning has been used for cloning neurotransmitter receptors like the substance K receptor, and peptide hormone receptors like the TSH-releasing hormone receptor. Expression of mRNA in a frog oocyte, and screening of ligand-induced membrane ion flux or depolarization was followed by selection, amplification, and sequencing of the relevant cDNA. Expression-cloning in the Cos cell line has been used for sequencing hormone receptors like the glucagon receptor.

4.2.2 Functional Domains of Tyrosine Kinase-Linked Receptors

Tyrosine kinase-linked receptors belong to the superfamily of single-transmembrane segment receptors that include receptors with catalytic activity like tyrosine kinase, serine-threonine kinase, guanylate cyclase and phosphotyrosine phosphatase in their cytoplasmic domain (Table 4.1). Activation of these receptors and their intrinsic or associated enzymes induces intracellular signals via phosphorylation or dephosphorylation of proteins or by formation of cGMP. More than 50 members of this family are known and include polypeptide growth factor, cytokine, and peptide hormone receptors. The family can be subdivided depending on the structure and function of the cytoplasmic domain which specifies the nature of the intracellular signaling mechanism (Table 4.2). Protein tyrosine kinase-containing receptors are typified by those for epidermal growth factor (EGF), insulin, insulin-like growth factor I (IGF-I), platelet-derived growth factor (PDGF), and nerve growth factor (NGF). Membrane receptors for growth hormone (GH), prolactin, erythropoietin, granulocyte-macrophage colony-stimulating factors and granulocyte colony-stimulating factor, interferons-α, -β, -γ, and interleukins (IL) IL-2, IL-3, IL-4, IL-5, IL-6, and IL-7 are devoid of intrinsic enzyme activity in the cytoplasmic domain, but associate with cytoplasmic tyrosine kinases like the Janus (JAK) family, and other membrane proteins, to form multisubunit receptor complexes. Receptors with intrinsic serine-threonine kinase activity include the transforming growth factor β (TGF-β) receptor type 1 and 2. Receptors that contain guanylate cyclase activity bind atrial natriuretic peptide (ANP). The tumor necrosis factor (TNF) p55 receptor and nerve growth factor (NGF) p75 receptor are devoid of intrinsic enzyme activity and their signaling mechanism is yet unknown. Finally, a family of membrane proteins has a receptor-like structure which contains phosphotyrosine phosphatase activity in its cytoplasmic domains, but no extracellular ligands have yet been identified. The structure and function of the two families of tyrosine kinase-linked receptors will be described in detail, whereas the other families will only be summarized in this chapter.

4.2.2.1 Tyrosine Kinase Receptor Family

The family of tyrosine kinase-linked receptors is characterized by a large extracellular domain with either a characteristic disulfide cross-linked region or an IgG-like domain, a single hydrophobic transmembrane domain, and a large cytoplasmic domain with the catalytic tyrosine kinase (Figure 4.1). One traverse of the lipid bilayer provides a minimum exposure of the receptor to the membrane lipids and facilitates receptor mobility, aggregation, and internalization. The tyrosine kinase-containing receptors constitute a large group of receptors which can be divided into seven classes based on a comparison of their individual structures. These include EGF and neu (or HER-2) receptors, insulin and IGF-1 receptors, PDGF receptors α and β, CSF-1 and kit receptors, FGF receptors, NGF (or trk) receptors, and hepatocyte growth factor (HGF) or scatter factor receptors. Figure 4.2 shows the three classes of receptor tyrosine kinases that were the first to be cloned: EGF receptors, insulin receptors, and PDGF receptors.

The first class is represented by the EGF receptor in which the hormone binding and tyrosine kinase domains are contained in a single transmembrane peptide chain. The configuration of the ATP binding site and the tyrosine kinase domain is generally similar to that of

TABLE 4.1
Superfamily of Single-Transmembrane Segment Receptors: Structural and Functional Classification

Receptor family	Subunit composition	Transduction system	Ligands
	Monomers or	The binding subunit itself is:	All are polypeptides:
(A) Tyrosine kinase receptors	homodimers or posttranslational heterotetramers or	(A) A ligand-stimulated tyrosine kinase	(A) Mitogenic growth factors; insulin
(B) Tyrosine kinase-linked receptors	native heterodimers or heterotrimers	(B) Not of known enzymatic activity associating with a cytoplasmic tyrosine kinase	(B) Growth hormone; prolactin; cytokines
(C) Guanylate cyclase receptors		(C) A ligand-stimulated guanylate cyclase	(C) Natriuretic peptides
(D) Serine/threonine kinase receptors		(D) A ligand-stimulated serine/threonine kinase	(D) Transforming growth factor β
(E) Tyrosine phosphatase receptors		(E) Intrinsic tyrosine phosphatase	(E) Unknown

Modified from Barnard, E.A., *Trends Biochem. Sci.,* 1992;17:368-374.

other members of the Src tyrosine kinase superfamily. The extracellular domain contains cysteine-rich domains that appear to be important for hormone binding, although these exist in two interrupted regions in the EGF receptor. There is evidence that the EGF receptor is inactive in its monomeric form and that transmission of the ligand signal requires receptor dimerization.

The second class, including the homologous insulin and IGF-I receptors, are the most complex, with a heterotetrameric structure consisting of two α- and two β-subunits joined by disulfide cross-bridges. The α-subunits are entirely extracellular and contain a cysteine-rich region that is believed to be involved in hormone binding. The β-subunits possess an extracellular domain, a transmembrane domain, and an intracellular domain which contains an ATP binding site and a catalytic kinase domain. The α- and β-subunits are synthesized as part of a single receptor precursor molecule which undergoes proteolytic processing to form the two subunits in a manner analogous to synthesis of insulin from proinsulin.

The PDGF receptors form a third structural group of tyrosine kinase receptors. They contain ligand-binding and tyrosine kinase activities in a single peptide chain, but possess a different type of extracellular cysteine-rich structure which is believed to form IgG-like repeats. In addition, the tyrosine kinase domain is interrupted by an insert of about 100 amino acids which is unrelated to other tyrosine kinases. Two types of PDGF receptors have been cloned: PDGF receptor α and PDGF receptor β. They show about 60% sequence identity and different binding specificity towards the three types of PDGF dimers: PDGF AA, AB, and BB. The monomeric PDGF receptor is inactive, but is activated after ligand-induced dimerization resulting in formation of three PDGF receptor dimers αα, ββ, and αβ. PDGF AA binds only to PDGF receptor αα, whereas PDGF BB binds with high affinity to PDGF receptor ββ and with lower affinity to PDGF receptor αα. PDGF AB interacts with all three PDGF receptor dimeric complexes. PDGF receptor α and receptor β show differences in their cellular actions and the PDGF receptor ββ is more potent in stimulating cell division and chemotaxis than is PDGF αα. Thus, the existence of three PDGF dimers, as well as the three dimeric PDGF receptor complexes, provides possibilities for varying the cellular effects.

The group of fibroblast growth factor (FGF) receptors include four single-chain receptors which show some relationship to the PDGF receptor class. They are characterized by an

TABLE 4.2
Single-Transmembrane Segment Receptors

Tyrosine Kinase Receptor Family

Epidermal growth factor	Platelet-derived growth factors A and B
Neu-differentiation factor	Colony-stimulating factor-1
Insulin	(macrophage-colony-stimulating factor)
Insulin-like growth factor I	Nerve growth factors (neurotrophins)
Fibroblast growth factors	Hepatocyte growth factor (scatter factor)

Tyrosine Kinase-Linked Receptor Family

Growth hormone	Granulocyte-macrophage-colony-
Prolactin	stimulating factor
Placental lactogen	Granulocyte-colony-stimulating factor
Erythropoietin	Interferons α, β, and γ
Interleukin-2	Tumor necrosis factor: p75
Interleukin-3	Leukemia inhibitory factor
Interleukin-4	Oncostatin
Interleukin-5	Ciliary neurotrophic factor
Interleukin-6	
Interleukin-7	

Guanylate Cyclase Receptor Family

Atrial natriuretic peptide: type A, B, and C

Serine-Threonine Kinase Receptor Family

Transforming growth factor	Activin
β: type I and II	Inhibin

Tumor Necrosis Factor-Nerve Growth
Factor Receptor Family

Tumor necrosis factor: p55	Nerve growth factor: p75

Phosphotyrosine Phosphatase Receptor Family

Ligands unknown

extracellular domain with three IgG-like repeats, one transmembrane domain, and a cytoplasmic domain with a tyrosine kinase interrupted by a small insert of 14 amino acids. The sequence of the extracellular domain may vary depending on alternative splicing; resulting in several receptor subtypes with varying ligand specificity. Ligands for these receptors include nine members of the FGF family which are widespread in the organism.

The group of colony-stimulating factor-1 (CSF-1) receptors includes the c-kit oncogene product and are distantly related to PDGF and FGF receptors. They have IgG-like domains in their extracellular portion and a kinase insert in their cytoplasmic portion. The NGF receptor group includes three members: trk A, trk B, and trk C, named after the c-trk oncogene product which was found to bind NGF. Trk receptors are single-chain polypeptides with cysteine-rich, leucine-rich, and IgG-like regions in the extracellular domain, a single transmembrane domain, and a cytoplasmic domain with a tyrosine kinase interrupted by an insert. Trk receptors bind five members of the NGF (or neurotrophin) family: NGF, brain-derived neurotrophic factor (BDNF), and neurotrophin-3, -4, and -5, all of which are widespread in the nervous system.

The HGF receptor binds to the c-met oncogene product. This is a two-chain, disulfide-linked polypeptide with an extracellular α-subunit and a transmembrane β-subunit with a

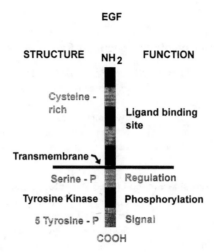

FIGURE 4.1 Structure and function of receptor tyrosine kinases. The EGF receptor is a single-polypeptide chain with 1186 residues and an approximate molecular weight of 170,000 Da. The receptor is composed of an extracellular region of 622 amino acids with two cysteine-rich domains and a ligand-binding region. The transmembrane region is 22 amino acids of hydrophobic nature. The intracellular portion is 542 amino acids and has three functional domains: the regulatory domain with serine and threonine residues that are phosphorylated leading to inactivation of the receptor; the tyrosine kinase domain that is activated by EGF binding and dimerization of receptors; the C-terminal domain with five tyrosine residues that are phosphorylated by the receptor tyrosine kinase and are involved in signal transduction via association with SH2 domain proteins.

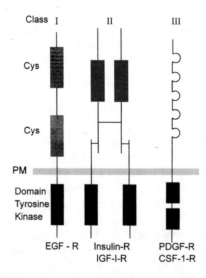

FIGURE 4.2 Structure of single-transmembrane segment receptor tyrosine kinases. Three classes are shown; class I is represented by the EGF receptor; class II by insulin and IGF-1 receptors; class III by PDGF and CSF–1 receptors. The shaded rectangles in EGF and insulin receptors represent cysteine-rich regions. Disulfide bonds in these regions are thought to have an important role in establishing the structure of the ligand binding site. The circles in the PDGF receptor represent IgG-like repeats. The black rectangles in all three classes represent the tyrosine kinase domain, which is interrupted by an insert in PDGF receptors.

TABLE 4.3
JAK Tyrosine Kinases in Cytokine Receptor Signaling

Cytokine receptor	Cell/tissue response	Tyrosine kinase		
		JAK1	JAK2	TYK2
Interferon-α/β	Cell arrest	+	?	+
Interferon-γ	Immune response	+	+	?
Interleukin-3	Hematopoietic cell proliferation	?	+	?
Granulocyte/macrophage-CSF	Granulocyte/macrophage differentiation	?	+	?
Erythropoietin	Induction of erythropoiesis	?	+	?
Granulocyte-CSF	Proliferation and differentiation of various cells,	+	+	?
Interleukin	particularly hematopoietic cells	+	+	+
Leukemia-inhibitory factor		+	+	?
Oncostatin	Growth inhibition of tumor cells	+	+	?
Ciliary neurotrophic factor	Neuronal cell proliferation and differentiation	+	+	?
Growth hormone	Growth, mammary gland differentiation, carbohydrate/lipid metabolism	?	+	?
Prolactin	Lactogenesis, gonadal cell function, B/T-cell proliferation	+	+	?

Modified from Ziemiecki, A., Harber, A.G., and Wieks, A.F., *Trends Cell Biol.*, 1994; 4:207-212.

cytoplasmic tyrosine kinase domain: a structure that is reminiscent of the insulin receptor. The HGF receptor is synthesized as a single polypeptide chain inactive precursor that is cleaved into an active two chain molecule.

4.2.2.2 Tyrosine Kinase-Linked Receptor Family

A large group of single-transmembrane segment receptors is characterized by the absence of enzymatic activity in the binding subunit. Receptors for GH, prolactin, cytokines, hematopoietic factors, and ciliary neurotrophic factor (CNTF) are related by sequence homology of the extracellular domain, whereas known motifs of signaling proteins such as kinases and phosphatases are absent in the cytoplasmic domain. These receptors are composed of several subunits which form active homologous or heterologous oligomers. The complex of two identical or different subunits binds its ligand with high affinity, whereas the single subunits bind with lower affinity. The high affinity, multisubunit receptors induce tyrosine phosphorylation by coupling with cytoplasmic tyrosine kinases of the Janus kinase family, of which three members are known: JAK1, JAK2, and TYK2. JAK kinases are characterized by the possession, in addition to a *bona fide* kinase domain, of a kinase-related domain, and have been named after Janus, the Roman god of gateways that had two faces. JAK kinases associate with several cytokine receptors and are involved in their signal transduction (Table 4.3).

The GH receptor is a 130-kDa protein consisting of 620 amino acids divided into a 246-residue extracellular domain, a single-transmembrane domain of 24 amino acids and an intracellular domain of about 350 residues (Figure 4.3). The extracellular domain possesses several potential sites of N-linked and O-linked glycosylation, as in most membrane receptors, but there are no cysteine-rich regions or obvious repeating structures. Although the GH receptor is tyrosine-phosphorylated, elucidation of its primary structure showed that the intracellular domain bears no resemblance to receptors of known functional type. The difference between the apparent molecular weight (130 kDa) and the predicted amino acid molecular weight by composition (70 kDa) is thought to be due to a high level of glycosylation and covalent association of the receptor with ubiquitin. When expressed in mammalian cells,

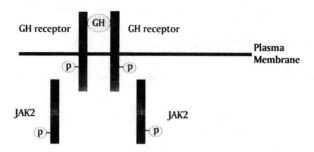

FIGURE 4.3 Structure of single-transmembrane segment receptors that form homologous dimers; the growth hormone (GH) receptor. One GH molecule binds to identical binding sites on the extracellular domains of two GH receptors that form a homodimer. The intracellular domains associate with a tyrosine kinase of the Janus kinase family, JAK2. Encircled P denotes potential tyrosine phosphorylation sites on the intracellular portion of GH receptor and JAK2.

the human GH receptor binds only human GH, whereas the rabbit receptor binds human GH, bovine GH, and ovine prolactin, and this correlates well with the known species specificity of GH. The extracellular domain of the GH receptor has been expressed in a soluble, secreted form and its three-dimensional structure determined by X-ray crystallography. The GH receptor was crystallized in its ligand-bound form, and the structure revealed that the extracellular domain forms a symmetrical dimer which associates with one GH molecule. GH has two distinct receptor-binding sites which interact with the same ligand-binding region on the two binding sites in the dimer. It appears that formation of the GH receptor homodimer is needed for high affinity binding of GH and the activation of cellular responses. This was supported by the finding that a GH mutant with inactivation of one of the two binding sites acted as an antagonist to GH.

The prolactin receptor is also a single-transmembrane polypeptide with 209 amino acids on the extracellular face, but only 58 amino acids in the cytoplasm. It has four homologous regions in the extracellular domain, but only one homologous region in the intracellular domain. Like the GH receptor, the prolactin receptor has no known functional signaling elements. In mammalian tissues there is a larger form of the prolactin receptor, highly homologous to the GH receptor. Also, as a result of alternative splicing, secretory forms of both the GH receptor and the prolactin receptor exist that contain no transmembrane or intracellular domains.

Cytokines and hematopoietic growth factors, a large family of protein mediators, regulate proliferation, differentiation, and functions of various lineages in the immune and hematopoietic system of receptors. Cloning of the receptors for erythropoietin, IL-2, IL-3, IL-4, IL-5, IL-6, and IL-7, colony-stimulating factors for granulocytes and macrophages (abbreviated GM-CSF, G-CSF, M-CSF), leukemia inhibiting factor, oncostatin, ciliary neurotrophic factor (CNTF), tumor necrosis factor (TNF) (p75), and interferon-α, -β, and -γ revealed that they consist of two distinct subunits: α-subunits and β-subunits. For two groups of cytokine receptors including, IL-3, IL-5, and GM-CSF as well as IL-6, leukemia inhibiting factor, oncostatin, and CNTF receptors, the α-subunit is cytokine-specific whereas the β-subunit is common among the three members of each group. The mature α-subunits are glycoproteins of 60 to 80 kDa with a short cytoplasmic domain of about 50 amino acids, Each α-subunit binds its specific cytokine with low affinity (K_d = 2 to 100 nM). The β-subunit, a glycoprotein of about 120 to 140 kDa, has an extracellular domain with two segments of the conserved motif of the hematopoietic growth factor receptors and a large cytoplasmic domain without any known motif of signaling proteins. Only one type of β-subunit (common β or β_c) is present in IL-3, IL-5, and GM-CSF receptors. Although β_c does not bind any cytokine by itself, it forms high affinity receptors (K_d = 100 pM) with an α-subunit. The $\alpha\beta$ heterodimer

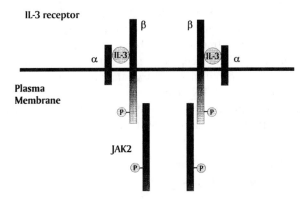

FIGURE 4.4 Structure of single-transmembrane segment receptors that form heterologous dimers; the interleukin-3 (IL-3) receptor. IL-3 binds to the high affinity IL-3 receptor complex composed of one α-subunit and one β-subunit. The ligand-receptor complex aggregates with another αβ heterodimer and associates with two cytoplasmic tyrosine kinases of the JAK family. Encircled P are tyrosine phosphorylation sites on receptor β-subunits and JAK2

aggregates with another αβ dimer and associates with two JAK2 kinases to form a signaling complex (Figure 4.4). IL-6, leukemia inhibiting factor, and CNTF receptors have specific α-subunits with an IgG-like domain and the common motif of the hematopoietic growth factor receptors of four cysteines. A 130-kDa glycoprotein known as gp130 is involved in the formation of the high affinity receptor, and represents a common subunit in these receptors.

4.2.2.3 Other Single-Transmembrane Segment Receptors

Guanylate cyclase receptors are characterized by the cytoplasmic guanylate cyclase that catalyzes the formation cyclic GMP from GTP. The deduced amino acid sequence of guanylate cyclase derived from cloned cDNAs predicts a single-transmembrane domain. In mammals, three types of guanylate cyclase receptors have been cloned, of which receptor type A binds atrial natriuretic peptide (ANP), and receptor types B and C bind peptides homologous to ANP, i.e., natriuretic peptides B and C (abbreviated BNP and CNP). The receptor guanylate cyclases are members of a superfamily of proteins that include the cytoplasmic form of guanylate cyclase.

Serine-threonine kinase receptors include TGF-β receptors type I and II, activin, inhibin, Müllerian-inhibiting substance, and bone morphogen receptors. These receptors have large extracellular domains containing a cysteine-rich region, a single-transmembrane domain, and a cytoplasmic serine-threonine kinase with two inserted sequences. The kinase is homologous to other serine-threonine kinases like protein kinases A and C. Transmission of the TGF-β signal requires heterodimerization of type I and type II TGF-β receptors and activation of the type I receptor serine-threonine kinase via transphosphorylation by a constitutively active type II receptor kinase. The signal pathway is not yet clear because downstream substrates of the receptor kinase have not yet been identified.

A group of membrane-bound phosphotyrosine phosphatases have receptor-like structures with a large extracellular domain containing a cysteine-rich, glycosylated region which forms a putative ligand-binding site, a single-transmembrane domain, and a cytoplasmic domain with two tandem tyrosine phosphatases. Eight members with some sequence homology have been cloned, including CD45, a lymphocyte common antigen. The regulation of the phosphatase activity is unknown because no extracellular ligands have yet been identified. The extracellular domain has regions with similarity to cell adhesion molecules, suggesting that they may be involved in cell aggregation.

Two receptors for TNF-α and -β (p55), and NGF (p75) are related by structural homology. These are single-transmembrane segments and monomeric receptors with no known signaling sequence in their cytoplasmic portion. It should be emphasized that TNF also binds to a p75 receptor, a member of the cytokine receptor family, and that NGF binds to the trk receptor tyrosine kinase, which are involved in signal transduction of TNF and NGF, respectively. Recent studies suggest that the p55 TNF receptor and p75 NGF receptor may be involved in apoptosis and mediate the cytotoxic actions of TNF and effects of NGF on programmed cell death during the development of the nervous system.

4.3 SIGNALING VIA TYROSINE KINASE-LINKED RECEPTORS

4.3.1 ACTIVATION OF RECEPTOR-LINKED TYROSINE KINASES

Tyrosine kinase activation is a key event in the intracellular signal transduction of tyrosine kinase receptors like EGF, PDGF, FGF, NGF, IGF-I, and insulin receptors and receptors linked with cytoplasmic tyrosine kinases like GH, prolactin, cytokine, and hematopoietic growth factor receptors. The initial signal transduction of these receptors involves dimerization, kinase activation, and tyrosine phosphorylation (Figure 4.5). Tyrosine kinase-linked receptors exist as inactive monomers in the plasma membrane, with the exception of the insulin and IGF-I receptors which are inactive disulfide-linked heterotetramers. Four different mechanisms are involved in dimerization of the receptor and activation of its associated tyrosine kinase: (1) a monomeric, monovalent ligand (like EGF) binds two receptors leading to dimerization; (2) a dimeric, bivalent ligand (like PDGF) sequentially binds two receptors that associate in a dimer; (3) a monomeric, bivalent ligand (like insulin) binds a dimeric (or heterotetrameric) receptor leading to kinase activation; and (4) a monomeric, bivalent ligand (like GH) binds two receptors through different receptor-binding regions leading to the formation of a dimer. The ligand-induced dimerization is followed by activation of the tyrosine kinase and rapid phosphorylation of the cytoplasmic receptor domain and intracellular substrates.

Receptor autophosphorylation occurs through a *trans*-mechanism in which one tyrosine kinase phosphorylates the other in the dimer. The role of autophosphorylation in signal transfer is phosphorylation of individual tyrosine residues in the cytoplasmic domain of the receptor. These phosphotyrosines serve as highly selective docking sites that bind cytoplasmic signaling molecules involved in the pleiotropic responses to growth factors and insulin. In the insulin receptor, autophosphorylation of three tyrosines in the kinase domain regulates kinase activity and leads to a 20-fold increase. This is also true for the homologous IGF-I receptor, as well as for the unrelated HGF receptor. Insulin and IGF-I receptor tyrosine kinases phosphorylate the insulin receptor substrate-1, which serves as a docking protein and interacts with a number of signaling molecules.

The receptor tyrosine kinase is an allosteric enzyme in which the extracellular domain is the regulatory subunit and is linked by the transmembrane domain to the cytoplasmic domain with its catalytic subunit. In the inactive state, the extracellular domain inhibits the tyrosine kinase activity. This inhibition is released by ligand binding, by removal of the extracellular domain by proteolytic cleavage, or by expression of truncated receptor tyrosine kinases as in oncogenes. Mutations in the transmembrane region of some receptors can also activate the tyrosine kinase. This suggests that ligand binding and receptor dimerization induces a conformational change of the transmembrane domain that is propagated to the cytoplasmic domain of the receptor, a phenomenon that has been confirmed using conformationally sensitive antibodies.

Several observations indicate that receptor tyrosine kinase activation is necessary for signal transduction by growth factors and insulin. Overexpression of normal receptor tyrosine kinases in cells increases the sensitivity and responsiveness for a number of biological effects.

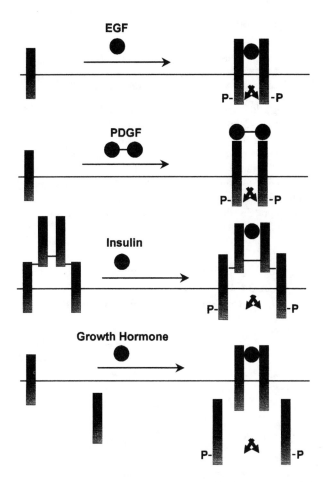

FIGURE 4.5 Receptor tyrosine kinase activation by dimerization. Four models of ligand-induced dimerization of receptors and activation of tyrosine kinase are shown. (1) EGF, a monomeric, bivalent ligand binds to an inactive receptor leading to dimerization, activation of tyrosine kinase, and transphosphorylation of tyrosine residues. (2) PDGF, a dimeric, bivalent ligand binds to an inactive monomeric receptor leading to cross-linking, kinase activation, and transphosphorylation. (3) Insulin, a monomeric, bivalent ligand binds to an inactive covalent dimeric (heterotetrameric) receptor leading to kinase activation and autophosphorylation. (4) Growth hormone, a monomeric, bivalent ligand binds to inactive monomeric receptors leading to dimerization and association with cytoplasmic JAK tyrosine kinases, kinase activation, and tyrosine phosphorylation.

Kinase-inactive receptors mutated at the ATP binding site retain ligand-binding activity, are internalized and mediate ligand degradation, but fail to stimulate biological effects including membrane transport, cytoskeletal organization, ribosomal protein S6 activation, glycogen synthesis, and DNA synthesis. Microinjection into cells of monoclonal antibodies to the kinase domain of the insulin and EGF receptors decreases the effects of insulin and EGF on both the kinase activity and biological responses. Finally, genetic or acquired alterations of tyrosine kinase activity are associated with various disorders in humans or experimental animals. Loss of function results in developmental defects or hormone resistance. Gain of function results in hyperplastic or malignant growth disorders.

4.3.2 SH2 AND SH3 DOMAIN PROTEINS IN SIGNAL TRANSDUCTION

Two domains in the Src tyrosine kinase have been identified in an increasing number of cellular proteins based on their amino acid sequence homology. These have been termed Src

Src Tyrosine Kinase

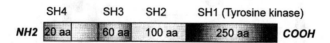

FIGURE 4.6   Src homology domains. Src contains four domains that have been found in a variety of cellular proteins involved in intracellular signal transduction. The SH1 domain is 250 amino acids (aa) and represents the catalytic domain of the tyrosine kinase that is common to the superfamily of src-like tyrosine kinases including membrane receptors, cytoplasmic and nuclear tyrosine kinases. The SH2 domain of approximately 100 amino acids and the SH3 domain of 60 amino acids are common to proteins with putative signaling functions. The SH2 domain binds tyrosine-phosphorylated regions of target proteins, frequently linking activated growth factor receptors to signal molecules. The SH3 domain binds proline-rich motifs in proteins often connected with small G proteins. The SH4 domain contains signals for myristylation and palmitylation.

TABLE 4.4
SH2 and SH3 Domain-Containing Proteins

Enzymes	
Src	Tyrosine kinase
Abl	Tyrosine kinase
PLC-γ	Phospholipase
GAP	Ras GTP-ase activator
SHPTP-1 and -2	Tyrosine phosphatase
Adaptors	
p85	Phosphoinositol-3-kinase
GRB-2	Ras exchange factor
SHC	Signal complex factor
IFSG-3	Transcription factor
Structural Proteins	
Spectrin	Cytoskeleton
Myosin	Cytoskeleton
Tensin	Cytoskeleton

homology 2 and 3 domains, or SH2 and SH3 domains (Figure 4.6). The Src homology 1 (SH1) domain is the catalytic region of the Src tyrosine kinase that is common to all tyrosine kinases. The N-terminal domain of Src with signals for myristylation and palmitylation represents the Src homology 4 (SH4) domain. SH2 domain-containing proteins can be divided into three classes based on their function: (1) enzymes like Src tyrosine kinase, Abl tyrosine kinase, phospholipase C-γ, Ras GTPase-activating protein (GAP), SH2 domain phosphotyrosine phosphatases-1 and -2 (SHPTP-1 and -2); (2) adaptor molecules like p85-subunit of phosphotidylinositol-3-kinase, growth factor receptor-binding protein-2 (GRB-2), SH2-containing sequence protein (SHC), and interferon-stimulated gene factor-3 (IFSG-3); and (3) structural proteins like spectrin, myosin, and tensin (Table 4.4). The SH2 domain protein interacts with specific phosphotyrosine motifs on cellular proteins leading to an increase of its enzymatic activity, molecular interactions, or cytoskeletal changes.

The signal transduction of receptor tyrosine kinases involves two rate-limiting steps: (1) interaction of specific phosphotyrosine-containing peptide sequences with SH2 domain-containing proteins like Src tyrosine kinase, phospholipase C-γ, the regulatory subunit p85 of phosphatidylinositol-3-kinase, SH2-containing sequence protein, and growth factor receptor-binding protein-2; (2) tyrosine phosphorylation of some signaling molecules like phospholipase C-γ, Src tyrosine kinase, SH2-containing sequence protein, and SH2 domain phosphotyrosine phosphatase-1. Autophosphorylation on specific tyrosine residues allows the receptor tyrosine kinase to select a repertoire of SH2 domain-containing proteins. For example, the EGF receptor contains five tyrosine residues in the carboxyl-terminal tail of the receptor that are phosphorylated. Each individual phosphotyrosine residue binds specific SH2 domain-containing regulatory molecules like phospholipase C-γ, phosphatidylinositol-3-kinase, Ras GTP-activating protein, growth factor receptor-binding protein-2, SH2-containing sequence protein, and SH2 domain phosphotyrosine phosphatase-2.

The structural basis for the specificity of the interaction between tyrosine-phosphorylated proteins and SH2 domain proteins has established a general principle: phosphotyrosine-containing peptides as short as four amino acids bind to SH2 domains with high affinity. The specificity is determined by a motif of three amino acid residues carboxyl-terminal for the phosphotyrosine. For example, the p85 subunit of phosphatidylinositol-3-kinase binds to phosphotyrosine-methionine-proline-methionine in PDGF receptors; growth factor receptor-binding protein-2 binds phosphotyrosine-isoleucine-asparagine-glutamine in EGF; phospholipase C-γ binds phosphotyrosine-leucine-isoleucine-proline in EGF and PDGF receptors. The binding affinity of different phosphopeptides for a given SH2 domain varies by 100-fold. The X-ray crystallographic structures of the SH2 domains in a complex with the specific phosphotyrosine tetrapeptides have provided an exact structural model of the interaction.

The phosphotyrosine-containing peptide binds a SH2 domain and selects a signal transduction pathway in a large repertoire of SH2 domain-containing proteins. The different phosphotyrosine docking sites on a receptor tyrosine kinase may bind multiple SH2 proteins in a "signal transfer complex" and the signaling function of the receptor will be determined by the sum of phosphotyrosine-SH2 domain interactions (Figure 4.7). As SH2 domains show overlapping specificity towards phosphotyrosine motifs, they may compete for the same docking sites on a receptor. Some SH2 domain proteins, like the SH2-containing sequence protein and the SH2 domain phosphotyrosine phosphatases-1 and -2, are phosphorylated on tyrosine residues and may propagate the signal via interaction with other SH2 domain proteins. Thus, receptor tyrosine kinases produce several types of intracellular signals that are integrated in a "signaling network". The nature of the final biological response depends not only on the distribution of the receptors and their intracellular signaling components but also on the exact "combination" of signals generated. In the case of tyrosine kinases, which act through phospholipase C-γ, phosphotidylinositol-3-kinase, growth factor receptor-binding protein-2, and other proteins, we might postulate that different ligands produce different combinations of effect. For example, PDGF has a combination of 25-50-25-0, whereas insulin has a combination of 0-0–50-25. In a cell expressing each of these signaling molecules, the exact combination of events allows for overlapping but distinct physiological effects.

Several SH2 domain proteins contain one or more SH3 domains. Their function is less clear, but recent evidence show that SH3 domains are involved in the activation of small Ras-like G-proteins. Growth factor receptor-binding protein-2 has two SH3 domains that interact with two characteristic polyproline sequences in Ras guanine nucleotide-releasing protein, leading to activation of Ras. The elucidation of the X-ray crystallographic structure of the SH3 domain may lead to further understanding of this interaction. Thus, two steps of protein-protein interactions involving SH2 and SH3 domains transmit the signal from the active receptor tyrosine kinase to Ras activation.

4.3.3 RAS AND RECEPTOR TYROSINE KINASE SIGNAL TRANSDUCTION

The Ras family of proteins, including c-Ras, H-Ras, K-Ras, and N-Ras are expressed in many cell types. Ras proteins are members of a superfamily of small GTP-binding proteins, including Rho, Ral, Rab, Rac, Rad, and Rap that have 30 to 55% homology to Ras. All Ras-related

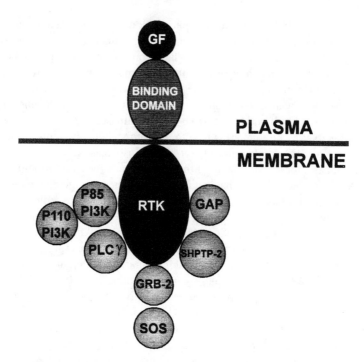

FIGURE 4.7 Signal transfer complex of receptor tyrosine kinases (RTK). Growth factor interacts with the extracellular binding domain and activates the receptor tyrosine kinase leading to autophosphorylation of tyrosine residues on the C-terminal domain of the receptor. The phosphotyrosine residues function as docking sites that bind various signaling proteins via interaction with their SH2 domains. These proteins include the regulatory p85 subunit of phosphoinositol 3-kinase (PI3K), phospholipase C-γ (PLC-γ), GTPase-activating protein (GAP), SH2 domain phosphotyrosine phosphatase-2 (SHPTP-2), and growth factor receptor-binding protein-2 (GRB-2). The SH2 domain proteins may interact with other proteins like the catalytic p110 subunit of PI3K or son-of-sevenless (SOS) protein that acts as a Ras GDP/GTP exchange factor. All proteins in the complex may be involved in the propagation of the signals leading to the ultimate effects.

proteins bind guanine nucleotides (GTP and GDP) and possess intrinsic GTPase activity. The biochemical properties of Ras are similar to those of the larger, heterotrimeric G-proteins involved in the signal transduction through seven-transmembrane segment receptors (see Chapter 8). Ras is anchored to the plasma membrane via prenylation at its carboxyl-terminus. Ras is active in its GTP-bound form and inactive in its GDP-bound form. Activation of Ras by exchange of bound GDP for GTP is facilitated by a Ras guanine nucleotide-releasing factor (also named GDP-GTP exchange factor or GDP-releasing factor). Inactivation of Ras by hydrolysis of bound GTP to GDP and P_i is catalyzed by the intrinsic GTPase following its activation by Ras GTPase-activating protein.

The role of Ras has been an enigma, but recent evidence has revealed that Ras is involved in signal transduction of receptor tyrosine kinases in mammalian cells. Microinjection of neutralizing Ras antibodies reverses the transformed phenotype of H-Ras-transformed cells and blocks PDGF- and insulin-induced mitogenesis. A dominant negative mutant of Ras inhibits EGF, PDGF, FGF, NGF, and insulin actions. Overexpression of c-Ras increases the sensitivity to several growth factors and insulin. Genetic and developmental studies in two lower animal species: the nematode *Caenorhabditis elegans* and the fruitfly *Drosophila melanogaster,* revealed that activation of receptors homologous with the mammalian EGF receptor leads to activation of Ras. Two molecules homologous to mammalian growth factor receptor-binding protein-2 and Ras guanine nucleotide-releasing protein were involved, and

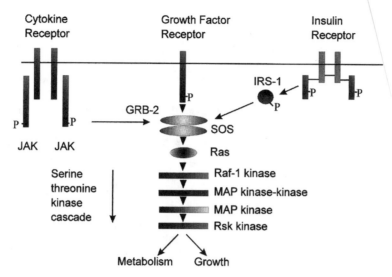

FIGURE 4.8 Signal pathway of receptor-activated tyrosine kinases. Activation of receptor-linked tyrosine kinases by cytokines, growth factors, and insulin induces receptor autophosphorylation. The complex of growth factor receptor-binding protein-2 (GRB-2) and son-of-sevenless (SOS) guanine nucleotide releasing protein is recruited to the plasma membrane by the receptor via SH2 domain-phosphotyrosine interaction. SOS activates Raf kinase which initiates a phosphorylation cascade: mitogen-activated protein (MAP) kinase-kinase, MAP-kinase, and p90[rsk] kinase, leading to cellular effects on metabolism and cell growth.

the latter was named "son-of-sevenless" (abbreviated SOS) as the protein mediates the signal of the "sevenless" receptor tyrosine kinase in *Drosophila* during eye development. The direct interaction between growth factor receptor-binding protein-2 and son-of-sevenless protein in EGF receptor activation of Ras has also been demonstrated in mammalian systems.

Growth factor and insulin receptors stimulate a cytoplasmic serine-threonine kinase that is essential for induction of cell proliferation and has been termed mitogen-activated protein (MAP) kinase. The activation of MAP kinase is the result of stimulation of a protein kinase cascade including Raf kinase and MAP kinase-kinase. The link between the receptor tyrosine kinase and Raf kinase appears to be activated Ras that interacts directly with Raf kinase. This represents one common signal transduction pathway by receptor tyrosine kinases (Figure 4.8). Growth factor, cytokines, or insulin activate receptor tyrosine kinases and protein phosphorylations at the membrane level. Growth factor receptor-binding protein-2 binds to specific phosphotyrosine motifs in the cytoplasmic domains. Ras guanine nucleotide-releasing protein (i.e., son-of-sevenless protein) is translocated to the membrane in a preexisting complex with the growth factor receptor-binding protein-2 and activates membrane-bound Ras by GDP-GTP exchange. Ras activates Raf kinase, which initiates a phosphorylation cascade including activation of MAP kinase-kinase, MAP kinase, and S6 protein kinase.

In summary, the signal transduction by receptor tyrosine kinases can be described by three paradigms:

1. *Activation by tyrosine phosphorylation.* Phosphorylation of a single tyrosine residue on phospholipase C-γ increases its hydrolysis of phosphatidylinositol-4,5-bisphosphate to inositol triphosphate and diacylglycerol.
2. *Activation by conformational change.* Interaction with a specific phosphotyrosine peptide changes the conformation of the regulatory p85 subunit of phosphatidylinositol-3-kinase and activates its catalytic p110 subunit.

3. *Activation by translocation.* The Ras guanine nucleotide-releasing protein, son-of-sevenless, is associated with growth factor receptor binding protein-2 and translocated to the plasma membrane where it activates Ras.

These three paradigms represent concurrent signaling pathways which are cooperative as well as redundant.

The interaction between phosphotyrosinepeptide motifs and SH2 domains in the signal transduction of receptor tyrosine kinases illustrates two simplifying principles of biology: the principle of redundancy and the principle of diversity. The principle of redundancy means that a simple mechanism or module is selected as a building block and used over and over again in many systems. The principle of diversity utilizes the concept that there are many ways of achieving the same goal, for example, stimulating glycogen metabolism or generating cell division. It is clear that the SH2 domain-signaling mechanism is highly redundant in evolution and that the SH2 domain-containing proteins and interactions show a rich diversity in cellular regulation.

4.4 FURTHER READING

Argetsinger, L.S., Campbell, G.S., Yang, X., et al., Identification of JAK2 as a growth hormone receptor-associated tyrosine kinase, *Cell,* 1993;74:237-244.

Barbacid, M., Ras genes, *Annu. Rev. Biochem.,* 1987;56:779-827.

Bokoch, G.M., Der, C.J., Emerging concepts in the Ras superfamily of GTP-binding proteins, *FASEB J.,* 1993;7:750-759.

Bourne, H.R., Sanders, D.A., McCormick, F., The GTPase superfamily: conserved structure and molecular mechanism, *Nature,* 1991;349:117-127.

Carpenter, G., Receptors for epidermal growth factor and other polypeptide mitogens, *Annu. Rev. Biochem.,* 1987;56:881-.

Chardin, P., Camonis, J.H., Gale, N.W., et al., Human SOS1: a guanine nucleotide exchange factor for ras that binds to GRB2, *Science,* 1993;260:1338-1343.

Ebina, Y., Ellis, L., Jarnagin, K., Edery, M., Graf, L., Clauser, E., Ou, J., Masiarz, F., Kan, Y.W., Goldfine, I.D., Roth, R.A., Rutter, W.J., The human insulin receptor cDNA. The structural basis for hormone-activated transmembrane signalling, *Cell,* 1985;40:747-758.

Egan, S.E., Weinberg, R.A., The pathway to signal achievement, *Nature,* 1993;365:781-783.

Garbers, D.L., Guanylate cyclase, a cell surface receptor, *J. Biol. Chem.,* 1989;264:1903.

Hall, A., The cellular functions of small GTP-binding proteins, *Science,* 1990;249:635-640.

Hanks, S.K., Quinn, A.M., Hunter, T., The protein kinase family. Conserved features and deduced phylogeny of the catalytic domain, *Science,* 1990;241:42–52.

Koshland, D.E., Jr., The two-component pathway comes to eukaryotes, *Science,* 1993;261:532.

Longo, N., Shuster, R.C., Griffin, L.D., Langley, S.D., Elsas, L.J., Activation of insulin receptor signaling by a single amino acid substitution in the transmembrane domain, *J. Biol. Chem.,* 1992;267:12416-12419.

Miyajima, A., Hara, T., Kitamura, T., Common subunits of cytokine receptors and the functional redundancy of cytokines, *Trends Biochem. Sci.,* 1992;17:378-382.

Morgan, D.O., Roth, R.A., Acute insulin action requires insulin receptor kinase activity. Introduction of an inhibitory monoclonal antibody into mammalian cells blocks the rapid effects of insulin, *Proc. Natl. Acad. Sci. U.S.A.,* 1987;84:41-45.

Murakami, M.S., Rosen, O.R., The role of insulin receptor autophosphorylation in signal transduction, *J. Biol. Chem.,* 1991;266:22653-22660.

Nicola, N.A., Hemopoietic cell growth factors and their receptors, *Annu. Rev. Biochem.,* 1989;58:45-47.

Pawson, T., Gish, G.D., SH2 and SH3 domains: From structures to function, *Cell,* 1992;71:358-362.

Pazin, M.J., Williams, L.T., Triggering signaling cascades by receptor tyrosine kinases, *Trends Biochem. Sci.,* 1992;17:374-378.

Ullrich, A., Schlessinger, J., Signal transduction by receptors with tyrosine kinase activity, *Cell,* 1990;61:203-212.

Velazquez, L., Fellous, M., Stark, G.R., Pellegrini, S., A protein tyrosine kinase in the interferon α/β signaling pathway, *Cell,* 1992;70:313-322.

Yarden, Y., Escobedo, J.A., Kuang, W.-J., Yang-Feng, T.L., Daniel, T.O., Tremble, P.M., Chen, E.Y., Ando, M.E., Harkins, R.N., Francke, U., Fried, V.A., Ullrich, A., Williams, L.T., Structure of the receptor for platelet-derived growth factor helps define a family of closely related growth factor receptors, *Nature,* 1986;323:226-232.

Ziemiecki, A., Harper, A.G., Wieks, A.F., JAK protein tyrosine kinases: their role in cytokine signalling, *Trends Cell Biol.,* 1994;4:207-212.

Section III

Ligand Binding Studies of Receptors

5 Direct Measurement of Drug Binding to Receptors

Dennis G. Haylett

CONTENTS

0-8493-9227-6/96/$0.00+$.50
© 1996 by CRC Press, Inc.

5.1 INTRODUCTION

In this chapter we look at ways in which the binding of ligands to macromolecules can be directly investigated. Although most interest centers on the interaction of drugs and hormones with receptors, the approach can be applied to any similar situation, for example the combination of drugs with ion channels or membrane transport systems. The binding of ligands, including drugs, to plasma proteins has been studied for 50 years or so, but binding to the much smaller amounts of protein (e.g., receptors) in cell membranes is more recent, becoming feasible only when suitable radioactively labeled ligands became available. The first rigorous study of drug binding to receptors was that by Paton and Rang, who investigated ^{3}H-atropine binding to muscarinic receptors in smooth muscle. The use of radiolabeled drugs in **radioligand binding studies** is now common and for many pharmaceutical manufacturers forms an essential part of the screening process, providing a rapid and quantitative means of determining the affinity of new drugs for a wide range of receptors. Labeling with radioisotopes is usually chosen because very small quantities, often as little as 1 fmol, can be readily and accurately measured. There also is interest in the measurement of ligand concentration by fluorescence, but this, of course, requires the availability or novel synthesis of ligands with suitable fluorescent moities, and currently this method requires substantially higher ligand concentrations. Fluorescent probes do, however, have a particular utility in kinetic experiments where the changes in fluorescence that occur on binding are detectable immediately and thus allow very good time resolution.

5.1.1 Objectives of Radioligand Binding Studies

These include:

- The measurement of **dissociation equilibrium constants**. This is of particular value in receptor classification and in the study of structure/activity relationships, where the effects of changes in chemical structure on affinity (and efficacy) are explored.
- The measurement of **association and dissociation rate constants.**
- The measurement of **receptor density**.

The recognition and quantification of receptor subtypes may also be possible if subtype-selective ligands are available. Changes in receptor density occurring under different physiological or pathological conditions can also be investigated. Examples include the reduction in β-adrenoreceptor density which occurs with the use of β-agonists in the treatment of asthma (down-regulation) and the increase in β-adrenoreceptor numbers in cardiac muscle in response to thyroxine. The densities of receptors may be measured either directly in tissue samples or in intact tissues by quantitative autoradiography. Autoradiography, in which a picture of the distribution of the radiolabel in a section of tissue is obtained by placing a photographic film in contact with the tissue, has provided valuable information on the distribution of many receptors in the brain. The possibility that the radiolabel will dissociate from the receptors during the fixation process may be avoided by using ligands which bind covalently. Photoaffinity labels, which initially bind to the receptors reversibly, but which can be converted by light-activation to a species which binds covalently, have proven useful for such investigations. Irreversible radioligands are also of use in the purification of receptors. Here the radioactivity permits the receptors to be tracked through the various purification steps, for example in the fractions eluting from separation columns.

Finally, it may be possible to obtain information on the mechanisms of action of agonists from the shapes of binding curves. For example, as discussed later, the binding of some agonists is affected by GTP, immediately suggesting the involvement of G-proteins in the transduction mechanism.

5.1.2 NOMENCLATURE

Compared with the conventions adopted in discussing the relationship between drug concentration and response (see Chapter 1), in ligand binding studies a rather different terminology has evolved.

R:	denotes the binding site, most often a true **R**eceptor, but quite commonly the term "receptor" is applied indiscriminately to any binding site.
L:	is the radiolabeled **L**igand, whose binding is directly measured. L may be an *agonist or antagonist* or indeed a channel blocker, etc.
I:	is used for an **I**nhibitor of the binding of L: again this could be an agonist or an antagonist.
B:	is often used to denote the amount of radioligand bound, B_{max} being the maximum binding capacity.
K_L, K_I:	are the dissociation equilibrium constants for binding of L and I (reciprocals of affinity constants).
K_d:	is also used more generally for the dissociation equilibrium constant of any ligand.

5.1.3 SPECIFICITY OF BINDING

An all-important consideration in binding studies is the extent to which the measured binding of a radioligand represents association with the receptor or other site of interest. In functional studies there is no difficulty — the response can only be elicited by the binding of an agonist to the receptor and for an antagonist to inhibit the response to an agonist it must also bind to the receptor (or to a site coupled to it). Invariably, in binding studies there is uptake of the radioligand by other tissue components (unless, of course, binding to a purified, soluble protein is under investigation). The binding to the receptor is normally termed **specific binding,** whereas the binding to nonreceptor tissue components is referred to as **nonspecific binding**. Nonspecific binding may be attributable to:

1. Ligand bound to other sites in the tissue, e.g., other receptors, enzymes, or membrane transporters. For example, some muscarinic antagonists will also bind to histamine receptors, and some adrenoreceptor ligands will also bind to the neuronal and extraneuronal uptake mechanisms for noradrenaline. Such uptake might of course be properly considered "specific", but it is not the binding of primary interest to the investigator. Unlike other sources of nonspecific binding, this binding will be saturable, though it may be hoped that it will be of lower affinity and so will increase in an approximately linear fashion over the concentration range of ligand used. If the characteristics of nonspecific binding of this sort are well established, it may be possible to eliminate it by the use of selective blockers (e.g., by the use of specific inhibitors of the uptake–1 process for noradrenaline).

2. Distribution of ligand into lipid components of the preparation (e.g., cell membranes) or uptake into intact cells or membrane vesicles.
3. Free ligand which is not separated from bound ligand during the separation phase of the experiment. Included in this category would be ligand bound to a filter or trapped in the membrane or cell pellet during centrifugation.

Unlike 1 above, nonspecific binding arising from 2 and 3 will be nonsaturable and will increase linearly with radioligand concentration. Nonspecific binding of types 1 and 2 and radioligand trapped in pellets should increase in proportion to the amount of tissue used in the binding reaction; binding to filters and to the walls of centrifuge tubes should not. If the investigator is fortunate, in that nonspecific binding in category 1 is linear over the range of radioligand concentrations used, then 1, 2, and 3 simply combine to constitute a single nonspecific component. Nonspecific binding is usually estimated by measuring the binding of the radioligand in the presence of an agent which is believed to bind selectively to the receptor, at a concentration which is calculated to prevent virtually all specific binding without appreciable modification of nonspecific binding (further details are provided in Section 5.3.4).

5.2 TYPES OF RADIOLIGAND BINDING EXPERIMENTS

Four kinds of ligand binding studies will be discussed:

- Saturation
- Kinetic
- Competition
- Retardation

5.2.1 SATURATION EXPERIMENTS

These experiments directly examine the binding of the radioligand at equilibrium and can provide estimates of K_L and B_{max}. Initially we consider the simple reaction:

$$R + L \rightleftharpoons RL \tag{5.1}$$

This represents binding in isolation and would be applicable to the binding of a competitive antagonist (or a channel blocker) which produces insignificant structural change in the receptor. (The case for an agonist which must produce such a change, often an isomerization, in order to generate the active state is considered later.) The binding at equilibrium is given by the following equation (equivalent to Equation 1.2):

$$[RL] = [R]_{TOT} \cdot \frac{[L]}{K_L + [L]} \tag{5.2}$$

Alternatively:

$$B = B_{max}, \frac{[L]}{K_L + [L]} \tag{5.3}$$

Typical units for B are picomoles per milligram protein, picomoles per milligram dry tissue, etc. A curve of B vs. [L] has the form of a rectangular hyperbola, exactly equivalent to the curve describing receptor occupancy presented in Chapter 1, Figure 1.1.

It is convenient at this point to consider nonspecific binding. Ideally, nonspecific binding should be entirely independent of specific binding, so that the total uptake of radioligand by the tissue should be the simple sum of the two. If we can assume that the nonspecific binding is a linear function of the ligand concentration, then the observed binding will be given by:

$$B = B_{max}, \frac{[L]}{K_L + [L]} + c.[L] \qquad (5.4)$$

where c is a constant. The relationship between total, specific, and nonspecific binding is indicated in Figure 5.1.

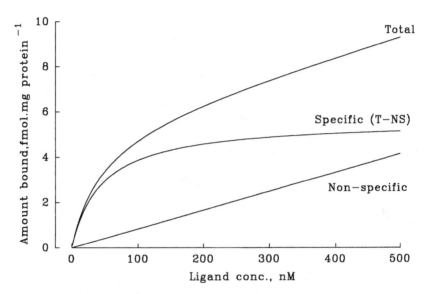

FIGURE 5.1 The binding of a radioligand to a receptor preparation normally involves a "nonspecific" component in addition to the "specific" receptor binding. In principle, at least, "specific" binding can be estimated from the total binding (T) by subtracting "nonspecific" binding (NS). (Theoretical curves with B_{max} = 5.6 fmol/mg protein, K_L = 45 nM, and c = 0.0083 fmol/nM.)

In practice "total" and "nonspecific" binding are measured over a range of concentrations of L which will allow specific binding to approach saturation. The analysis of saturation experiments to obtain estimates of K_L and B_{max} is described later.

It is useful now to recall the **Hill coefficient**, which has been discussed in detail in Chapter 1. In binding studies the Hill coefficient, n_H, is a convenient means of describing the steepness of the plot of specific binding against the log of the ligand concentration, generally without any attempt to define the underlying mechanism. In the simplest case, a plot of specific binding against [L] is analyzed to provide a fit of the following equation (equivalent to Equation 1.6):

$$B = B_{max}, \frac{[L]^{n_H}}{K_L^{n_H} + [L]^{n_H}} \qquad (5.5)$$

Thus, n_H would be unity for a simple bimolecular reaction following the law of mass action. If n_H is greater than 1 the plot of specific binding against log [L] will be "steep" and if less than 1 it will be "shallow". Under these circumstances a Hill plot (see Chapter 1) would have slopes either greater or less than unity.

5.2.1.1   Multiple Binding Sites

It is of course quite possible that there may be more than one kind of "specific" binding site for the radioligand. This may represent the presence of receptor subtypes (for example, subtypes of 5HT receptors, adrenoreceptors, etc.), or the binding sites might be functionally quite different. For example, some receptor ligands may also be channel blockers (e.g., tubocurarine) or inhibitors of transmitter uptake (e.g., phenoxybenzamine). The question then arises as to whether or not the sites are interacting or noninteracting. If there are only two sites and they do not interact, an additional term can simply be added to the binding equation. For total binding:

$$B = B_{max_1} \cdot \frac{[L]}{K_{L_1} + [L]} + B_{max_2} \cdot \frac{[L]}{K_{L_2} + [L]} + c.[L] \qquad (5.6)$$

where subsubscripts 1 and 2 specify the two sites. (Further terms can be added for additional components.) The curve for specific binding will no longer be a simple rectangular hyperbola, though whether distinct components can be distinguished by eye will depend on the difference in the K_L values and on the number of observations and their accuracy. Theoretical curves are shown in Figure 5.2. For relatively small differences in the K_L values of the two sites, the curve appears to have a single component, but analysis would show it to have a low Hill coefficient.

The separate components are revealed more clearly when a logarithmic scale is used for the radioligand concentration. Thus deviations from sigmoidicity are quite evident in Figure 5.2 (right-hand side).

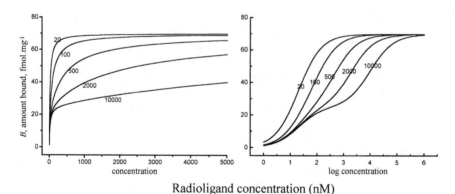

Radioligand concentration (nM)

FIGURE 5.2   Theoretical curves for the specific binding of a radioligand to a preparation containing two classes of binding site. A high affinity component with a B_{max} of 25 fmol/mg has a fixed K_L of 20 nM. The second component, with a B_{max} of 45 fmol/mg is given K_L values varying between 20 and 10,000 nM, as indicated. The K_L values for the two sites must differ considerably before the existence of two components becomes obvious. (Data displayed using both linear and logarithmic concentration scales.)

5.2.1.2   Interacting Sites

There are some instances, for example the nicotinic acetylcholine receptor, where the binding site is duplicated on identical subunits incorporated into a multimeric protein. There is then the possibility that binding to one site may influence binding to the other. The two sites could in principle behave in an identical fashion, but it is more likely that incorporation of the subunits into the asymmetrical multimer (a heteropentamer for the nicotinic receptor) introduces constraints which lead to different affinities for ligands. Of particular importance is the likelihood that occupation of one site by the ligand will increase or decrease the affinity for binding to the other, i.e., show positive or negative cooperativity. The following provides the simplest representation of this situation:

$$R + L \overset{K_1}{\rightleftharpoons} RL + L \overset{K_2}{\rightleftharpoons} RL_2 \; (\overset{K_3}{\rightleftharpoons} RL_2^*) \tag{5.7}$$

In this scheme the two binding sites are considered identical. RL_2^* is the active state produced when L is an agonist. The shape of the binding curve depends on the relative magnitudes of K_1 and K_2. If $K_1 > K_2$ there will be positive cooperativity (i.e., binding to the first site will increase affinity for the second) and if $K_1 < K_2$ there will be negative cooperativity. Figure 5.3 illustrates the shapes of the binding curves predicted for different ratios of K_1 to K_2.

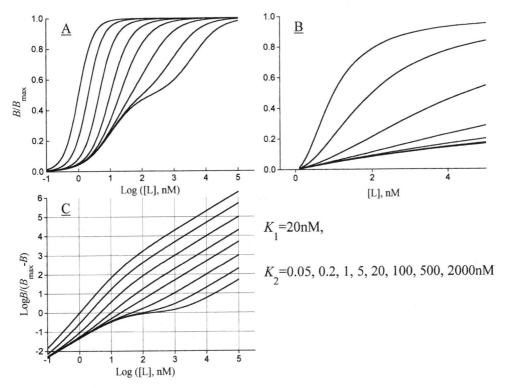

FIGURE 5.3 Binding of a radioligand to a protein containing two identical binding sites. (Scheme shown in Equation 5.7, but ignoring isomerization.) Binding of the first ligand molecule is given a K_1 of 20 nM. The K_2 value for binding of a second ligand molecule is given a range of values to represent varying degrees of cooperativity, from strongly positive (0.05 nM) to strongly negative (2000 nM). As illustrated in A, for a logarithmic concentration scale, positive cooperativity steepens the curve, whereas negative cooperativity makes it shallower. Two components become quite evident for the larger values of K_2. In panel B the linear concentration scale has been expanded to show the S-shaped foot of the binding curve, indicative of positive cooperativity. The Hill plot, C, shows that with a large degree of positive cooperativity n_H approaches 2 for low concentrations of radioligand.

In "competition" experiments, also, it is possible that the binding of the radioligand is inhibited not by competition at a common site, but by the inhibitor affecting the binding remotely through interaction with a different part of the receptor molecule(i.e., by an allosteric action).

5.2.1.3 Agonists

The foregoing discussion of saturation experiments considered the binding step in isolation. However, for agonists to produce a tissue response there must be some change in the receptor (isomerization), for example a conformational change to open an integral ion channel or to promote association with a G-protein. The complications arising with agonists will now be discussed.

5.2.1.3.1   The del Castillo-Katz Model of Receptor Activation

This model, represented below, has already been discussed in Chapter 1, Section 1.4.4.

$$A + R \underset{}{\overset{K_1}{\rightleftharpoons}} AR \underset{}{\overset{K_2}{\rightleftharpoons}} AR^* \tag{5.8}$$

In a ligand binding study the measured binding includes AR^* as well as AR. The relevant equation is

$$B_{(AR+AR^*)} = B_{max} \cdot \frac{[A]}{\left(\dfrac{K_1 K_2}{1 + K_2}\right) + [A]} \tag{5.9}$$

In this equation, A has been used in preference to L to emphasize that an *agonist* is being considered. The equation retains the form of a rectangular hyperbola, 50% occupancy occurring when $[A] = K_1 K_2/(1+K_2)$. $K_1 K_2/(1+K_2)$ is thus an *effective* equilibrium constant. The important point to note is that binding measurements do not give an estimate of K_1 alone. The effective "equilibrium constant", $K_1 K_2/(1+K_2)$, is smaller than K_1, so the isomerization step increases "affinity" (in effect, dragging the receptor into the occupied state).

Another complication is receptor **desensitization**. Desensitization of the nicotinic acetylcholine receptor is attributed to the receptor, especially in its activated form, changing spontaneously to a desensitized, inactive state. A simple representation is given in the following scheme:

$$A + R \rightleftharpoons AR + A \rightleftharpoons A_2R \rightleftharpoons A_2R^*$$
$$\updownarrow \qquad \updownarrow \qquad \quad \updownarrow \qquad \quad \updownarrow$$
$$A + R_D \rightleftharpoons AR_D + A \rightleftharpoons A_2R_D \rightleftharpoons A_2R_D^*$$

This is based on the Katz-Thesleff cyclic model of desensitization, modified to incorporate the binding of two molecules of acetylcholine and including an isomerization step. It is evident from this scheme that the agonist-receptor complexes are of several different forms and the equations describing the binding are correspondingly complex. For the nicotinic acetylcholine receptor it is found that agonist binds to the desensitized receptor (R_D) with high affinity.

5.2.1.3.2   The Ternary Complex Model of Receptor Activation

The following model has already been introduced in Chapter 1 (Section 1.4.6):

$$A + R \rightleftharpoons AR + X \rightleftharpoons ARX \tag{5.10}$$

ARX, comprising three reacting species, is the **ternary complex**. This scheme is often used to describe G-protein-mediated responses when X is replaced by G, but is clearly an oversimplification. For example, it does not include the additional states introduced by the binding of GTP and GDP. From the point of view of ligand binding studies we need to note that measured binding will include both AR and ARX. The equation which gives the bound concentration (AR + ARX) at equilibrium is complex (and in the case of G-protein-coupled responses will also have to take into account the concentrations of receptors and G-protein, as discussed in Chapter 1, and of GTP and GDP). A particular feature of the binding of agonists to receptors which couple to G-proteins is that the concentration of GTP will affect the binding curve. The binding of agonists often exhibits components with high and low affinities and GTP is found to increase the proportion in the low affinity state. This will be considered further when discussing competition experiments.

5.2.2 Kinetic Studies

Both the onset of binding, when the radioligand is first applied, and offset, when dissociation is promoted, can be studied directly. The relevant kinetic equations outlining the theory for the simple bimolecular interaction of ligand with receptor are presented in Chapter 1, Section 1.3.

5.2.2.1 Measurement of the Dissociation Rate Constant, k_{-1}

To measure the dissociation rate constant all that is necessary, in principle, is first to secure a satisfactory occupancy of the receptors by the radioligand and then to prevent further association, either by adding a competing agent in sufficient concentration or by lowering [L] substantially by dilution. The amount of drug bound to the receptors is measured at selected times after initiating net dissociation and, for the simple model considered in Sections 1.2 and 1.3 of Chapter 1, will show an exponential decline.

$$\text{RL} \xrightarrow{k_{-1}} \text{R} + \text{L} \tag{5.11}$$

$$B_{\text{t}} = B_0 . e^{-k_{-1}t} \tag{5.12}$$

$$\log_e B_t = \log_e B_0 - k_{-1}t \tag{5.13}$$

B_0 and B_t are the amounts bound initially (at $t = 0$) and at specific times (t) after initiating dissociation. A plot of $\log_e B_t$ against t is linear with a slope of $-k_{-1}$; k_{-1} may thus be estimated directly from the slope of this plot or may be obtained by nonlinear least-squares curve fitting to Equation 5.12. It is always desirable to plot $\log_e B_t$ against t to detect any nonlinearity, which might reflect either the presence of multiple binding sites or the existence of more than one occupied state of the receptor.

5.2.2.2 Measurement of the Association Rate Constant, k_{+1}

For the simple bimolecular reaction involving a single class of binding site the onset of binding should also contain an exponential term. Thus:

$$B_t = B_\infty \cdot \left(1 - e^{-k_{on}t}\right) \tag{5.14}$$

where:

B_t = the binding at time t.
B_∞ = the binding at equilibrium.
k_{on} = the observed onset rate constant.

However, as shown in Chapter 1, k_{on} is not a simple measure of k_{+1}, rather:

$$k_{on} = k_{-1} + k_{+1}[L] \tag{5.15}$$

Equation 5.14 can be converted into a linear form:

$$\log_e\left(\frac{B_\infty - B_t}{B_\infty}\right) = -k_{on}t \tag{5.16}$$

so that k_{on} can be obtained from the slope of the plot of the left-hand side of the equation against t.

Once k_{on} is known, k_{+1} can be estimated in at least three different ways. Firstly, an independent estimate of k_{-1} can be determined from dissociation studies as described above, whence $k_{+1} = (k_{on} - k_{-1})/[L]$. Secondly, k_{on} can be measured at several different concentrations of L and a plot of k_{on} against [L] constructed in which, according to Equation 5.15, k_{+1} is given directly by the slope. This plot will also provide an estimate of k_{-1} (intercept). Thirdly, it is possible to perform a simultaneous nonlinear least-squares fit of a family of onset curves (obtained by using different concentrations of L), the fitting routine thus providing estimates of k_{+1}, k_{-1}, and B_{max}. (Problem 5.2 provides an opportunity to calculate binding rate constants.)

If there are multiple binding sites, or the ligand-receptor complex isomerizes, then the onset and offset curves will be multiexponential. It is generally assumed that nonspecific binding will occur rapidly, and this should certainly be so for simple entrapment in a membrane or cell pellet. If, however, specific binding is very rapid or nonspecific binding particularly slow (possibly reflecting uptake of the ligand by cells), then the time course of nonspecific binding also needs to be determined in order to allow an accurate assessment of the onset of specific binding. Note too that the onset of ligand binding will be slowed in the presence of an inhibitor and this phenomenon is employed in **retardation** experiments (discussed in Section 5.2.4).

5.2.3 COMPETITION EXPERIMENTS

Of course, saturation experiments are only possible when a radiolabeled form of the ligand of interest is available. Competition experiments on the other hand are particularly useful in allowing the determination of dissociation constants for unlabeled drugs which compete for the binding sites with a ligand which *is* available in a labeled form. This approach has been widely adopted by the pharmaceutical industry as a rapid means of determining the affinity of novel compounds for a particular receptor for which a well-characterized radioligand is available.

In competition experiments a fixed amount of radioligand, generally at a concentration below K_L, is equilibrated with the receptor preparation in the presence of a range of concentrations of the unlabeled inhibitor, I. In these studies, the amount of radioligand bound is usually plotted against log[I]. Figure 5.4 provides an example for the simple case where the radioligand and inhibitor compete reversibly for a single class of site.

In this illustration the constant level of nonspecific binding has not been subtracted, whereas in most published studies it would be. The amount of nonspecific binding could of course be defined by applying high concentrations of the inhibitor itself, but if the competing agent is expensive or in short supply it is possible to employ another well-characterized inhibitor for the same purpose. The two main features of this curve are its position along the concentration axis and its slope. The position along the concentration axis is conventionally indicated by the **IC$_{50}$: the concentration of inhibitor which reduces the specific binding by 50%.** The predicted relationship (see also Equation 1.39) between the amount of specific binding in the presence of I (B$_I$) and [I] is given by:

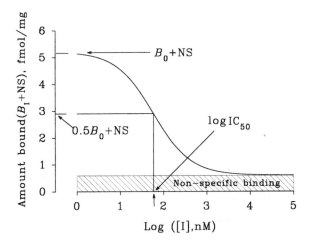

FIGURE 5.4 In this illustration of a competition experiment, a fixed concentration of radioligand, in the absence of inhibitor, produces specific binding of B_0. The specific binding in the presence of a competitive inhibitor is denoted by B_I. A constant amount of nonspecific binding is assumed to be present. The concentration of inhibitor which reduces specific binding by 50% is referred to as the IC_{50}.

$$B_I = B_{max} \cdot \frac{[L]}{K_L\left(1 + \frac{[I]}{K_I}\right) + [L]} \tag{5.17}$$

Provided that a value for K_L is available it is possible to use this equation to obtain a value for K_I, the dissociation equilibrium constant for the inhibitor, by nonlinear least-squares analysis of the displacement curve. Alternatively, K_I can be calculated from the IC_{50}, which may be obtained by simple interpolation by eye, from a Hill plot, or by fitting a curve to an equation of the type:

$$B_I = B_0\left(1 - \frac{[I]}{[I] + IC_{50}}\right) \tag{5.18}$$

where B_0 is the specific binding observed in the absence of competing ligand.

5.2.3.1 Relationship Between K_I and IC_{50}

B_0 is given by Equation 5.3:

$$B_0 = B_{max}, \frac{[L]}{K_L + [L]}$$

and, by definition, when $[I] = IC_{50}$, $B_I = 0.5\, B_0$, therefore (from Equation 5.17):

$$B_{IC_{50}} = B_{max} \cdot \frac{[L]}{K_L\left(1 + \frac{IC_{50}}{K_I}\right) + [L]} \tag{5.19}$$

$$= 0.5 \cdot B_{max} \cdot \frac{[L]}{K_L + [L]}$$

by cancellation and rearrangement:

$$K_{\mathrm{I}} = \mathrm{IC}_{50} \cdot \frac{K_{\mathrm{L}}}{K_{\mathrm{L}} + [\mathrm{L}]} = \frac{\mathrm{IC}_{50}}{\left(1 + \dfrac{[\mathrm{L}]}{K_{\mathrm{L}}}\right)} \tag{5.20}$$

The term $1 + [\mathrm{L}]/K_{\mathrm{L}}$ is often referred to as the Cheng-Prusoff correction. It is clear from this analysis that the IC_{50} does not give a direct estimate of K_{I} unless [L] is very low, when IC_{50} tends to K_{I}. Just as with saturation experiments, the situation will be complicated by the presence of different classes of binding sites (e.g., receptor subtypes) and by the involvement of G-proteins in agonist binding.

5.2.3.2   Multiple Binding Sites

The effect of multiple binding sites on displacement curves will be determined by the relative affinities of the radioligand and displacing agent for the different sites. Considering the simple situation where the radioligand exhibits the same affinity for each of two sites (e.g., propranolol for β-adrenoreceptors), the displacement curve for an inhibitor will show two components only if the K_{I} values for the binding of the inhibitor for the two sites are sufficiently different, and if the measurements of displacement are accurate and made over an adequate range of concentrations of I (see also Figure 5.2 and Section 5.4.4).

5.2.3.3   G-Protein-Linked Receptors

As already mentioned, GTP affects binding of agonists to G-protein-coupled receptors, and this has been much studied because of the light it can throw on the mechanism of action of such receptors. These receptors often exhibit two states which bind agonists with different affinities. The interactions of G-proteins with receptors are discussed in Chapter 8 and here it is only necessary to note that the high affinity form of the receptor is that coupled to the G-protein. In the simplest model, when GTP replaces GDP on the α-subunit the G-protein splits to release the α-GTP and βγ-subunits which mediate the cellular effects of the agonist. The receptor then dissociates, reverting to the low affinity state. Hence in the absence of GTP a significant proportion of the receptors will be in the high affinity state, but in its presence most will adopt the low affinity state. The resulting "GTP shift" is illustrated in Figure 5.5. Note that it applies only to the binding of agonists since antagonists do not promote coupling of the receptors to the G-protein.

5.2.4   RETARDATION EXPERIMENTS

It is useful to consider a particular variant of competitive binding experiment which has been used especially to investigate the nicotinic acetylcholine receptor. In essence, it is possible to determine the dissociation equilibrium constant for a reversible competitive inhibitor by the reduction it produces in the rate of binding of an irreversible radioligand (e.g., α-bungarotoxin). In practice, the time-course of binding of the irreversible ligand is studied in the absence and presence of the inhibitor. The expected outcome is shown in Figure 5.6.

When the irreversible ligand is applied by itself, the change in the proportion of sites occupied, p_{LR}, with time will be given by:

$$\frac{\mathrm{d}p_{\mathrm{LR}}(t)}{\mathrm{d}t} = k_{+1}[\mathrm{L}]\{1 - p_{\mathrm{LR}}(t)\} \tag{5.21}$$

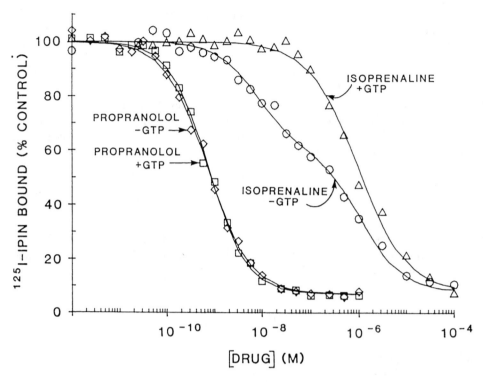

FIGURE 5.5 Effect of GTP on the competition binding curves of isoprenaline and propranolol. Membranes prepared from L6 myoblasts were incubated with ^{125}I-iodopindolol (50 pM) in the presence of either (—)-isoprenaline or (—)-propranolol with or without 100 μM GTP for 90 min at 25°C. GTP has no effect on the binding of the antagonist but shifts the curve for displacement by the agonist to the right (by abolishing the high affinity component of binding). (Reproduced from Wolfe, B.B. and Molinoff, P.B., *Handbook of Experimental Pharmacology*, Trendelenburg, U. and Weiner, N., Eds., Springer-Verlag, Berlin, 1988. With permission.)

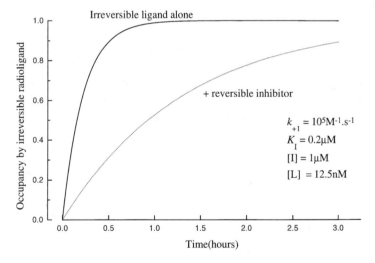

FIGURE 5.6 Retardation experiment. A reversible inhibitor will slow down the rate of association of an irreversible ligand with its receptor. These curves have been constructed according to Equation 5.26 using the numerical values indicated in the figure. These have been chosen to illustrate the effect of an antagonist, such as tubocurarine, on the binding of α-bungarotoxin to the nicotinic receptor of skeletal muscle.

$(1 - p_{LR}(t)$ is the proportion of receptors remaining free and available to bind with L.) If $p_{LR} = 0$ at $t = 0$ the solution is

$$p_{LR}(t) = 1 - e^{-k_{+1}[L]t} \qquad (5.22)$$

This equation is the application of Equation 1.14 to an irreversible ligand, i.e., $k_{-1} = 0$, and in the long run all of the receptors will be occupied so that $p_{LR}(\infty)$ is unity. The rate constant for equilibration is thus given by $k_{+1}[L]$. For the case where binding is studied in the presence of an inhibitor, Equation 5.21 becomes:

$$\frac{dp_{LR}(t)}{dt} = k_{+1}[L]\{1 - p_{LR}(t) - p_{IR}(t)\} \qquad (5.23)$$

where (p_{IR} is the proportion of receptor sites occupied by the inhibitor. The rate of association is slowed because the concentration of free binding sites has been reduced through occupation by I. If we assume that I equilibrates rapidly with the available sites:

$$p_{IR}(t) = \{1 - p_{LR}(t)\} \cdot \frac{[I]}{K_I + [I]} \qquad (5.24)$$

Substituting in Equation 5.23:

$$\frac{dp_{LR}(t)}{dt} = k_{+1}[L]\left\{1 - p_{LR}(t) - \left(1 - p_{LR}(t)\right) \cdot \frac{[I]}{K_I + [I]}\right\} \qquad (5.25)$$

$$= k_{+1}[L]\left(1 - p_{LR}(t)\right)\left(1 - \frac{[I]}{K_I + [I]}\right)$$

The solution for $p_{LR} = 0$ at $t = 0$ is:

$$p_{LR}(t) = 1 - e^{-k_{+1}[L]\left(1 - \frac{[I]}{K_I + [I]}\right)} \qquad (5.26)$$

The onset rate constant (cf Equation 5.22) is reduced by the factor $1 - [I]/(K_I + [I])$. If the rate constants for binding of the irreversible ligand are determined in the absence and presence of the inhibitor and denoted k_0 and k_I, respectively, then:

$$\frac{k_0}{k_I} = \frac{k_{+1}[L]}{k_{+1}[L]\left(1 - \frac{[I]}{K_I + [I]}\right)} = \frac{[I]}{K_I} + 1 \qquad (5.27)$$

Thus for a given concentration of I an estimate of its equilibrium constant can be determined.

5.3 PRACTICAL ASPECTS OF RADIOLIGAND BINDING STUDIES

The majority of binding studies estimate the amount of binding by the separation of bound from free ligand, using either centrifugation or filtration, followed by measurement of the quantity bound. The separation step can, however, be avoided if a suitable fluorescent ligand is available since the change in fluorescence which occurs on binding can be measured directly in the mixture. The separation stage can also be avoided in *scintillation proximity assays*. These assays are applicable to ligands containing radioisotopes (e.g., tritium) which produce low-energy β-particles which travel only a very short distance (≈ 10 μm) in aqueous solution. The receptor preparation is immobilized on microbeads which contain scintillant molecules. The scintillant molecules are able to detect β-radiation emanating from radioligand bound to receptors located on the bead surface (and thus in close proximity), but will not respond to radiation from the relatively remote radioligand molecules free in the aqueous solution. For this technique to be used it is necessary to be able to couple the receptor preparation to the bead in a way which does not interfere with the binding of the ligand. Provided this can be done, scintillation proximity counting provides a simple method of detecting binding and can, furthermore, be used to follow the time-course of binding while the reaction mixture remains in the scintillation counter.

5.3.1 RECEPTOR PREPARATIONS

Most receptors (with the exception of the steroid receptors that influence DNA transcription) are located on the cell surface, and purified cell membranes are thus an obvious choice of preparation. When a tissue is homogenized, however, any membrane fraction isolated may well contain membranes from intracellular organelles in addition to cell membranes from all the cell types present in the tissue. Thus "brain" membranes will contain membranes not only from neurones but also from glia, as well as the smooth muscle and endothelial cells of blood vessels. It may, however, be possible to prepare membranes from pure cell preparations, e.g., cell lines in culture or cells obtained by disaggregation of the tissue with enzymes, and subsequently subjected to purification by differential centrifugation. More recently, binding studies have been performed on membranes from cell lines transfected with cloned human receptor genes and a wide range of such cloned receptors is now available for routine drug screening.

A feature of cell disruption is that it may expose receptors that were not originally on the cell surface. Some of the receptors will have been in the process of insertion while others may have been endocytosed. This would lead to an overestimate of the cell surface receptor density. On the other hand, cell membranes may form vesicles which can have either an outside-out or inside-out orientation. Cell-surface receptors in inside-out vesicles will not bind the ligand unless it can penetrate the vesicle. It is usually necessary to wash membrane preparations several times to remove endogenous material which might affect the binding (e.g., proteolytic enzymes, endogenous ligands). One important advantage of cell membranes is that often the preparation can be stored deep-frozen for many weeks without any change in binding properties.

The use of cell membranes can be criticized on the grounds that the receptors have been removed from their natural environment and will no longer be subject to cellular control mechanisms; for example, the phosphorylation of intracellular domains may be modified. These problems can be avoided by using intact cells for binding studies. Tissue "slices" (e.g., brain, heart) are used, as are cells isolated from dissected tissue by collagenase or trypsin digestion. Permanent cell lines in culture can also be used. There is, however, some concern that the application of proteolytic enzymes to aid the disaggregation of tissues might modify the receptors. When using intact cells there is also the possibility that some ligands will be transported into the cells, leading to a higher nonspecific binding. Furthermore, some cells may contain enzymes which metabolize the radioligand. Since cells need to be maintained under physiological conditions to remain viable, binding results are more likely to reflect the true *in vivo* situation.

Studies on purified, soluble receptors are much less common and are subject to the uncertainty that removal from the lipid environment of the cell membrane may modify binding.

5.3.2 The Radioligand

Although nonlinear least-squares methods allow complex binding curves to be analyzed, single-component curves will yield more precise estimates of the binding parameters. If it is not possible to avoid multiple components, the curves will be more satisfactorily analyzed if the individual components of the binding exhibit substantially different dissociation equilibrium constants. There is thus an obvious advantage in using **selective** radioligands which have greater affinity for one type of binding site. A **high affinity** is also desirable since it allows the binding to be studied at low concentration which, other things being equal, will reduce nonspecific binding. A high ratio of specific to nonspecific binding will reduce the errors in the estimated parameters. A high affinity, however, also has consequences for the rate at which the binding reaches equilibrium. The association rate constant, k_{+1}, has an upper limit, determined by collision theory, of about 10^8 M^{-1} s^{-1}, from which it follows that ligands with high affinities must have very low k_{-1} values. From Equations 5.12 and 5.15 it is seen that this will lead to both a slow onset (at the low concentrations of L which would be used) and a slow offset of binding. A slow rate of offset is advantageous in the separation of bound from free ligand by filtration, where it is important to ensure that the washing steps do not cause significant dissociation. The radioligand should also have a **high specific activity** so that very small quantities of bound ligand can be accurately measured. The specific activity, simply defined as the amount of radioactivity, expressed in becquerels or curies per mol of ligand, is dependent on the half-life of the isotope used and on the number of radioactive atoms incorporated into the ligand molecule. A radioisotope with a short half-life decays rapidly so that there are many disintegrations in unit time, resulting in a high specific activity.

The isotopes used most frequently for labeling are ^{125}I and ^3H, with half-lives of 60 days and 12.3 years, respectively (labeling with ^{14}C, with a half-life of 5760 years, would result in a low specific activity). Ligands labeled with single atoms of either ^{125}I or ^3H will have maximum specific activities of 2200 or 29 Ci/mmol, respectively. There is a basic difference between labeling with ^3H and with ^{125}I, namely that with ^3H the radioisotope can replace H atoms in the molecule with only insignificant changes in the chemical properties; indeed, it would be possible to replace several H by ^3H without a significant change in chemical properties but with a useful gain in specific activity. In contrast, most natural ligands and nearly all drugs do not contain an iodine atom which can be replaced by ^{125}I. Instead it is necessary to produce an iodinated derivative which *will* have different chemical properties, and quite likely a different affinity for the receptor. (Mainly for this reason, it is usual to incorporate only one atom of ^{125}I in each ligand molecule.) It is, therefore, necessary to check that the radioiodinated derivative retains the desired properties of the parent compound. With radioiodine it is possible to achieve 100% isotopic labeling, since it is possible to obtain pure ^{125}I and to separate the labeled ligand from both unincorporated $^{125}I^-$ and noniodinated parent compound.

It is obviously important to ensure that the label is associated only with the intended ligand. Potential problems include the possibilities that contaminating substances might also have been labeled and that the radioligand suffers chemical modification during storage. Highly radioactive ligands can suffer radiation damage. The presence of radioactive impurities will almost certainly lead to a reduction in the ratio of specific to nonspecific binding.

For many receptors both hydrophilic and hydrophobic radioligands are available. In some cases the hydrophobic ligands have been found to give higher estimates of B_{max}, suggesting that they have access to receptors within the cell which are denied to hydrophilic ligands. This is exemplified by the greater B_{max} values observed for the muscarinic receptor ligand ^3H-scopolamine (tertiary amine) compared with ^3H-N-methylscopolamine (quaternary ammonium). These differences in access to receptors can be exploited to study receptor internalization.

5.3.3 Incubation Conditions

5.3.3.1 Incubation Medium

Binding to intact cells must of necessity be performed in a physiological solution and the results obtained are hence more likely to correlate with functional studies. It would be wise to avoid the inclusion of protein (e.g., albumin) since protein may well bind the radioligand to a significant extent, and this would not be detected by measurement of the radioactivity of the supernatant obtained by centrifugation. Binding to membranes, by contrast, is quite often performed in a simple buffer solution, for example 20 or 50 mM Tris or Hepes buffers. It is clear, however, that the affinity of some ligands for receptors is increased in solutions of low ionic strength.

This effect has been clearly demonstrated for muscarinic cholinergic receptors. In principle, it could be avoided by including sufficient NaCl to make the incubation medium isotonic with the appropriate physiological solution. Particular ions have been shown to have effects on certain receptor systems. Mg^{++}, for example, commonly affects binding to G-protein-coupled receptors, which is in keeping with its known effects on G-protein activation (see Chapter 8). The ionization of weakly acidic or basic groups in both receptor and ligand will be affected by pH and is likely to modify binding. Accordingly, binding studies should be done at physiological pH, if at all possible.

5.3.3.2 Temperature

Temperature has effects on both the rates of reaction and equilibrium constants. A rise in temperature will increase the rates of both association and dissociation, as shown in Table 5.1 for the binding of ^{3}H-flunitrazepam to rat brain membranes.

TABLE 5.1
Effect of Temperature on the Kinetics of [^{3}H]-Flunitrazepam Binding to Rat Brain Homogenates

Temp. (°C)	k_{+1} ($M^{-1}.s^{-1}$)	k_{-1} (s^{-1})	K_D (nM)
0	7.3×10^5	7.3×10^{-4}	1.0
22	4.6×10^6	1.0×10^{-2}	2.2
35	1.1×10^7	5.9×10^{-2}	5.3

From Speth, R.C., Wastek, G.J., and Yamamura, H.A., *Life Sci.*, 24, 351, 1979. With permission, Elsevier Science, Inc.

The effect on the equilibrium constant is less because the changes in both k_{+1} and k_{-1} are in the same direction. It has been found for some receptors that the effect of temperature on affinity is greater for agonists than for antagonists. Table 5.2 illustrates the results for binding to β-adrenoreceptors obtained by Weiland et al.

The difference in the effect of temperature on agonist as compared with antagonist binding was thought to reflect the structural changes in the receptor (isomerization) which occurs only with agonists. More recent investigations of this issue, however, have not confirmed the generality of this conclusion.

In the light of these results, it might seem best to measure binding only at the relevant physiological temperature. However, conducting the incubation at low temperature has some

TABLE 5.2
K_I Values for Inhibition of ^{125}I-Iodohydroxybenzylpindolol Binding to β-Adrenoreceptors in Turkey Erythrocyte Membranes at 1°C and 37°C

	K_I (nM) 37°C	K_I (nM) 1°C	$\dfrac{K_I(37°C)}{K_I(1°C)}$
Agonists			
Isoprenaline	254	11	23.3
Noradrenaline	2680	48	55.5
Adrenaline	5230	326	16
Antagonists			
Propranolol	1.6	0.59	2.6
Pindolol	4.5	1.5	2.95
Atenolol	5300	2530	2.09

Note: The binding curves for both agonists and antagonists were unaffected by GTP.

Data from Weiland et al., *Nature*, 281, 114, 1979. With permision.

advantages. For example, proteolytic damage to the receptor and breakdown of the ligand, if it is chemically unstable, will be reduced during very long incubations (though this advantage may of course be offset by the longer incubation time needed for equilibration).

5.3.3.3   Duration of Incubation

Equilibrium studies clearly require an incubation period which is long enough to allow equilibration to be achieved. As discussed above, the time required will be longer at lower temperatures. It is critically dependent on the affinity of the ligand for the receptor. As outlined earlier, the rate constant for the onset of binding is given by $k_{-1} + k_{+1}[L]$. If k_{+1} is given a value of 10^7 M^{-1}s^{-1}, it can be estimated that to achieve 97% of equilibrium for a ligand with a K_L of 100 pM would require 1 h at 37°C and as much as 58 h at 0°C . The effect of a competing drug is to slow the rate of equilibration. These considerations demonstrate the desirability of conducting pilot kinetic studies **before** any detailed equilibrium measurements are made.

5.3.3.4   Amount of Tissue

The aim should be to employ sufficient material to give a good ratio of specific to nonspecific binding without causing significant **depletion** of the radioligand. Nonspecific binding that is associated with binding to the filter is likely to be a fixed amount at any given ligand concentration, so increasing the amount of receptor present should increase the signal-to-noise ratio. A large concentration of receptor may, however, bind a substantial fraction of the radioligand present and so reduce the free concentration. Such depletion is an important consideration. If the free ligand concentration can be measured directly then this should be done, and the concentration so obtained is that applicable to the equations presented in this chapter. An alternative, if [L] cannot be measured, is to derive equations which allow for depletion arising from both specific and nonspecific binding. Such equations have been presented by Birdsall and Hulme, but some of the assumptions made are necessarily over-simplifications. It is preferable to try to design the study so that depletion is kept to an insignificant level (say, <5%) and so can be ignored.

5.3.4 Methods of Separating Bound From Free Ligand

For particulate receptor preparations (intact cells or membranes), it is usual to separate bound from free ligand by either **centrifugation** or **filtration**. (For soluble receptor preparations, equilibrium dialysis using a semipermeable membrane, or gel filtration can be employed.)

5.3.4.1 Filtration

At a time determined by the design of the experiment, the reaction mixture is either tipped or drawn by suction onto the filter and the supernatant immediately filtered under vacuum. The filter, often made of glass fiber, must of course retain all of the receptor preparation but at the same time allow a rapid separation. It is also necessary to check for binding of ligand to the filter. There are several examples in the literature of "specific", saturable binding of radioligand to filters. The receptor preparation retained by the filter is normally washed two or three times with a small volume of incubation buffer which does not contain the radioligand, in order to remove superficial radiolabel. It is essential to minimize any dissociation of bound ligand during these washes. This can be achieved by using only a few, rapid washes and by washing with buffer at a low temperature. Commercially available filtration systems now allow many samples to be handled simultaneously. Commonly used filtration equipment does not, however, allow the supernatant to be collected for the determination of the free ligand concentration.

5.3.4.2 Centrifugation

Incubation is often performed in small plastic tubes which can be centrifuged directly to form, within seconds, a cell or membrane pellet. The supernatant can then be either tipped off or removed by suction. The radioactivity of the supernatant can be measured to determine the free ligand concentration. Any supernatant remaining on the surface of the pellet or tube can be reduced by washing, again using cold buffer. Most receptors will be within the pellet and will not be exposed to the wash solution, so that dissociation should be limited. It is obviously important that washing does not disturb the pellet, causing loss of receptors. In some experiments using intact cells, separation has been achieved by conducting the incubation over a layer of oil of appropriate density. At the desired time, the cells are centrifuged through the oil layer, leaving virtually all the supernatant on top. Supernatant and oil are then removed by suction and no washing step is needed. If plastic tubes are used, the tip of the tube containing the pellet can be cut off, thus reducing further any counts due to radioligand attached to the tube wall.

Finally, the bound radioligand (on the filter or in the pellet) is quantified using standard methods for measuring radioactivity (usually scintillation counting).

5.3.5 Determination of Nonspecific Binding

Nonspecific binding is estimated by setting up additional incubation mixtures which, in addition to the radioligand, also include enough of a displacing agent to greatly reduce the "specific" receptor binding. Since most of the displacing agents employed to define nonspecific binding act competitively, it is necessary to use a concentration which is 100 to 1000 times larger than its K_d to ensure that higher concentrations of the radioligand do not overcome the inhibition. It is also important to check that the displacing agent does not reduce nonspecific binding. This is likely to be more of a problem if a nonlabeled form of the radioligand itself is used; preference should, therefore, be given to a chemically distinct displacing agent. Extra reassurance can be obtained if similar values for nonspecific binding are estimated using more than one displacing agent. This is often the case in competition experiments where several competing drugs produce an identical maximal inhibition of binding, thus providing a reliable estimate of the residual nonspecific binding.

5.4 ANALYSIS OF BINDING DATA

There are essentially two steps in the analysis of binding experiments:

- Preliminary inspection and analysis of the data to try to establish a model which adequately describes the binding. For example, multiple components or exhibit cooperativity may be identified.
- Estimation of the model parameters, e.g., B_{max}, K_L with some indication of the errors associated with the estimates.

It is always desirable to plot the data in terms of the amount of radioligand bound as a function either of the radioligand concentration (saturation experiments) or inhibitor concentration (competition experiments). A logarithmic concentration scale usually provides a clearer picture of the relationship, deviations from a simple monotonic curve being more obvious. It is also common to use linearizing transformations of the binding curves, both to reveal binding complexities and to provide initial estimates of binding parameters. Various linear transformations have been used to analyze saturation experiments, as will now be outlined.

5.4.1 SCATCHARD PLOT

Equation 5.3 can be rearranged to give:

$$\frac{B}{[L]} = \frac{B_{max}}{K_L} - \frac{B}{K_L} \tag{5.28}$$

The Scatchard plot is bound/free ($B/[L]$, y-axis) vs. bound (B, x-axis). (The Eadie-Hofstee plot is bound vs. bound/free.) If this equation is applicable (i.e., the binding represents a simple bimolecular interaction) the data points will fall on a straight line, the slope will be $-K_L^{-1}$ and the intercept on the x-axis (when $B/[L] = 0$) will give B_{max}. See Figure 5.10 for a Scatchard plot of the data provided in problem 5.1. Curved Scatchard plots can indicate positive or negative cooperativity or the presence of sites with different affinities for the ligand.

The Scatchard plot has, in the past, been the main means of obtaining estimates of K_L and B_{max}, but it is only reliable if the data are very good and a straight line is obtained. It should be noted that simple linear regression should not be applied to the Scatchard plot since B with its associated error occurs in both variables. Linear regression of Scatchard plots systematically overestimates K_d and B_{max}. Because nonlinear Scatchard plots are even more difficult to handle, there is often a strong temptation to fit straight lines to plots which clearly are not straight. Nonlinear least-square methods (see below) are much to be preferred for the estimation of parameters with their confidence limits.

5.4.2 LINEWEAVER-BURK PLOT

This double-reciprocal plot is based on another rearrangement of Equation 5.3:

$$\frac{1}{B} = \frac{K_L}{B_{max}} \cdot \frac{1}{[L]} + \frac{1}{B_{max}} \tag{5.29}$$

A plot of $1/B$ vs. $1/[L]$ will give a straight line providing that Equation 5.3 applies, from which when $1/B = 0$, $1/[L] = -1/K_L$ and when $1/[L] = 0$, $1/B = 1/B_{max}$. A Lineweaver-Burk plot is shown in Figure 5.10, where it may be compared with the Scatchard plot of the same data. The double-reciprocal plot spreads the data very poorly, is inferior to the Scatchard plot, and is rarely employed in binding studies.

5.4.3 HILL PLOT

This has already been discussed in detail in Chapter 1 and earlier in this chapter. Yet another rearrangement of Equation 5.3 gives:

$$\frac{B}{B_{max} - B} = \frac{[L]}{K_L}, \tag{5.30}$$

$$\log\left(\frac{B}{B_{max} - B}\right) = \log[L] - \log K_L$$

The Hill plot is $\log (B/(B_{max} - B))$ vs. $\log [L]$. As noted earlier, it is the slope of the Hill plot (the Hill coefficient, n_H) which is of particular utility. If the equation holds, a straight line of slope $= 1$ should be obtained. A value greater than unity may indicate positive cooperativity and a slope less than unity either negative cooperativity or, commonly, the presence of sites with different affinities. The data of Problem 5.1 are also presented as a Hill plot in Figure 5.10.

5.4.4 ANALYSIS OF COMPETITION EXPERIMENTS

Equation 5.18, describing competitive binding, can also be transformed into the form of a Hill plot:

$$\log\left(\frac{B_I}{B_0 - B_I}\right) = \log IC_{50} - \log[I] \tag{5.31}$$

For simple competitive interaction at a single class of site, a plot of $\log (B_I/(B_0 - B_I))$ vs. $\log[I]$ will be linear with a slope of -1 and intercept on the x-axis of $\log IC_{50}$. This estimate of IC_{50} can be used to derive a value for K_I as discussed earlier. A different plot, equivalent to the Eadie-Hofstee plot for saturation experiments, has also been used to reveal more complex binding characteristics in competition experiments. Figure 5.7 provides an example of the analysis of a competition study in which two sites are indicated.

A plot of B vs. $\log[I]$ (Figure 5.7, A and B) might initially suggest two components, but the scatter of the observations would counsel caution. The Hill plot (Figure 5.7D) reveals a slope (by linear regression) of -0.629 (significantly different from -1), which is not consistent with simple 1:1 competition at a single binding site but is instead suggestive of multiple binding sites or negative cooperativity. An Eadie-Hofstee plot (Figure 5.7C) is clearly non-linear. Nonlinear least-squares analysis (see next section) of the data is shown in Figure 5.7, A and B. In B a single component is fitted using Equation 5.18, but with the terms raised to the power n_H. The fit is quite reasonable and yields an n_H of -0.648, close to the value from the Hill plot. A closer fit, Figure 5.7A, (predictably) is obtained to a two-component model (in which n_H is constrained to one) according to:

$$B_I = B_{0(1)}\left(\frac{IC_{50(1)}}{IC_{50(1)} + [I]}\right) + B_{0(2)}\left(\frac{IC_{50(2)}}{IC_{50(2)} + [I]}\right) \tag{5.32}$$

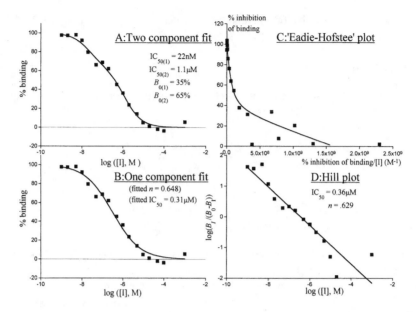

FIGURE 5.7   Analysis of a competition experiment in which the binding of a radiolabeled β-adreno-receptor antagonist (^{125}I-iodopindolol) is inhibited by a β$_1$-β$_2$ selective antagonist. The four panels indicate various ways in which the data can be analyzed: see text. (The data for the figure has been extracted from Figure 4, Chapter 7 of Wolfe, B.B. and Molinoff, P.B., *Handbook of Experimental Pharmacology,* Trendelenburg, U. and Weiner, N., Eds., Springer-Verlag, Berlin, 1988.).

5.4.5 NONLINEAR LEAST-SQUARES METHODS OF DATA ANALYSIS

As already noted, with the advent of powerful microcomputers and software incorporating appropriate fitting routines, binding data can be readily analyzed by means of nonlinear least-squares fitting procedures. It is beyond the scope of this chapter to give a full description of this method. In essence, however, the procedure first requires the selection of an expression which is believed to represent the system being investigated. Initial guesses are then made of the unknown parameters, e.g., K_L and B_{max}, and using these guesses the expected binding is calculated corresponding to the ligand concentration at each datum point. The deviations of the observed points from the calculated points are squared and added together. Thus:

$$\text{Sum of squares} = \sum w\left(B_{obs} - B_{calc}\right)^2 \tag{5.33}$$

where:

B_{obs} is the measured binding.
B_{calc} is the binding calculated using the guesses.
w   is a weighting factor. This allows the investigator to give more or less weight to particular data points according to their perceived reliability. Where each datum point has an associated standard error it is quite common, for example, to weight inversely with the variance.

The program then makes systematic changes to the guessed values and recalculates the sum of squares, repeating this process until the sum of squares reaches a minimum, i.e., the **least-squares estimate** is obtained. Many of the programs will also produce estimates of the standard deviation of the estimated values. The process is described in more detail in Colquhoun's textbook, *Lectures on Biostatistics,* and its application to binding studies has been considered specifically by Wells (see Further Reading Section). *Sigmaplot* (Jandel) and *Origin* (Microcal) are examples of commercially available graphing and curve-fitting programs. A program designed specifically for the analysis of ligand binding experiments is *Ligand* (Biosoft).

Closer least-squares fits can obviously be obtained by adopting more complicated models involving extra parameters. The use of more complicated models can, of course, be more readily justified if there is independent supporting evidence available, e.g., knowledge of multiple binding sites from functional studies.

5.5 RELEVANCE OF RESULTS FROM BINDING STUDIES

Binding studies are done independently of any biological response and it is obviously desirable to have some check that the binding is occurring to a relevant or identifiable site. Thus, wherever possible, the binding results should be compared with results from functional studies. This can be achieved most easily for competitive antagonists. In this case Schild plots (see Chapter 1) can provide an estimate of affinity from the shift of concentration/response curves which should correspond to the K_d obtained in binding studies. Hulme and Birdsall provide an excellent illustration of such a correlation for muscarinic receptors, and a further example is provided in Figure 5.8, which compares functional and binding studies of potassium channel blockers.

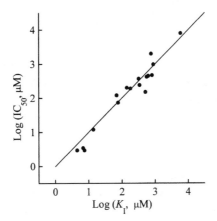

FIGURE 5.8 Correlation between the abilities of various compounds to inhibit [^{125}I]-monoiodoapamin binding to guinea-pig hepatocytes (K_I values, abscissa) and their abilities to inhibit the K^+ permeability increase induced by angiotensin II in these cells (IC$_{50}$ values, ordinate). The straight line is that expected for direct equivalence. The measurements are highly correlated, suggesting that the compounds do indeed produce their effects by binding to the apamin-sensitive K^+ channels. (Data from Cook, N.S. and Haylett, D.G., *J. Physiol.*, 358, 373, 1985. With permission.)

It will clearly be more difficult to establish such relationships when there are subtypes of a receptor in a tissue. In these circumstances, the availabilty of agents which exhibit selectivity for subtypes will assist the interpretation.

5.6 PROBLEMS

These problems are provided to afford an opportunity for the reader to analyze binding data of different sorts. The problems do not require nonlinear least-squares analysis, but this would be recommended to those with access to appropriate facilities. The analysis of each set of data is discussed in detail in the next section.

PROBLEM 5.1: SATURATION BINDING

The following data are from an experiment measuring ^{125}I-monoiodoapamin binding to guinea-pig hepatocytes. Conditions were such that depletion of radioligand was negligible over the whole of the concentration range studied.

TABLE 5.3
Data for Problem 5.1

Radioligand conc. ([L], pM)	Amount bound (fmol/mg dry tissue)	
	Total	Noninhibitable
20	0.110	0.018
50	0.224	0.046
100	0.351	0.071
150	0.495	0.143
200	0.557	0.180
300	0.708	0.275
500	0.942	0.462
1000	1.530	0.900
1500	1.920	1.310

1. Plot specific (inhibitable) binding against [L]. Make initial estimates of K_L and B_{max} from this graph.
2. Construct a Scatchard plot of the data and derive new estimates of K_L and B_{max}.
3. Construct a Hill plot ($\log[B/(B_{max} - B)]$ vs. $\log [L]$). What can be concluded from the slope of this plot?

PROBLEM 5.2: KINETICS

The onset of binding of radiolabeled apamin to guinea-pig hepatocytes was studied for three concentrations of the ligand over a 200-s period and provided the following results:

TABLE 5.4
Data for Problem 5.2

Time, s	Specific binding (fmol/mg dry tissue)		
	[L] = 30 pM	[L] = 100 pM	[L] = 300 pM
5	0.025	0.071	0.165
10	0.029	0.112	0.294
15	0.041	0.135	0.340
20	0.063	0.166	0.392
30	0.063	0.218	0.460
50	0.098	0.257	0.481
100	0.102	0.260	0.503
200	0.112	0.270	0.488

These data are plotted in Figure 5.9 and indicate how the rate constant for onset of binding increases with the ligand concentration.

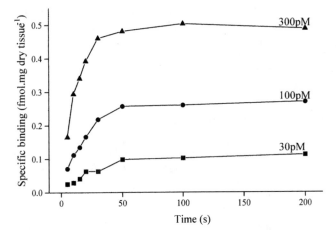

FIGURE 5.9   Plot of the data for Problem 5.2.

For each set of results the expected binding is given by:

$$B_t = B_\infty \left(1 - e^{-\left(k_{-1} + k_{+1}[L]\right)t}\right) \tag{5.34}$$

Estimate k_{+1} and k_{-1} from the data (see Section 5.2.2.2).

PROBLEM 5.3: COMPETITION EXPERIMENT

The binding of three concentrations of ^{125}I-labeled iodohydroxybenzylpindolol (IHYP) to membranes from turkey erythrocytes was studied in the absence and presence of a range of sotalol concentrations. The following are the results:

TABLE 5.5
Data for Problem 5.3

[Sotalol], M	Total binding (fmol/mg protein)		
	[IHYP] = 30 pM	[IHYP] = 100 pM	[IHYP] = 300 pM
0.0	34.0	56.2	75.1
1.0×10^{-8}	33.8	57.0	74.0
3.2×10^{-8}	32.5	55.3	74.6
1.0×10^{-7}	31.0	55.0	73.8
3.2×10^{-7}	26.2	51.8	69.6
1.0×10^{-6}	20.0	42.6	67.0
3.2×10^{-6}	9.7	26.3	50.6
1.0×10^{-5}	4.2	13.0	35.0
3.2×10^{-5}	3.0	7.9	22.5
1.0×10^{-4}	1.9	5.0	12.5
3.2×10^{-4}	1.4	3.8	11.9
1.0×10^{-3}	1.2	3.5	10.0

Plot the total amount of IHYP bound against log [sotalol] and draw smooth curves by eye through each set of points. Estimate the IC_{50} for each curve. Given that the K_L for IHYP is 37 pM, calculate K_I from each IC_{50}. (See Equation 5.20.)

Tabulate the specific binding for each set of data and construct Hill plots (Equation 5.31). Are the results consistent with a single population of receptors? Compare the IC_{50}s from these plots with your previous estimates.

5.7 FURTHER READING

First rigorous study of radioligand binding.

Paton, W. D. M. and Rang, H. P., The uptake of atropine and related drugs by intestinal smooth muscle of the guinea-pig in relation to acetylcholine receptors, *Proc. R. Soc. B*, 163, 1, 1965.

Scintillation proximity method.

Udenfriend, S., Gerber, L., and Nelson, N., Scintillation proximity assay; A sensitive and continuous isotopic method for monitoring ligand/receptor and antigen/antibody interactions, *Anal. Biochem.*, 161, 494, 1987.

Effect of ionic strength on ligand binding.

Birdsall, N. J. M., Burgen, A. S. V., Hulme, E. C., and Wells, J. W., The effects of ions on the binding of agonists and antagonists to muscarinic receptors, *Br. J. Pharmacol.*, 67, 371, 1979.

Comprehensive treatment of theoretical and practical aspects of radioligand binding experiments.

Hulme, E. C. and Birdsall, N. J. M., Strategy and tactics in receptor binding studies, in *Receptor-Ligand Interactions. A Practical Approach*, Ed., Hulme, E. C., IRL Press, Oxford, 1992, chap. 4.

Parameter estimation, including nonlinear least-squares methods.

Colquhoun, D., *Lectures on Biostatistics*, Clarendon Press, Oxford, 1971.
Wells, J. W., Analysis and interpretation of binding at equilibrium, in *Receptor-Ligand Interactions. A Practical Approach*, Ed., Hulme, E. C., IRL Press, Oxford, 1992, chap. 11.

5.8 SOLUTIONS TO PROBLEMS

PROBLEM 5.1: SATURATION DATA

The raw data are plotted in Figure 5.10A. The top two points of the specific data might suggest that B_{max} has been reached by about 1000 pM, with a value between the measured values at 1000 and 1500 pM, say 0.62 fmol/mg dry wt. An estimate of K_L can be obtained by reading from the graph the ligand concentration which produces binding of 0.5 B_{max} (i.e., 0.31 fmol/mg dry wt Equation 5.3). This estimate will depend on how the curve has been drawn, but is likely to be around 120 pM.

A Scatchard plot of the data is shown in Figure 5.10C. For convenience, the fitted line is the regression of B/F on B (though as noted earlier, this is statistically unsound) and provides an estimate for B_{max} (x-intercept) of 0.654 fmol/mg dry wt and an estimate for K_L (−1/slope) of 132 pM. A Lineweaver-Burk (double reciprocal) plot is provided for comparison in Figure 5.10D. Linear regression gives another estimate for B_{max} (1/y-intercept, see Equation 5.29) of 0.610 fmol/mg dry wt. The estimate of K_L from this plot (slope $\times B_{max}$) is 114 pM.

To construct the Hill plot (Figure 5.10E) it was assumed that B_{max} was 0.654 fmol/mg dry wt — the Scatchard value. The slope of the plot is 1.138 with a standard deviation of

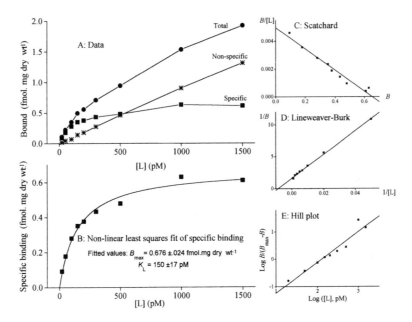

FIGURE 5.10   Analysis of the saturation data provided for Problem 5.1 (see accompanying text).

0.12, so it would not be unreasonable to suppose n_H was indeed 1 and so consistent with a simple bimolecular interaction. Figure 5.10B shows a nonlinear least-squares fit of the specific binding to Equation 5.3 (giving all points equal weight). The least-squares estimates are 0.676 fmol/mg dry wt for B_{max} and 150 pM for K_L. (Estimates of the standard errors of these values are noted in the figure.) A nonlinear least-squares fit of the *total* binding data to Equation 5.4 gave $B_{max} = 0.686$ fmol/mg dry wt and $K_L = 151$ pM. The data for Problem 5.1 were in fact generated by setting the points randomly about a curve with $B_{max} = 0.68$ fmol/mg dry wt and $K_L = 150$ pM.

Both the Scatchard and double reciprocal plots, in this case, underestimate both parameters. The latter plot being particularly inaccurate.

PROBLEM 5.2: KINETIC DATA

A graphical analysis, which allows the determination of k_{+1} and k_{-1} from the given data, is described in Section 5.2.2.2. For each set of data it is necessary to determine k_{on}. These values can be obtained from the semilogarithmic plots of $\ln((B_\infty - B_t)/B_\infty)$ vs. t. But what value should be taken for B_∞? Estimates can be made by eye from the data, and for Figure 5.11C the B_∞s for 30 and 100 pM have been taken as the highest recorded values, and for 300 pM as the mean of the values at 100 and 200 s.

In plotting Figure 5.11C, the points beyond 50 s have been ignored since the errors in $(B_\infty - B_t)$ become proportionately very large. Linear regressions have been fitted to the three lines giving k_{on} estimates of 0.0377 s^{-1} (30 pM), 0.0572 s^{-1} (100 pM) and 0.0765 s^{-1} (300 pM). Nonlinear least-squares fits, using Equation 5.14, were also made of each set of data (using *Origin*) and the fitted curves are shown in Figure 5.11A. The fitted values for B_∞ were 0.110 ± 0.005, 0.269 ± 0.006, and 0.494 ± 0.006 fmol/mg dry wt and for k_{on} 0.0351 ± 0.004, 0.0518 ± 0.003, and 0.0828 ± 0.003 s^{-1}. These latter values have been plotted against [L] in Figure 5.11B and linear regression gives a slope ($\equiv k_{+1}$) of 1.72×10^{-4} pM^{-1} s^{-1} (=1.7 × 10^8 M^{-1} s^{-1}) and intercept ($\equiv k_{-1}$) of 0.032 s^{-1}. (All three curves were also fitted simultaneously to Equations 5.14 and 5.15 using a nonlinear least-squares program (D. Colqhoun, unpublished) and provided values for k_{+1} and k_{-1} directly: $k_{+1} = 1.63 \times 10^{-4}$ pM^{-1} s^{-1}, $k_{-1} = 0.034$ s^{-1}.)

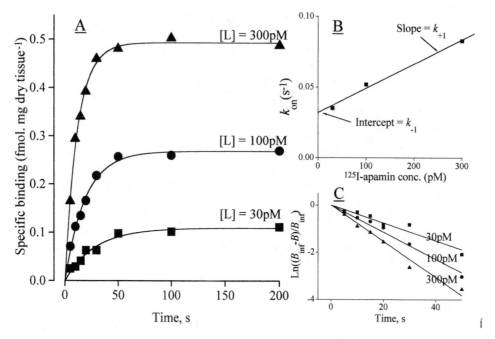

FIGURE 5.11   Analysis of the kinetic data provided for Problem 5.2 (see accompanying text).

PROBLEM 5.3: COMPETITION DATA

The individual plots of the data will produce curves equivalent to that in Figure 5.4, the nonspecific binding, of course, increasing with radioligand concentration. IC_{50}s can be read from the curves directly (taking account of nonspecific binding) or can be obtained from Hill plots for specific binding (see Equation 5.31). Hill plots of the data are presented in Figure 5.12, the points for concentrations outside 3×10^{-7} to 3×10^{-4} M being excluded because of the large errors associated with them.

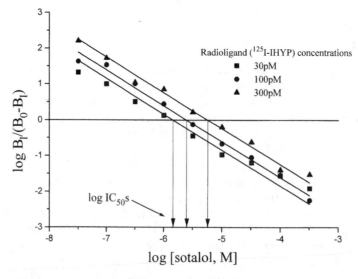

FIGURE 5.12   Hill plots of the results of the competition experiment used for Problem 5.3. The fitted lines have been constrained to have a slope of −1. IC_{50} values are given by the x-intercepts and can be used to determine K_I for the binding of sotalol (see accompanying text). The IC_{50} values, as expected from Equation 5.20, increase with the radioligand concentration.

The lines are seen to be straight, and linear regression indicates slopes not significantly different from -1. The fitted lines have therefore been constrained to have a slope of -1. The x-intercepts corresponding to the IC_{50}s are 1.43 μM, 2.48 μM, and 5.74 μM. (Compare these with estimates obtained by direct interpolation on the plots of the raw data.) Nonlinear least-squares fits of each set of data to Equation 5.18 provided IC_{50} estimates of 1.20 ± 0.07 μM, 2.51 ± 0.13 μM, and 6.17 ± 0.45 μM. K_Is can be obtained from the IC_{50}s using Equation 5.20. Taking K_L as 37 pM gives K_I values of 0.66, 0.68, and 0.68 μM, respectively, which as expected are very similar. The data for this problem were actually generated using a starting value for K_I of 0.68 μM.

Section IV

Signal Transduction Systems

6 Introduction to Signal Transduction

John C. Foreman

CONTENTS

6.1 INTRODUCTION

In Chapter 1 of this book a brief introduction was given to the history of the development of the concept of the drug or hormone receptor. The early views about receptors were based on the idea that the receptor is a specific binding site on the cell surface for a drug or hormone. It was also recognized that the interaction of the ligand with its specific receptor would bring about a change in cellular response. Chapters 2, 3, and 4 of the book describe how the application of molecular biology to the study of receptor macromolecules has provided considerable insight into the structure of receptors. The molecular biology of receptors has revealed information not only about the structure of the ligand binding site in the receptor molecule but also about the components of the receptor which begin the transduction of the information provided by the ligand-receptor interaction into a cellular response.

It is perhaps not surprising, especially with hindsight, that the structure of the receptor determines not only the specificity of its interaction with a ligand but also the specificity with respect to the transduction system employed for starting the cellular response. Although evidence from molecular biology supports the concept, it was already recognized before the advent of molecular biological techniques that particular receptors were associated with specific transduction systems. For example, the β-adrenoreceptor invariably appeared to be associated with the activation of adenylyl cyclase and the elevation of the intracellular messenger, cyclic AMP.

The concept of a receptor has changed: it now includes not only the structural and functional characteristics of the ligand binding site but also the signal transduction system with which it is associated. The ligand binding site of the receptor can be studied quantitatively by measurement of the interaction of agonists and antagonists in a functional system (Chapter 1). The ligand binding site can also be studied quantitatively on a membrane preparation by measuring the binding of a labeled ligand and its displacement by other

0-8493-9227-6/96/$0.00+$.50
© 1996 by CRC Press, Inc.

selective ligands (Chapter 5). In Chapters 2, 3, and 4 the different types of receptors were presented on the basis of molecular structure and this is as much connected with signal transduction as it is with the ligand binding site. The purpose of of this chapter is to present in some detail the signal transduction systems which are related to the main classes of membrane receptors, and to present very simply the basic schemes for signal transduction which will be elaborated upon in subsequent chapters. Intracellular receptors, such as those for the steroid hormones, have not been incorporated into this book.

6.2 THE RELATIONSHIP BETWEEN STRUCTURE AND SIGNAL TRANSDUCTION

On the basis of structure and signal transduction mechanisms, it is possible to construct four broad categories of receptors:

- Membrane proteins which act as ion channels and also carry the binding site for the ligand which operates the channel (Figure 6.1a). An example is the nicotinic receptor for acetylcholine.
- Membrane proteins which carry the binding site for the ligand and transmit information to the cell by interacting with and activating a heterotrimeric G-protein (Figure 6.1b). An example is the β-adrenoreceptor.
- Membrane proteins which carry the binding site for the ligand and either possess or associate with an enzyme activity (Figure 6.1c). Examples are the receptors for atrial natriuretic peptide and insulin.
- Intracellular proteins which bind the ligand and interact with DNA. Examples are the receptors for steroid hormones (Figure 6.1d).

Within these broad categories, the signals which are generated can differ. For example, G-protein activation can generate inositol trisphosphate (IP_3) and diacylglycerol (DAG) to provide an intracellular calcium signal and a signal dependent upon the activation of protein kinase C. However, G-protein activation can also stimulate adenylyl cyclase to generate a cyclic AMP signal. The difference between these two receptor-G-protein signal transduction systems arises from the different G-proteins which couple to the receptor (see Chapter 8).

In contrast, the same signal may be generated by receptors which fall into different members of these broad categories. For example, a calcium signal arising from IP_3 formation can result both from the activation of a G-protein-coupled receptor and also from the receptor-enzyme category (see below).

6.3 SIGNALS AND SECOND MESSENGERS

The concept of a "second messenger" arose from studies of the mechanism of action of the β-adrenoreceptor on liver cells. Cyclic AMP was shown to be formed when adrenaline acted at this receptor, and the idea was that the water-soluble cAMP transmitted, as the "second message", the information from the adrenaline-receptor interaction on the outside of the cell (first message) to the intracellular response elements. We now know that the mechanism is more complex than this, and continued use of the words "second messenger" can be confusing because there are many steps in the information transfer. Signal transduction is a better term for the process.

Signals can be transmitted either by amplitude or by frequency modulation: that is, the response is governed by either the size of the signal or by the change in frequency of the signal. In both cases, there must be a process for generating the signal and also a process for terminating its action. Intracellular molecules which play a major, early role in signal transduction are

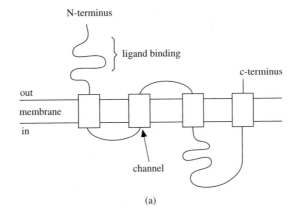

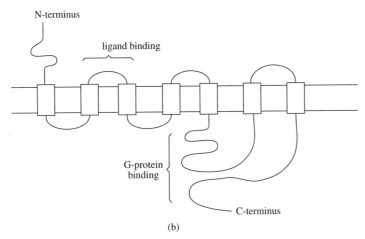

FIGURE 6.1 The four broad structural categories of receptor showing the N- and C-termini of the polypeptide chains and the regions which are involved with ligand binding and with the initiation of signal transduction: a, receptor with an integral ion channel; b, receptor which initiates the signal through heterotrimeric G-protein activation.

cAMP, cGMP, calcium, and diacylglycerol. In the chapters which follow there are examples of signal modulation where the ligand-receptor interaction affects the termination of the signal as well as examples where the ligand-receptor interaction affects the generation of the signal.

Interestingly, but perhaps not surprisingly, these signal transduction molecules can be formed by ligand interaction with receptors in different categories.

6.3.1 CALCIUM AND DIACYLGLYCEROL

A rise in the intracellular concentration of calcium is recognized as an important signal in a very wide variety of biological processes. The source of the calcium causing the rise in the intracellular concentration can be the extracellular medium or an intracellular store. If the source is extracellular, the membrane, which is normally impermeable to calcium, must be made more permeable by the opening of a channel which conducts calcium ions. In some cases, depolarization of the membrane opens voltage-sensitive calcium channels to allow calcium to enter the cell down an electrochemical gradient. In other cases, the ligand-receptor interaction generates a chemical signal which opens membrane channels through which calcium can enter the cell. For example, it has been proposed that inositol tetrakisphosphate (IP_4) can provide such a chemical signal to open membrane channels for calcium. Another

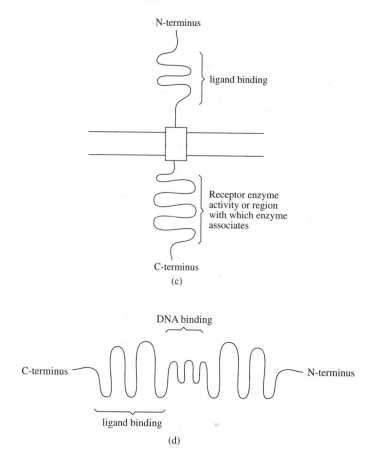

Figure 6.1 (continued)   c, receptor with an integral or associated enzyme activity; d, intracellular receptor which binds to DNA.

calcium channel opened through a ligand-receptor interaction is the so-called calcium release activated channel (I_{CRAC}), where the ligand-receptor interaction causes emptying of intracellular calcium stores and, in some undefined way, the emptying of these stores causes a membrane calcium channel to open.

Intracellular stores of calcium can be released to cause a rise in the intercellular concentration of calcium. The properties and behavior of these stores is discussed in Chapter 10. Inositol trisphosphate (IP_3) is a principal signal in the cell for release of calcium from intracellular stores. IP_3 is formed by the action of phospholipase C on phosphatidylinositol bisphosphate (PIP_2), and at the same time diacylglycerol (DAG) is formed. Diacylglycerol is also a signaling molecule which activates protein kinase C (Chapter 11). IP_3, and hence a calcium signal, is generated through two different receptor categories as outlined above (Figure 6.2). In one case, interaction of a ligand with a seven-transmembrane segment receptor linked to a G-protein (G_q) causes the activation of phospholipase Cβ. The phospholipase then splits PIP_2 into IP_3 and DAG. In the other case, interaction of the ligand with a tyrosine kinase receptor causes the activation of phospholipase Cγ which generates IP_3 and DAG from PIP_2.

6.3.2 CYCLIC NUCLEOTIDES

The role of cAMP as a signal transducer was one of the first functions to be established. The ligand-receptor interaction activates adenylyl cyclase through a G-protein (G_s) and the cAMP

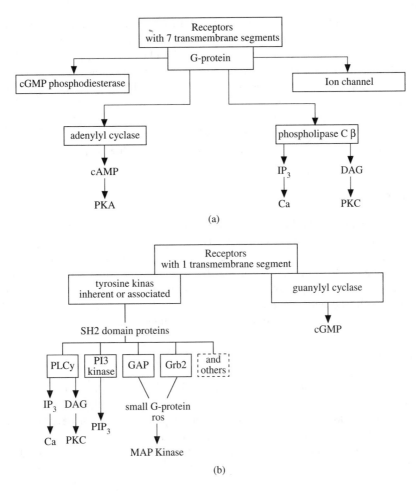

FIGURE 6.2 Diagram illustrating the diversity of signals that can be generated by the seven- or the one-transmembrane segment receptors.

generated activates protein kinase A (PKA) which phosphorylates effector proteins. Shortly after the discovery of cAMP, cGMP was identified, and it was initially believed that the cGMP generating system was exactly analogous to the cAMP system. Now, very important differences between these two cyclic nucleotide signal transducers have been revealed. Adenylyl cyclase is a membrane-bound enzyme activated by a G-protein which couples to the seven-transmembrane segment class of receptors (Figure 6.2). In contrast, guanylyl cyclase exists as a soluble, cytoplasmic enzyme as well as a membrane-bound enzyme — the soluble enzyme responding to the redox state of the cell and the membrane enzyme being an integral part of a receptor belonging to the one transmembrane segment class (Figure 6.2).

6.3.3 TYROSINE KINASE RECEPTORS

These receptors belong to the one-transmembrane segment category which is associated with an enzyme activity. It is also a category where there has been recent rapid progress in the understanding of the signal transduction mechanisms. The ligands for the receptors in this category, where the enzyme activity is a tyrosine kinase, activate the receptors by cross-linking of ligand binding sites. In some cases the tyrosine kinase activity is an integral part of the receptor, but in other cases a separate protein with tyrosine kinase activity interacts with the receptor protein when the ligand has bound. The receptor protein is phosphorylated at tyrosine residues, and the signal is then conveyed by the interaction of the receptor with intracellular proteins which recognize the membrane domains with phosphorylated tyrosines.

Proteins which recognize the receptor domains with phosphorylated tyrosines all appear to possess identical structural features, called SH2 (sequence homology 2) domains, through which the recognition takes place. The SH2 domain-containing proteins are heterogeneous with respect to function (Figure 6.2) and include phospholipase Cγ and phosphatidylinositol-3-kinase (PI-3-kinase). The implication is that receptors of this type can generate diverse signals. Another feature of this type of receptor is that in many but not all cases a small G-protein-like ras is part of the signal transducing pathway (Figure 6.1 and Chapter 13).

6.3.4 ION CHANNELS

We have seen that one of the broad categories of receptors comprises an ion channel and ligand binding site in the same protein. It needs to be pointed out that ion channels can be opened by receptors of the other broad classes. Seven-transmembrane segment receptors linked to G-proteins also open ion channels: for example, the muscarinic receptor opens potassium channels. The one-transmembrane segment receptors may also open ion channels. For example, the ligand activates phospholipase A_2 which generates arachidonic acid, and the eicosanoids formed cause channel opening (see Chapter 13).

6.4 SUMMARY

The purpose of this chapter has been to emphasize that signal transduction systems are part of the concept of a receptor. The main signal transducing systems have been introduced in simple terms and it has been shown how the same type of signal can be generated from receptors belonging to the different structural categories.

In the following seven chapters, the various signal transducing systems will be described in more detail.

7 Receptors Linked to Ion Channels: Activation and Block

Alasdair J. Gibb

7.1   INTRODUCTION

Many measurements in pharmacology rely on a chain of events following receptor activation to produce a measurable response: for example, contraction of the smooth muscle of a piece of guinea-pig ileum in response to muscarinic receptor activation by acetylcholine. This means that the relationship between receptor occupancy and response is likely to be complex and mechanisms of drug action in such systems are often difficult to define.

In contrast to this, agonist responses at ligand-gated ion channels and drug effects at ion channels are often more amenable to mechanistic investigation because the response (ionic

0-8493-9227-6/96/$0.00+$.50

current through open ion channels when measured with voltage or patch-clamp techniques) is directly proportional to receptor activation. This is a great advantage and has allowed electrophysiological techniques to be used to study ion channel activation and drug block of ion channels in great detail.

This chapter deals mainly with information that can be obtained from equilibrium, or at least steady-state recordings of ion channel activity. However, a great deal of information has also been obtained from kinetic studies of ion channels where the aim has been to determine values for the rate constants in a receptor mechanism. In general, only equilibrium constants can be determined from equilibrium studies.

7.1.1 RESPONSE TO RECEPTOR ACTIVATION

Activation of the ligand-gated ion channel receptors causes opening of the ion channel which forms a central pore through the receptor structure. Ions such as Na^+ and K^+ and possibly also Ca^{++}, depending on the ionic selectivity of the channel, flow though cationic channels which are formed by nicotinic AChRs, glutamate receptors, $5HT_3$ receptors, or ATP receptors. These ionic currents are generally excitatory and lead to depolarization of the cell. Chloride, with some contribution from HCO_3^- ions, is the main charge carrier through GABA and glycine receptor channels and these currents are generally, but not always, inhibitory.

The ligand-gated ion channel receptors mediate fast synaptic transmission at the neuro-muscular junction and throughout the central and peripheral nervous system. In addition, where the receptor channels are permeable to Ca^{++}, they are involved in the control of the intracellular Ca^{++} concentration and hence feed into many of the transduction mechanisms which involve Ca^{++} as a second messenger. Ca^{++} influx through glutamate receptors of the NMDA (*N*-methyl-D-aspartate) subtype is thought to be particularly critical in the processes of synaptogenesis and control of the strength of synaptic connections in the brain, while excess Ca^{++} influx through NMDA receptor channels is thought to be the main cause of neuronal cell death during hypoxia or ischemia in the brain.

Over the past 40 years, the development of electrophysiological techniques has allowed the effects of agonists and antagonists at the ligand-gated ion channel receptors to be studied with great precision. This has been particularly useful in studies of the mechanism of action of drugs because the result of receptor activation (current through the ion channel) can be measured directly, and channel opening is directly linked to receptor activation. Thus, it should be no surprise that the first physically plausible mechanism for receptor activation was the result of electrophysiological studies of AChR activation. Those experiments were performed by Katz and co-workers in the Biophysics Department at University College, London almost 40 years ago.

7.2 AGONIST MECHANISMS

The simplest agonist mechanism which can be used to describe activation of the ligand-gated ion channel receptors is that first suggested by del Castillo and Katz for activation of nicotinic AChRs at the neuromuscular junction.

$$A + R \underset{k_{-1}}{\overset{k_{+1}}{\rightleftharpoons}} AR \underset{\alpha}{\overset{\beta}{\rightleftharpoons}} AR^* \qquad (7.1)$$

This mechanism makes the vital point that receptor activation must represent a step (most likely several steps) subsequent to agonist binding (see also Chapter 1). However, this mechanism does not allow for the fact that there is now considerable functional, biochemical, and structural evidence that there are two ACh binding sites on nicotinic acetylcholine receptors of muscle and electric organs and it is probably the case that other ligand-gated ion channels such as the glutamate and GABA receptors also require binding of two agonist molecules for efficient activation of the receptor. At present, the mechanism most commonly applied to AChR activation is as follows:

$$A + R \underset{k_{-1}}{\overset{2k_{+1}}{\rightleftharpoons}} AR + A \underset{2k_{-2}}{\overset{k_{+2}}{\rightleftharpoons}} A_2R \underset{\alpha}{\overset{\beta}{\rightleftharpoons}} A_2R^* \qquad (7.2)$$

Here the microscopic association and dissociation rate constants for each step in the receptor activation mechanism are given, where k_{+1} and k_{+2} refer to agonist binding, k_{-1} and k_{-2} to agonist dissociation, and β and α are the rate constants for channel opening and closing, respectively. The factor of 2 before k_{+1} and k_{-2} occurs because the mechanism assumes that either of the two agonist binding sites can be occupied or vacated first. In addition, note that the two sites are equivalent before agonist binding.

7.2.1 EVIDENCE FOR NONIDENTICAL AGONIST BINDING SITES

The agonist binding sites on the receptor are some distance from the ion channel and outside the membrane. They are in pockets formed mainly by the two α-subunits and the adjacent δ- and ϵ-subunits. Thus the environment of the two binding sites is unlikely to be identical because of the nonidentical adjacent subunits. However, experimental evidence demonstrating nonequivalence of the two binding sites has not been consistent.

The best evidence for the binding sites being different comes from studies of the Torpedo AChR, where both binding studies and patch-clamp studies of cloned receptors expressed in fibroblasts suggest that there is on the order of a 100-fold difference in affinity for ACh between the two sites. Similar experiments on the BC3H1 cell line suggest that there is also heterogeneity of the agonist binding sites on this embryonic mouse muscle AChR. In contrast, some experiments have found no evidence for a large difference between ACh binding at the two sites on frog endplate AChRs.

At present, this issue has not been resolved and further functional and structural work continues to address this question. However, it should be noted that the presence on a receptor of two agonist/antagonist binding sites, which may be different, adds considerably to the complexity of the results expected from binding studies or dose-ratio experiments such as the Schild method.

7.2.2 APPLICATION OF THE TWO-BINDING-SITE MECHANISM

Equation 7.2 has proved to be a good description of AChR activity in a wide range of experimental situations, and more recently has been used as a starting point in developing mechanisms to describe the activation of other ligand-gated ion channels such as glutamate receptors and GABA receptors.

Expressions relating the equilibrium occupancy of any state in this mechanism to agonist concentration can be derived as described in Chapter 1 (e.g., Equation 1.26). If we define the equilibrium constants for agonist binding as $K_1 = k_{-1}/k_{+1}$ and $K_2 = k_{-2}/k_{+2}$ and a constant E describing the efficiency of channel opening (equivalent to *efficacy*) as $E = \beta/\alpha$, then the equilibrium occupancy of the open state (A_2R^*) will be

$$p_{A_2R^*} = \frac{[A]}{[A] + \dfrac{1}{E}\left\{[A] + K_2\left(2 + \dfrac{K_1}{[A]}\right)\right\}} \qquad (7.3)$$

It is instructive to write this equation in the form analogous to that for a single agonist binding site mechanism since this form illustrates the dependence of p_{A_2R*} (at low agonist concentrations) on the square of the agonist concentration, which steepens the dose-response curve.

$$p_{A_2R*} = \frac{[A]^2}{\dfrac{K_1K_2}{E} + [A]\left\{[A] + \dfrac{[A]}{E} + \dfrac{2K_2}{[E]}\right\}} \tag{7.4}$$

The equilibrium occupancy of the open state of an ion channel is usually referred to as the p_{open} and is the fraction of time that a single channel is open, or equally, the fraction of a population of channels that are open at equilibrium. For a two-binding-site agonist mechanism, the relationship between the p_{open} and the agonist concentration (p_{open} curve) has the familiar sigmoid shape (when the agonist concentration is plotted on a logarithmic scale) of a dose-response curve, but is steeper than for a single binding site mechanism.

7.2.3 HILL COEFFICIENTS AND COOPERATIVITY

In Chapter 1 (Sections 1.2.2 and 1.2.4) the Hill equation and the Hill coefficient, n, are described for a single agonist binding site mechanism. Hill coefficients greater than or less than unity are often interpreted as indicating positive or negative cooperativity, respectively, in the relationship between receptor occupancy and response. For example, positive cooperativity could arise due to amplification in a transduction mechanism mediated by G-proteins.

If the receptor has two agonist binding sites, the question arises as to whether binding of agonist at one site can influence the binding of the agonist at the other site. This is referred to as *cooperativity between agonist binding sites*. If binding at one site reduces the affinity at the second site, this is referred to as *negative cooperativity*, while if binding at one site increases the affinity at the second site this is termed *positive cooperativity*. Note that there may be cooperativity between agonist binding sites even although the unoccupied sites have the same affinity for the agonist. However, it is also possible that the two agonist binding sites are different before agonist binding occurs (on average, one site is then more likely to be occupied before the other), and in this case it is still possible for the binding of agonist at one site to influence binding at the other site.

The slope of the p_{open} curve for Equation 7.2 is more complex than for a single agonist binding site: Equation 7.4 does not have the same form as the Hill-Langmuir equation, and the Hill plot is not a straight line (as mentioned in Chapter 1, Section 1.2.4). This is because for the two-agonist binding site mechanism the Hill coefficient n depends on the agonist concentration.

$$n = 2\left(\frac{1+[A]/K_1}{1+2[A]/K_1}\right) \tag{7.5}$$

When $[A] \ll K_1$, then $n = 2$, but falls to $n = 1$ when $[A] \gg K_1$. In a study of AChR activation at the frog endplate, estimates made were of $EC_{50} = 15\ \mu M$, $K_1 = K_2 = 77\ \mu M$, and $n = 1.6$ at the EC_{50} concentration.

An approximation to the Hill plot is often used with agonist-response data for ligand-gated ion channels to suggest a lower limit for the number of agonist binding sites on the receptor. It turns out that for many (but not all) mechanisms, if $[A] \ll K_A$, then the slope of a plot of log(response) vs. log[A] approaches the number of agonist-binding reactions required for receptor activation. Figure 7.1 illustrates this using data recorded from a *Xenopus* oocyte expressing embryonic mouse muscle AChR receptors. In this example, the response being

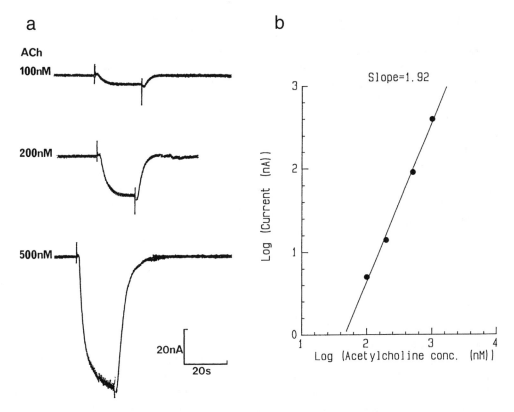

FIGURE 7.1 Macroscopic AChR responses and the Hill slope for AChR activation. (a) Current through AChR ion channels in response to increasing concentrations of ACh was recorded from a *Xenopus* oocyte which has been injected 3 days previously with cRNA [kindly supplied by Professor S.F. Heinemann, Salk Institute] for the α, β, γ, and δ subunits of the mouse muscle AChR. An inward current through the AChR ion channels is shown as a downward deflection of the trace. Small artifacts on the trace indicate the time when the solution flowing into the bath was changed from control to the indicated ACh concentrations, and then back to control. Currents were recorded with a two-microelectrode voltage clamp. The membrane potential was –60 mV and the recordings were made at room temperature. (b) The response (in nA) to increasing concentrations of ACh is plotted against ACh concentration (in nM) on log-log scales. The slope of the line (1.92) is an approximation to the Hill coefficient (when receptor occupancy is small) and suggests that two agonist molecules must bind to the receptor to produce efficient receptor activation.

measured is the summed current flowing through many thousands of open receptor channels in the oocyte membrane. At these low agonist concentrations ($[A] \ll K_A$), the slope of the plot (in this case, 1.92) suggests that the binding of two ACh molecules is necessary for receptor activation, and this correlates well with the known subunit stoichiometry of muscle AChRs of $\alpha_2 \beta\gamma\delta$ where the ACh binding sites are known to be formed mainly by the α-subunits.

7.2.4 HILL COEFFICIENT FOR HOMOMERIC RECEPTOR CHANNELS

Several functional receptors have been described in expression systems where the receptor is expressed from a single receptor subunit. Receptor subunits which form functional homomeric channels include the neuronal nicotinic $\alpha 7$ receptor, the $5HT_3$ receptor, some non-NMDA receptor subunits, NMDA receptors formed from the NR1 subunit, glycine receptor, and the P_{2X} ATP receptor. Based on analogy with the known structure of Torpedo AChRs, it is assumed that these functional receptors have a pentameric structure of five subunits surrounding a central ion channel pore. Such a structure suggests that there will be five agonist-binding sites on the receptor. What then, should we expect the Hill coefficient to be for these receptors? Hill coefficients for these receptors are generally found to be in the range from 1 to 3. Such measurements are complicated by receptor desensitization (see below). However, these results can be interpreted as indicating that in situations where there are five agonist binding sites on the receptor, perhaps only any two need be occupied for full receptor activation.

7.2.5 Receptor Desensitization

Desensitization can be defined as the tendency of a response to wane, despite the presence of a stimulus of constant intensity (e.g., constant agonist concentration). In the case of the nicotinic ACh receptor there is good evidence that desensitization results from a change in receptor conformation to an inactive refractory state. To describe this in terms of the AChR activation mechanism we could add a desensitized state to the scheme shown in Equation 7.2 to give

$$A + R \underset{k_{-1}}{\overset{2k_{+1}}{\rightleftharpoons}} AR + A \underset{2k_{-2}}{\overset{k_{+2}}{\rightleftharpoons}} A_2R \underset{\alpha}{\overset{\beta}{\rightleftharpoons}} A_2R^* \underset{2k_{-D}}{\overset{k_{+D}}{\rightleftharpoons}} A_2R_D \quad (7.6)$$

Here k_{+D} and k_{-D} are the rate constants for entry into and exit from the desensitized state A_2R_D. Investigation of the applicability to AChR desensitization of a range of mechanisms like the linear scheme in Equation 7.6 provided good evidence that linear schemes could not adequately account for AChR desensitization. In particular, it was noted that onset was often slower than offset of desensitization at agonist concentrations producing around 50% steady-state desensitization, and while the rate of onset was dependent on the nature of the agonist, offset was independent of the agonist. These results are not expected from linear schemes like Equation 7.6. It was concluded that a cyclic scheme such as the following was necessary:

$$\begin{array}{ccc} A + R & \overset{K_A}{\rightleftharpoons} & AR & \overset{\beta}{\rightleftharpoons} & A_2R^* \\ K_D' \updownarrow & & \updownarrow K_D & \\ A + R_D & \underset{K_A'}{\rightleftharpoons} & AR_D & \end{array} \quad (7.7)$$

Here the equilibrium constants for each reaction are given and only a single agonist binding step is shown for simplicity.

The desensitized state of the receptor has very high affinity for the agonist ($K_A' \ll K_A$) and receptors are more likely to desensitize when occupied by agonist ($K_D \ll K_D'$). These observations have important consequences for radioligand binding studies utilizing ligand-gated ion channel receptor agonists. Generally, because desensitization is fast relative to the time scale of a binding experiment, what is measured will be dominated by the equilibrium constant for binding of the agonist to the desensitized state of the receptor, and this may be of higher affinity by several orders of magnitude than the affinity of the agonist for the resting, nondesensitized receptor. This is simply another case of the results developed in Chapter 1, showing that, in general, the *apparent* affinity of agonists estimated by methods such as radioligand binding will be a function of all the equilibrium constants in a reaction mechanism.

Desensitization is probably a quite general receptor phenomenon although it varies widely in extent and rate of onset and offset. The scale and time course of AChR desensitization is illustrated in Figure 7.2, which shows responses to increasing concentrations of ACh of a patch

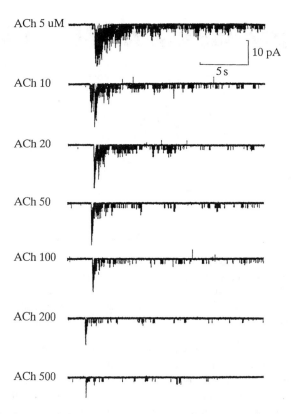

FIGURE 7.2 Activation of single AChR channels in an outside-out membrane patch. Responses to increasing concentrations of ACh of a membrane patch containing several AChRs. A small artifact near the beginning of each trace indicates the time when the solution flowing into the recording chamber was changed to the solution containing the indicated concentration of ACh. With increasing ACh concentration, it can be seen that the channels are activated more rapidly and that receptor desensitization becomes increasingly more rapid such that the peak response is reduced at the higher ACh concentrations. Once the response to agonist has reached a steady state, probably more than 90% of the receptors in the patch are desensitized. It is then possible to see individual "clusters" of channel openings which reflect periods when single AChRs briefly exit from a desensitized state and undergo repeated activation by the agonist ACh, before reentering the desensitized state again. Identification of these clusters provides a means of directly observing and measuring the p_{open} for the receptor at high agonist concentrations, as illustrated in Figure 7.3.

of cell membrane containing several AChRs. Two things are obvious: firstly, during each ACh application the response rises rapidly to a peak and then wanes to a level where the trace can be seen stepping between single-channel current levels. Secondly, it can be seen that with increasing ACh concentration, the peak response does not simply become greater. Instead, it first increases and then decreases due to the increasing rate of onset of desensitization.

7.2.6 DETERMINATION OF THE P_{OPEN} CURVE

Due to the occurrence of desensitization, the shape of the full relationship between agonist concentration and response cannot be determined from experiments like those illustrated in Figure 7.1. In practice, the most accurately determined part of the macroscopic dose-response curve is at the low concentration limit where the effects of desensitization on the dose-response curve are small.

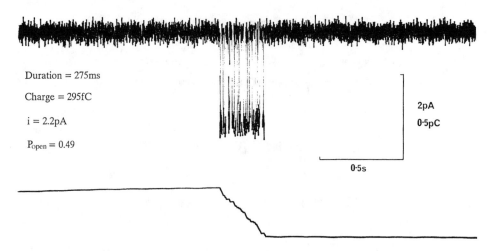

FIGURE 7.3 Measurement of receptor p_{open} during clusters of AChR channel openings in an outside-out patch expressing mouse muscle AChR as described for Figure 7.1. The upper trace shows a single cluster of AChR channel openings activated by 10 μM ACh. The lower trace shows a trace of the output from an analogue integrator circuit. The duration of the cluster is 275 ms and the charge passed was 295 fC. The average single-channel current was 2.2 pA, giving a p_{open} for this cluster of 0.49.

Single-channel recording provides a way around the problem of desensitization because periods when all the receptors in the membrane patch are desensitized are obvious as long stretches of recording where no channel openings occur. Desensitization has therefore been used to provide a means of obtaining groups of successive openings, all due to the activity of a single AChR, referred to as "clusters". The desensitized periods are simply discarded and the channel p_{open} measured during the clusters of activity between desensitized periods.

In each trace in Figure 7.2, after several seconds of exposure to ACh it becomes possible to identify individual clusters of AChR channel openings. Analysis of these clusters of channel openings, as illustrated in Figure 7.3, allows the relationship between ACh concentration and p_{open} to be determined.

Figure 7.3 shows an example of a cluster of AChR channel openings recorded from an outside-out membrane patch in the presence of 10 μM ACh. In principle, the p_{open} during the cluster is simple to calculate: the fraction of time the channel is open is the total time spent in the open state, divided by the duration of the cluster. However, the limited bandwidth of any recording system means that some short openings will be too short to be measured. Therefore, it is preferable to measure the charge passed during the cluster (since charge is not lost with filtering) and use the accumulated charge (the integral of the current during the cluster) to calculate the p_{open}.

$$p_{open} = \frac{charge\ passed\ during\ cluster\ (pC)}{single\ channel\ current\ (pA)\ \times\ cluster\ duration\ (s)} \qquad (7.8)$$

Using the method of integrating the charge passed during each cluster of channel activity, it is possible to determine accurately the p_{open} curve at high agonist concentrations. However, notice that this method depends on identification of clusters of channel openings where each cluster can be assigned as resulting unambiguously from the activity of a single receptor channel: at low p_{open} it is possible for two channels to be active during a cluster without giving any clear indication of double openings, but giving about double the true p_{open} for a single receptor. Therefore, the lower part of the p_{open} curve cannot be determined in this type of experiment. Ideally, the whole p_{open} curve should be determined from experiments where there is only one receptor present in the patch of membrane being recorded. In practice, this is extremely difficult to achieve because the density of receptors is too high in most cell membranes and there is no way to tell how many receptors are in the patch.

Figure 7.4 shows an example of a cluster of AChR channel openings and the p_{open} curve obtained from the same patch. It was possible to identify clusters clearly when the p_{open} was greater than about 0.4. The results are complicated by the presence of open channel block of the AChR channel by the agonist, ACh (see Section 7.33 and Equation 7.22). This causes the p_{open} to gradually decrease at high agonist concentrations, particularly above 1 mM. The maximum p_{open} for the patch illustrated in Figure 7.4a was 0.83 ± 0.01 ($n = 45$ clusters) and occurred at 200 μM ACh (Figure 7.4b). How should these results be interpreted? The p_{open} curve in Figure 7.4b was fitted with the relationship between p_{open} and ACh concentration predicted for the two-agonist binding site mechanism extended to allow for block of the open ion channel by ACh (Equation 7.34). This fitting allows estimates to be made for each of the equilibrium constants in the reaction mechanism.

a.

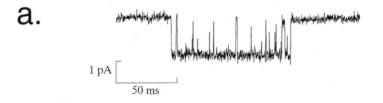

1 pA

50 ms

b.

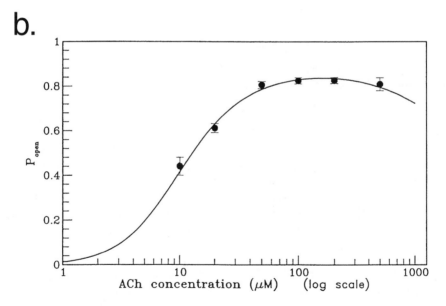

FIGURE 7.4 A p_{open} curve for mouse muscle AChR expressed in *Xenopus* oocytes. In (a) is shown a cluster of AChR channel openings activated in response to 200 μM ACh. The cluster $p_{open} = 0.87$. In (b) the relationship between cluster p_{open} and ACh concentration is shown. The data points show the mean ± SE ($n = 8$ to 82 clusters) at each ACh concentration. The solid line shows the fit of the data to the reaction mechanism given in Equation 7.24 where the agonist can both activate the receptor and block the open ion channel. The equilibrium constants for agonist binding to the two binding sites on the receptor were assumed to be equal (K_A) and were estimated to be 22 μM, the ratio of channel opening to closing rate constants (β/α) was 7.9, and the equilibrium constant for open channel block (K_B) was 4.9 mM. [Adapted from Gibb et al., 1990, *Proc. R. Soc.*, 242, 108-112.]

However, there is one difficulty with interpreting the results of fitting the p_{open} curve. The difficulty is that when the maximum p_{open} approaches unity, increasing β/α or decreasing K_A has a very similar effect on the p_{open} curve, both changes simply shifting it to the left. Thus β/α and K_A cannot be estimated independently when the maximum p_{open} is high. One solution to this is to estimate β/α separately and then fix this value when fitting the p_{open} curve to estimate K_A. Fortunately, estimates of β and α can be obtained from the analysis of bursts of single channel openings recorded at low agonist concentrations, as detailed below.

7.2.7 ANALYSIS OF SINGLE-CHANNEL RECORDINGS

Development of the single-channel recording technique was an enormous advance for studies of ion channel function. For the first time it became possible to ask detailed questions about the mechanism of activation and block of the ligand-gated ion channel receptors. It became possible to measure directly the duration of ion channel openings and closings and so avoid some of the most limiting assumptions which had been necessary when interpreting macroscopic current records. An interesting point is that although single-channel recordings are generally made at equilibrium, it is possible to obtain detailed information about the rates of channel opening and closing. This is because, in a sense, any single molecule is never at equilibrium but spends randomly distributed times in different conformational states. The mean length of time spent in individual states is dependent on the sum of the rates of all possible routes for leaving that state, and so measurement of channel open times and closed times provides information about the rate constants for transitions in a reaction mechanism. A complete description of the interpretation of single-channel data is beyond the scope of this chapter (See the Further Reading section).

7.2.8 ANALYSIS OF BURSTS OF ION CHANNEL OPENINGS

Equation 7.2 predicts that channel openings will occur in groups or *bursts*. Bursts of openings occur because each time the receptor reaches state A_2R, the channel may either open or an agonist molecule can dissociate from the receptor. When the agonist dissociation rate k_{-2} is similar to the channel opening rate β, the channel may open and close several times before agonist dissociation occurs, generating a burst of openings. The burst of openings and closings is also referred to as an *activation*, which can be defined as everything that occurs from the first opening following agonist binding until the end of the last opening before all agonist molecules dissociate from the receptor (obviously, occasions where the agonist binds and then dissociates without opening a channel are invisible). It is predicted that ligand-gated ion channel receptor activation would result in bursts of channel openings given what was known about fast synaptic transmission, and this idea has been used to interpret data from single-channel recordings of AChR channel openings.

From Equation 7.2 the mean open time is predicted to be the reciprocal of the rate constant for channel closing ($\tau_{open} = 1/\alpha$). For bursts recorded at very low agonist concentrations, the mean closed time within bursts, $\tau_g = 1/(\beta + 2k_{-2})$ and the mean number of gaps per burst, $N_g = \beta/2k_{-2}$. Using these two simultaneous equations it is then possible to calculate β and k_{-2}.

From recordings of bursts of mouse AChR channel openings at low concentrations of ACh (less than 1 μM) the duration of openings and closings and the number of closings per burst was measured. On average $\tau_{open} = 3.0$ ms, $\tau_g = 94$ μsec, and $N_g = 0.86$, giving $\alpha = 333$ s^{-1}, $\beta = 4919$ s^{-1}, and $k_{-2} = 2860$ s^{-1}. If we assume $k_{+2} = 2 \times 10^8$ M^{-1}s^{-1} then $K_A = 14$ μM. Thus $\beta/\alpha = 15$ and the maximum $p_{open} = \beta/(\alpha+\beta) = 0.94$. These values are consistent with those obtained from fitting the p_{open} curve in Figure 7.4. The ratio $\beta/(\alpha + \beta)$ indicates that ACh very efficiently activates the channel while the large value for β indicates that a high [ACh] will very rapidly (within a few hundred microseconds) activate the channel, as is observed during neuromuscular transmission.

7.3 ANTAGONISM OF ION CHANNEL RECEPTORS

The use of the Schild method for estimation of the dissociation equilibrium constant of a competitive antagonist is described in detail in Chapter 1. The great advantage of the Schild method lies in the fact that it is a null method: agonist <u>occupancy</u> in the absence or presence of antagonist is assumed to be equal when <u>responses</u> in the absence or presence of the antagonist are equal. Even when the relationship between occupancy and response is complex, the Schild method has been found to work well.

7.3.1 COMPETITIVE ANTAGONISM AND THE SCHILD EQUATION

Using the procedures outlined in Chapter 1, it is straightforward to show that the Schild equation is also obtained for competitive antagonism of ion channel receptors if there is a single agonist binding site. However, where there are two agonist binding sites to consider the situation is more complicated, as several new questions about the mechanism must be answered:

- Is the antagonist affinity for both binding sites equal? It is quite possible that even if the agonist has the same affinity for both sites, an antagonist will not.
- Can two antagonist molecules occupy the receptor at the same time?
- Does binding of the antagonist at one site influence the affinity of the other site for either agonist or antagonist?

The situation can be simplified by assuming the

- Agonist affinity at each site is the same.
- Antagonist affinity at each site is the same.
- Occupancy of one site by either agonist or antagonist does not influence the affinity of the second site for either agonist or antagonist.

Even with these simplifying assumptions, a mechanism to describe the simultaneous action of both agonist and antagonist at a two-binding-site receptor is complex:

$$
\begin{array}{ccccccc}
B + R + A & \underset{k_{-A}}{\overset{2k_{+A}}{\rightleftharpoons}} & B + AR + A & \underset{2k_{-A}}{\overset{k_{+A}}{\rightleftharpoons}} & A_2R & \underset{\alpha}{\overset{\beta}{\rightleftharpoons}} & A_2R^* \\
& k_{-B} \updownarrow 2k_{+B} & & k_{-B} \updownarrow k_{+B} & & & \\
B_2R \underset{k_{+B}}{\overset{2k_{-B}}{\rightleftharpoons}} B + BR + A & & \underset{k_{-A}}{\overset{k_{+A}}{\rightleftharpoons}} & BRA & & & (7.9)
\end{array}
$$

An expression for the equilibrium occupancy of $p_{A_2R^*}$ can again be obtained using the methods outlined in Chapter 1. A potential complication is that this mechanism contains a cycle and so the product of the reaction rates in both clockwise and anticlockwise directions should be equal in order to ensure that the principle of microscopic reversibility is maintained. In this case, microscopic reversibility is maintained. Thus:

$$
2k_{+A} \cdot k_{+B} \cdot k_{-A} \cdot k_{-B} = 2k_{+B} \cdot k_{+A} \cdot k_{-B} \cdot k_{-A} \qquad (7.10)
$$

In the presence of both agonist A, and antagonist B, p_{A_2R*} depends on both the agonist and antagonist concentration in quite a complicated fashion. However, the relationship is essentially an extension to Equation 7.3 and is arrived at as follows:

$$p_{B_2R} + p_{BR} + p_{BRA} + p_R + p_{AR} + p_{A_2R} + p_{A_2R*} = 1 \qquad (7.11)$$

1. The proportions of all forms of the receptor must add up to one.
2. When the system is at equilibrium, each individual reaction step in Equation 7.9 can be used to write down expressions for each form of the receptor in terms of the active form of the receptor, A_2R^*.

$$p_{A_2R} = \frac{1}{E} p_{A_2R*}, \quad p_{AR} = \frac{2K_A}{[A]E} p_{A_2R*}, \quad p_R = \frac{K_A^2}{[A]^2 E} p_{A_2R*} \qquad (7.12)$$

$$p_{BAR} = \frac{2[B]K_A}{K_B[A]E} p_{A_2R*}, \quad p_{BR} = \frac{[B]K_A^2}{2K_B[A]^2 E} p_{A_2R*}, \quad p_{B_2R} = \frac{[B]^2 K_A^2}{K_B^2[A]^2 E} p_{A_2R*} \qquad (7.13)$$

The relationship between p_{A_2R*} and both agonist and antagonist concentration can then be written as:

$$p_{A_2R*} = \frac{[A]}{[A] + \dfrac{1}{E}\left\{[A] + K_A\left[2 + \dfrac{2[B]}{K_B} + \dfrac{K_A}{[A]}\left(1 + \dfrac{[B]}{K_B}\right)^2\right]\right\}} \qquad (7.14)$$

It is clear from comparison of Equation 7.14 with Equation 7.3, reproduced below as Equation 7.15 with $K_A = K_1 = K_2$

$$p_{A_2R*} = \frac{[A]}{[A] + \dfrac{1}{E}\left\{[A] + K_A\left(2 + \dfrac{K_A}{[A]}\right)\right\}} \qquad (7.15)$$

that there is now no simple expression relating dose ratio to antagonist concentration. After equating occupancies in the absence and presence of the blocker and multiplying the agonist concentration in Equation 7.14 by the dose ratio, then r can be found from the expression

$$\left(2 + \frac{K_A}{[A]}\right) = \frac{1}{r}\left[2 + \frac{2[B]}{K_B} + \frac{K_A}{r[A]}\left(1 + \frac{[B]}{K_B}\right)^2\right] \qquad (7.16)$$

This expression can be rearranged to give a quadratic equation in r

$$\frac{2[A]}{K_A} + 1 = \frac{1}{r}\left(\frac{2[A]}{K_A} + \frac{2[A][B]}{K_A K_B}\right) + \frac{1}{r^2}\left(1 + \frac{[B]}{K_B}\right)^2 \qquad (7.17)$$

and this can be rearranged to have the standard form

$$r^2(a) + r(b) + (c) = 0 \tag{7.18}$$

whose two solutions are found from the equation

$$r_1, r_2 = \frac{-b \pm \sqrt{b^2 - 4ac}}{2a} \tag{7.19}$$

One solution is negative and the other is (perhaps surprisingly!) the familiar Schild equation.

$$r = \frac{[B]}{K_B} + 1 \tag{7.20}$$

More directly, it may be seen by inspection of Equations 7.14 and 7.15 that

$$\left(2 + \frac{K_A}{[A]}\right) = 2\left(\frac{1 + [B]/K_B}{r}\right) + \frac{K_A}{[A]}\left(\frac{1 + [B]/K_B}{r}\right)^2 \tag{7.21}$$

and so for the right and left sides of this equation to be equal

$$\frac{1 + [B]/K_B}{r} = 1 \tag{7.22}$$

and so the Schild Equation applies.

Thus, if we assume that the two binding sites are identical and independent then the Schild equation holds for the two-binding-site mechanism. If however, the antagonist binds with different affinity to each site then the dose ratio becomes a complex function of both agonist and antagonist concentrations and equilibrium constants. It is therefore not surprising that a parallel shift of the p_{open} curve with increasing concentration of antagonist is predicted not to be observed when the binding sites are different and so the dose ratio will depend on the response level at which it is measured. However, some simplifying assumptions can still be made. If the p_{open} is small ($[A] \ll K_A$), then an approximately parallel shift of the dose-response curve occurs and the dose ratio is

$$r \approx \sqrt{\left(1 + \frac{[B]}{K_{B1}}\right)\left(1 + \frac{[B]}{K_{B2}}\right)} \tag{7.23}$$

Here K_{B1} and K_{B2} are the equilibrium constants for the blocker at the two sites. In this situation the Schild plot is not linear: it has a slope of less than unity at antagonist concentrations around K_B (where $K_B = (K_{B1}K_{B2})^{1/2}$) and tends to unity at high or at low antagonist concentrations.

An example of the use of the Schild plot in examining the action of the antagonist tubocurarine on AChRs at the frog neuromuscular junction is shown in Figure 7.5. This figure illustrates an experiment where the net inward current measured in response to different concentrations of carbachol is plotted first in the absence (control) and then in the presence of increasing concentrations of tubocurarine. Recordings were made at two different

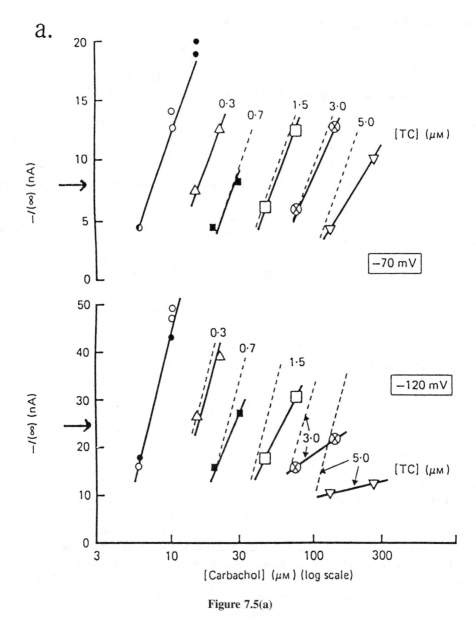

Figure 7.5(a)

membrane potentials and then the Schild plot for each membrane potential was constructed. The results illustrate that at −70 mV the Schild plot is linear and has a slope close to unity, suggesting competitive antagonism (without any distinction between binding sites for the antagonist). However, at a membrane potential of −120 mV the Schild plot is nonlinear and has a slope steeper than unity. This occurs because tubocurarine also blocks the open ion channel of the endplate AChR and when the membrane potential is made more negative, the positively charged tubocurarine molecule is attracted into the ion channel, resulting in a noncompetitive block of the receptor as discussed in the next section.

7.3.2 Ion Channel Block

The ion channel blocking mechanism has been widely tested and found to be important in both pharmacology and physiology. Examples are the block of nerve and cardiac sodium channels by local anesthetics, or block of NMDA receptor channels by Mg^{2+} and the anesthetic ketamine.

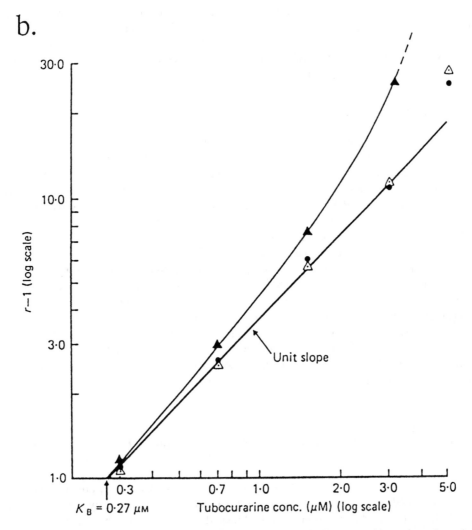

FIGURE 7.5 Use of the Schild method for estimation of the K_B of a competitive antagonist acting at a ligand-gated ion channel receptor. In (a) is shown log concentration-response curves for the equilibrium net inward current ($-I_{(\infty)}$) evoked by carbachol in the presence of increasing concentrations of tubocurarine (TC) at a membrane potential of -70 mV (upper panel) and at a membrane potential of -120 mV (lower panel). It can be seen that, except for the highest concentration of tubocurarine (5 μM), at -70 mV this antagonist produces an approximately parallel shift of the carbachol dose-response curve, as expected for competitive antagonism. However, in the same experiment at a membrane potential of -120 mV, the shift of the dose-response curves is far from parallel. This is because the positively charged tubocurarine molecule is being attracted into the AChR channel when the inside of the cell is made more negative. The dashed lines in the upper and lower panels show the responses predicted for pure competitive antagonism with $K_B = 0.27$ μM. Dose ratios were calculated at a response level of -8 nA at -70 mV and -24 nA at -120 mV. In (b) is shown the Schild plot of $\log(r-1)$ against log (tubocurarine concentration). The filled circles show equilibrium dose ratios at -70 mV, filled triangles show equilibrium dose ratios at -120 mV, and open triangles show the peak response at -120 mV. Because open channel block by tubocurarine is relatively slow to develop, when the peak response is measured mainly competitive antagonism is seen and the Schild slope is close to unity. The fact that both curves coincide at low antagonist concentrations (small dose ratios) suggests that the K_B for competitive binding to the receptor is independent of the membrane potential, as might be expected if the agonist binding site is outside the membrane potential field. (Adapted from Colquhoun, D., Dryer, F. and Sheridan, R.E., *J. Physiol.*, 293, 247-284, 1979. With permission.)

The channel block mechanism was first used quantitatively to describe block of the squid axon K^+ current by tetraethylammonium ions (TEA). The effects of channel blockers on synaptic potentials and synaptic currents were investigated, particularly at the neuromuscular junction, and the development of the single-channel recording technique allowed channel blockages to be observed directly for the first time.

7.3.3 A Mechanism for Channel Block

The idea that drugs could act by directly blocking the flow of ions through ion channels probably started, like any hypothesis, as some sort of abstract idea without any physical basis. It is easy to draw a cartoon with something like the plug in a sink, blocking the flow of water down the drainhole (ion channel). However, pharmacologists worth their salt would (hopefully!) want to convert the cartoon into a mechanism that is both physically plausible (i.e., does not contravene any of the accepted laws of physics) and provides quantitative predictions which can be tested experimentally.

Ideally, the aim would be to estimate the association and dissociation rate constants for each drug. This would then give the dissociation equilibrium constant (K_B) for drug binding. Just as in the use of the Schild method to quantify competitive antagonism, a quantitative estimate of the K_B for channel block allows comparison of different drugs and a pharmacological classification of the ion channels they bind to.

In other words, we could say that when an ion channel is open, the drug binding site is exposed. If a drug binds to that site, flow of ions through the channel is blocked. We might further suppose that the drug has to unblock before the channel can close normally. A standard mechanism used to describe channel block of ligand-gated ion channel receptors is then:

$$A + R \underset{k_{-1}}{\overset{2k_{+1}}{\rightleftharpoons}} AR + A \underset{2k_{-2}}{\overset{k_{+2}}{\rightleftharpoons}} A_2R \underset{\alpha}{\overset{\beta}{\rightleftharpoons}} A_2R^* + B \underset{k_{-B}}{\overset{[B]k_{+B}}{\rightleftharpoons}} A_2RB \quad (7.24)$$

where β and α are the channel opening and closing rates and k_{+B} and k_{-B} are the microscopic association and dissociation rate constants for blocking the channel by the drug B. Here [B] is indicated on the transition into the blocked state to remind the reader that the rate of this reaction depends on [B]. Notice that this mechanism does not take into account the possibility that a drug could bind to the channel in the closed (occupied or unoccupied) conformation.

With mechanisms like these it is often possible to simplify the analysis of the action of a channel blocker by assuming agonist binding is much faster than channel opening and closing and then combining several closed states together so that the mechanism approximates a three-state system.

$$A_2R \underset{\alpha}{\overset{\beta'}{\rightleftharpoons}} A_2R^* + B \underset{k_{-B}}{\overset{[B]k_{+B}}{\rightleftharpoons}} A_2RB \quad (7.25)$$

Notice that the channel opening rate is now denoted β'.

Since the channel can only open from the A_2R state the effective opening rate β' is obtained by multiplying the real opening rate β by the equilibrium occupancy of A_2R.

$$\beta' = p_{A_2R} \beta \quad (7.26)$$

7.3.4 Macroscopic Kinetics: Relaxations (e.g., Synaptic Currents) and Noise

Changes in the occupancy of the open channel state of the receptor as a function of time ($p_{A_2R^*}(t)$) in response to a perturbation of the receptor equilibrium can be used to obtain information about the rates of channel gating and interaction of drugs with ion channel receptors. The system is said to *relax* towards a new equilibrium. The time course of the *relaxation* is used to measure rates from the average behavior of many ion channels in a recording while *noise analysis* uses the frequency of the moment-to-moment fluctuations in occupancy of the open channel state at equilibrium to provide information about the rates in the receptor mechanism.

For k states, a relaxation (or noise spectrum) will contain k-1 exponential (or Lorentzian) components. Thus, the mechanism in Equation 7.26 above will have two states in the absence of blocker and so give rise to relaxations (or noise spectra) which can be fitted with single exponential (or Lorentzian) functions. Addition of the blocker creates an extra state (the blocked state), giving $k = 3$. For $k = 3$, the occupancy of the open state as a function of time will be described by two exponentials:

$$p_{A_2R^*}(t) = p_{A_2R^*}(\infty) + w_1 \exp\left(-\frac{t}{\tau_1}\right) + w_2 \exp\left(-\frac{t}{\tau_2}\right) \tag{7.27}$$

The reciprocals of the time constants, τ_1 and τ_2 are the rate constants λ_1 and λ_2. The weights of the exponentials (w_1 and w_2) are complicated functions of the transition rates in Equation 7.25. However, the rate constants are eigenvalues found by solving the system of differential equations which describe the above mechanism. Thus, λ_1 and λ_2 are the two solutions of the quadratic equation

$$\lambda^2 + b\lambda + c = 0 \tag{7.28}$$

where

$$-b = \lambda_1 + \lambda_2 = \alpha + \beta' + [B]k_{+B} + k_{-B} \tag{7.29}$$

and

$$c = \lambda_1\lambda_2 = \alpha k_{-B}\left[1 + \frac{\beta'}{\alpha}\left(1 + \frac{[B]}{k_{-B}/k_{+B}}\right)\right] \tag{7.30}$$

Notice that when β' is small (i.e., when the occupancy of A_2R is very small, as it will be if the agonist concentration is low), then

$$\lambda_1 + \lambda_2 = \alpha + [B]k_{+B} + k_{-B} \tag{7.31}$$

and

$$\lambda_1 + \lambda_2 = \alpha k_{-B} \tag{7.32}$$

With the simplifying assumption of a small β', the <u>sum</u> and the <u>product</u> of the rate constants measured in an experiment can be used to calculate k_{-B} and k_{+B} if α is known from experiments in the absence of the blocker. This is simply done by plotting the sum or the product of the measured rate constants against blocker concentration. From Equation 7.32, the product of the rate constants should be independent of blocker concentration with a value equal to αk_{-B} while the sum of the rate constants (Equation 7.31) will give a straight line with slope equal to k_{+B} and intercept of $\alpha + k_{-B}$. If the experimental data is consistent with these predictions, then the data points plotted in this way should lie on a straight line and this is then good evidence that the mechanism of action of the drug is to block the open ion channel.

The assumption that β' is very small has been used when studying the effects of channel blockers on synaptic currents since the transmitter concentration (and hence p_{A_2R}) is probably small during the decay phase of the current. During noise analysis experiments a low agonist concentration is used so that again, under these conditions β' should be small.

7.3.5 CHANNEL BLOCK AT EQUILIBRIUM

The relationship between p_{open} ($p_{control}$) and agonist concentration for the two-agonist-binding site mechanism is given in Equation 7.4 and reproduced below in a slightly different form.

$$p_{control} = \cfrac{1}{1 + \cfrac{1}{E} + \cfrac{2K_2}{[A]E} + \cfrac{K_1K_2}{[A]^2E}} \tag{7.33}$$

$$p_{control} = \cfrac{1}{1 + \cfrac{1}{E} + \cfrac{2K_2}{[A]E} + \cfrac{K_1K_2}{[A]^2E} + \cfrac{[B]}{K_B}} \tag{7.34}$$

Taking the ratio of $p_{control}/p_{blocker}$ gives this simple result

$$\frac{p_{control}}{p_{blocker}} = 1 + \frac{p_{control}}{K_B} \cdot [B] \tag{7.35}$$

When an open channel blocker is added, the p_{open} in the presence of the blocker ($p_{blocker}$) given above is a function of both agonist (A) and blocker (B) concentration.

Since the current recorded in a voltage clamp experiment is directly proportional to the channel p_{open}, the ratio of current in the absence of blocker to that in the presence of increasing concentrations of blocker can be used to calculate K_B. The experimental design is to obtain a fairly large response to agonist alone, and then calculate the ratio of this control response to responses to the same concentration of agonist in the presence of increasing concentrations of channel blocker. The ratio $p_{control}/p_{blocker}$ when plotted against [B] will be a straight line which intercepts the y-axis at 1 and has a slope of $p_{control}/K_B$. If $p_{control} = 1$, then the slope = $1/K_B$. If $p_{control}$ is known for a particular agonist concentration then obviously K_B can still be estimated. If we <u>assume</u> $p_{control} = 1$, then the calculated K_B will be greater than the true K_B: for example, by a factor of 2 if $p_{control} = 0.5$, by a factor of 10 if $p_{control} = 0.1$.

7.3.6 SINGLE-CHANNEL ANALYSIS OF CHANNEL BLOCK

Below is an outline of some of the information that can be obtained from single-channel data using fairly simple measurements such as the mean open time and mean shut time.

Open times.

Channel blockers will produce a reduction of the mean open time from

$$\tau_o = \frac{1}{\alpha} \tag{7.36}$$

in control to

$$\tau_o = \frac{1}{\alpha + k_{+B}[B]} \tag{7.37}$$

in the presence of blocker. This is calculated from the rule that the mean lifetime of any state is equal to the reciprocal of the sum of the rates for leaving that state.

Closed times.

Closed periods due to channel blockages have, from the same rule, a mean lifetime of

$$\tau_g = \frac{1}{k_{-B}} \tag{7.38}$$

Blockage frequency.

The frequency of blockages per second of open time is $k_{+B}[B]$, and so the mean <u>number</u> of blockages in each channel opening is simply the blockage frequency multiplied by the mean open time.

$$N_g = \frac{k_{+B}[B]}{\alpha} \tag{7.39}$$

Bursts of openings.

Where the channel blocker converts single openings into obvious bursts (e.g., local anesthetic block of nicotinic channels), the mean number of openings per burst is of course one more than the mean number of gaps (blockages).

$$N_o = 1 + \frac{k_{+B}[B]}{\alpha} \tag{7.40}$$

Notice that the mean total open time per burst will be

$$N_o\tau_o = \left(1 + \frac{k_{+B}}{\alpha}\right)\frac{1}{\alpha + k_{+B}[B]} \tag{7.41}$$

$$N_o\tau_o = \left(\frac{\alpha + k_{+B}[B]}{\alpha}\right)\frac{1}{\alpha + k_{+B}[B]} \tag{7.42}$$

$$N_o\tau_o = \frac{1}{\alpha} \tag{7.43}$$

This is an important result. The simple open channel block mechanism predicts that the total open time per burst is the same as the mean open time in the absence of blocker, even although openings are now chopped up by channel blockages. In fact, for channels which give bursts of openings in control recordings, the total open time per burst is constant in the presence or absence of blocker.

This result is also of importance because it shows that simple open channel blockers do not reduce the charge passed by the channel during each activation and so they will not reduce the charge injected at a synapse by a synaptic current. Instead, what they do is prolong the time over which the charge is injected, which can have quite dramatic effects on synaptic transmission.

$$\tau_b = \frac{1}{\alpha} + N_g \cdot \tau_g \tag{7.44}$$

$$\tau_b = \frac{1}{\alpha} + \frac{1}{k_{-B}} \cdot \frac{k_{+B}[B]}{\alpha} \tag{7.45}$$

$$\tau_b = \frac{1}{\alpha}\left(1 + \frac{[B]}{K_B}\right) \tag{7.46}$$

$$\tau_b = \frac{1}{\alpha} + \frac{1}{\alpha K_B} \cdot [B] \tag{7.47}$$

Burst length:
The mean burst length is found as shown above.

Thus a plot of the mean burst length vs. [B] will give a straight line of intercept $1/\alpha$ and slope $1/(\alpha K_B)$.

7.3.7 THE TIME SCALE OF CHANNEL BLOCK

Channel blockers are often divided into "slow", "intermediate", or "fast" blockers. This classification is based around the very wide range of values which have been found for the microscopic dissociation rate constant of different channel blockers.

Nearly all channel blockers have been found to have microscopic association rate constants (k_{+B}) in the range around 10^7 M^{-1} s^{-1}. In contrast, microscopic dissociation rate constants (k_{-B}) range over several orders of magnitude from around 10^5 s^{-1} (e.g., block of nicotinic receptor channels by ACh) to 0.01 s^{-1} for MK-801 (dizocilpine) block of NMDA channels. The mean lengths of the blockage gaps can therefore range from 10 μsec up to 100 s. It is only when the blockages are in the intermediate range, of the order of 1 ms in duration, that the gaps are easily detected in single-channel recordings. If the blocker is a slow blocker with very long blockage gaps, the data record looks as though the frequency of channel openings has decreased. If the blocker is fast, the single-channel amplitude appears decreased because the blocking and unblocking is too fast to be resolved.

7.3.8 USE DEPENDENCE OF CHANNEL BLOCKERS

It follows from the fact that the blocker is assumed to bind only to the activated state of the channel that the degree of block will be not only concentration dependent but also *use dependent*: in other words, the more the channels are activated, the more they become blocked.

It follows from the above discussion on the time scales of channel block that the degree of use dependence will be critically dependent on the microscopic dissociation rate constant. Slow blockers show extreme use-dependence and this is augmented with blockers which display the "trapping" phenomenon. Trapping occurs when the channel can close, and the agonist dissociates with the blocker still bound in the channel. The blocker is then trapped in the channel until the next time the receptor is activated. Important examples of trapping block are the action of hexamethonium at autonomic ganglia and the block of the NMDA receptor channel by MK801 or the anesthetic ketamine.

7.3.9 Voltage Dependence of Channel Block

One of the interesting results which arose from early voltage clamp experiments with channel blocking drugs is that the potency of the blocker was dependent on the membrane voltage. In contrast, this was found to be not the case for competitive antagonism at endplate nicotinic receptors (Figure 7.5). These results were interpreted as indicating that the acetylcholine binding site on the receptor (and therefore competitive block at that site by tubocurarine) is not influenced by the potential difference across the membrane, whereas if binding is affected by the membrane potential, then the binding site must be at a region of the protein which is part of the way across the electric field of the membrane.

Binding of a charged drug at a site within an electric field will be influenced by both chemical interactions (hydrogen bonding, etc., common to all drug-receptor interactions) and also by the electric field and charge on the drug.

The microscopic rate constants for association and dissociation at a site within an electric field (for block by charged drugs) are exponential functions of the membrane voltage:

$$k_{+B}(V) = k_{+B}(0)\exp\left(\frac{-\delta z F V}{2RT}\right) \tag{7.48}$$

$$k_{-B}(V) = k_{-B}(0)\exp\left(\frac{\delta z F V}{2RT}\right) \tag{7.49}$$

Here δ refers to the fraction of the membrane voltage which the blocking drug senses at the binding site and the sign on the δ is determined by whether the blocking drug approaches the binding site from inside or outside of the membrane. As expressed here, these equations describe the rate constants for block from the outside. The valence of the blocking drug is given as z and F, R, and T are the Faraday constant ($9.65 \times 10^4\,C\,mol^{-1}$), the gas constant ($8.32\,J\,K^{-1}\,mol^{-1}$), and the absolute temperature (293 K at room temperature), respectively. The voltage-dependence of the dissociation equilibrium constant is given by:

$$\frac{k_{-B}(V)}{k_{+B}(V)} = K_B(V) = K_B(0)\exp\left(\frac{\delta z F V}{2RT}\right) \tag{7.50}$$

From this relationship it can be seen that a semilogarithmic plot of $\ln K(V)$ vs. membrane potential will give a straight line with slope of $\delta z F/RT$ and intercept of $\ln K(0)$. The inverse of the slope gives the change in membrane voltage required to give an e-fold change in the equilibrium constant. It can be seen that the maximum slope will be obtained when $\delta = 1$. For a blocker with a single charge this will give a maximum slope of 25 mV for an e-fold change while for a divalent ion the maximum slope will be 13 mV for an e-fold change.

Figure 7.6 shows a diagrammatic representation of the energy barrier which a channel blocking drug might be supposed to overcome to reach its binding site within the channel.

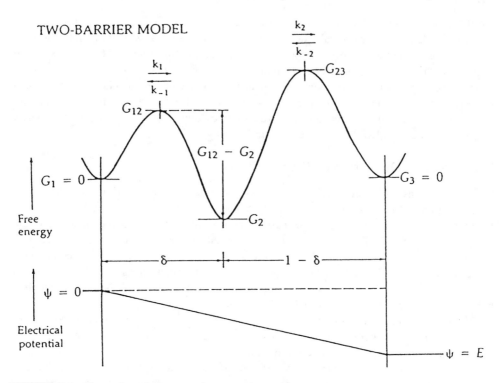

FIGURE 7.6 Shown is a diagrammatic representation of a two-energy barrier model which can be used to describe the energy barriers a channel blocking drug might be supposed to overcome to reach its binding site within the channel. This diagram allows for the possibility that the blocking drug could actually permeate the channel after binding rather that returning to the same side of the membrane it had originally come from. This generalized mechanism can be used to describe channel block from either side of the membrane, access to the binding site being dependent on the height of the energy barriers which the drug has to cross. The free energy G is shown relative to that outside the membrane. The transition rates k_1, k_{-1}, k_2, k_{-2} will depend on both the height of the energy barrier and the membrane potential and can be calculated as described by Hille (Adapted from *Ionic Channels of Excitable Membranes,* Hille, B., Ed., Sinauer Associates, Sunderland, MA, 1992. With permission.)

This diagram allows for the possibility that the blocking drug could actually permeate the channel after binding, rather than returning after dissociation to the same side it had originally come from. This generalized mechanism can be used to describe channel block from either side of the membrane, access to the binding site being dependent on the height of the energy barriers which the drug molecule has to cross. More generally, Figure 7.6 helps to illustrate the idea that the difference between permeation of an ion through the channel and block of the channel may be one of degree, and not necessarily a reflection of any fundamental difference in the way a permeant ion or blocker interacts with the channel protein.

7.4 CONCLUDING REMARKS

The material in this chapter has centered around the effects of drugs at receptors in the ligand-gated ion channel class. In particular, the aim has been to emphasize that a quantitative treatment of some simple mechanisms can allow experimentally testable predictions to be made for the effects of a drug, and estimates of the affinity of a drug for its binding site/sites on the receptor. In as far as quantifying the interactions of drugs with their receptors is at the heart of advances in the development of selective drugs and in the classification of receptors, this approach is likely to continue to be an essential part of pharmacology. This is particularly so for studies in the central nervous system where a bewildering array of receptor subtypes await the development of subtype-selective drugs in order that the functional and therapeutic significance of this receptor diversity can be determined.

7.5 PROBLEMS

Q1. An experiment in which single AChR ion channel currents were recorded at a membrane potential of −60 mV showed that the duration of individual channel openings followed a single exponential distribution. The mean open time was 5.0 ms. When the experiment was repeated in the presence of an antagonist, drug B, in a concentration of 10 μM, it was found that the mean open time was reduced to 2.5 ms, and that the channel openings were interrupted by brief shut periods with a mean duration of 1.0 ms such that openings were grouped into bursts. When the experiment was repeated at a membrane potential of −120 mV the mean open time was 10 ms in the absence of drug B but only 2 ms in its presence; the interruptions of the channel openings had become longer, lasting 2 ms on average at −120 mV.

These results are consistent with drug B being an open channel blocker.

(a) Calculate the microscopic association and dissociation rate constants and equilibrium constant for the action of drug B.

(b) What can you say about the probable site of action of drug B given that the drug has a single positive charge?

Hint: the reciprocal of the mean lifetime of an individual state is the sum of the rates (in s^{-1}) for __leaving__ that state.

Q2. With endplate nicotinic receptors it has been found that as well as activating the receptor, acetylcholine (ACh) blocks the ion channel. A possible mechanism to describe this situation might therefore be

$$
A + R \underset{k_{-1}}{\overset{k_{+1}}{\rightleftharpoons}} \underset{\text{closed}}{AR} \underset{k_{-2}}{\overset{k_{+2}}{\rightleftharpoons}} \underset{\text{open}}{AR^* + A} \underset{k_{-3}}{\overset{k_{+3}}{\rightleftharpoons}} \underset{\text{blocked}}{ARA} \tag{7.51}
$$

(a) Stating any assumptions you need to make, derive an expression for the equilibrium occupancy of the AR^* state (p_{AR^*}) in Equation 7.51.

(b) Write down expressions for the mean open time (τ_o) and mean duration of the blocked state (τ_b).

Hint: the mean lifetime of any state is equal to the reciprocal of the sum of the rates for leaving that state.

In experiments designed to test the mechanism in scheme (1), two high concentrations of ACh (300 μM and 800 μM) were tested in single-channel recording experiments and τ_o, τ_b, and the channel open probability (p_{open}) measured. The results were as follows:

TABLE 7.1

[ACh]	τ_o	τ_b	p_{open}
300 μM	0.2 ms	0.04 ms	0.5
800 μM	0.1 ms	0.04 ms	0.4

(c) Using a plot of $1/\tau_o$ vs. [ACh], calculate k_{-2} and k_{+3}. In addition, calculate k_{-3} from the duration of the blockages (τ_b) and hence calculate the equilibrium constant (K_3) for block of the channel by ACh. In other experiments values of $10^7 \, M^{-1} \, s^{-1}$, $10^4 \, s^{-1}$, and $10^4 \, s^{-1}$ were found for k_{+1}, k_{-1}, and k_{+2}, respectively.

(d) Using the expression you derived in (a), calculate the p_{AR*} you would expect at 300 μM and 800 μM ACh. How does this compare with the experimentally observed p_{open} given in Table 7.1? Suggest reasons why the calculated and observed p_{open} might be different.

Q3. A simple mechanism for competitive antagonism of a ligand-gated ion channel receptor would be as follows:

$$BR \underset{k_{+B}}{\overset{k_{-B}}{\rightleftharpoons}} B + R + A \underset{k_{-A}}{\overset{k_{+A}}{\rightleftharpoons}} AR \qquad (7.52)$$

(a) Derive an expression for the equilibrium occupancy of state AR given the concentration of antagonist [B] and agonist [A] and their microscopic rate constants for association and dissociation with the receptor.

In an experiment designed to measure k_{-B} and k_{+B}, the agonist was applied at a concentration of 100 μM (the equilibrium constant for the agonist is known to be 11 μM). Then, a step change in the antagonist concentration was made from zero to [B] and back to zero again. On application of the antagonist the response was observed to decline (relax) exponentially towards a steady-state level of block with time constant τ_{on}.

If it is assumed that equilibration with the agonist is much faster than equilibration with the antagonist then the relaxation time constants, τ_{on}, can be shown for Equation 7.1 to be described by the equation:

$$\tau_{on} = \frac{1}{p_{free} \, k_{+B}[B] + k_{-B}} \qquad (7.53)$$

where p_{free} is the fraction of receptors in state R before the antagonist is applied.

The antagonist was tested at three concentrations and the results were as follows:

TABLE 7.2

[B]	τ_{on}	Block at equilibrium
7.5 μM	0.4 s	62%
20 μM	0.2 s	83%
45 μM	0.1 s	95%

(b) Calculate the microscopic rate constants k_{+B} and k_{-B} and hence the equilibrium constant K_B. Using these and the equation you derived in part (a), calculate the percentage block (decrease in p_{AR}) expected at equilibrium for each of the antagonist concentrations used. How well do these calculated values agree with those observed experimentally?

Suggest possible reasons why the calculated equilibrium block might not agree with that observed experimentally. Describe what a single-channel recording of the receptor activity would look like at equilibrium in the presence of the agonist alone and in the presence of agonist plus antagonist.

7.6 FURTHER READING

Textbooks with relevant material

Sakmann, B. and Neher, E. (1995), *Single Channel Recording,* 2nd ed., Plenum Press, New York. (Many good articles that discuss methods and principles.)

Hille, B. (1992), *Ionic Channels of Excitable Membranes,* 2nd ed., Sinauer Associates, Sunderland, MA. (Chapter 7: Endplate Channels and Kinetics. Chapter 15: Channel Block Mechanisms.)

Ogden, D.C. (1994), Microelectrode techniques. *The Plymouth Workshop Handbook,* 2nd ed., Company of Biologists Ltd., Cambridge, U.K. (Excellent discussion of both methods and principles.)

References

Ascher, P. and Nowak, L. (1988), The role of divalent cations in the *N*-methyl-D-aspartate responses of mouse central neurones in culture, *J. Physiol.,* 399, 247-266.

Colquhoun, D. (1986), On the principles of postsynaptic action of neuromuscular blocking agents, in *New Neuromuscular Blocking Agents,* Kharkevich, D.A., Ed., Springer-Verlag, New York; *Handbuch Exp. Pharm.,* Vol. 79.

Colquhoun, D., Dreyer, F. and Sheridan, R.E. (1979), The actions of tubocurarine at the frog neuromuscular junction, *J. Physiol.,* 293, 247-284. (Endplate currents, voltage-jumps, and noise analysis of tubocurarine block: a slowly dissociating blocker.)

Colquhoun, D. and Ogden, D.C. (1988), Activation of ion channels in the frog end-plate by high concentrations of acetylcholine, *J. Physiol.,* 395, 131-159.

Colquhoun, D. and Sakmann (1981), Fluctuations in the microsecond time range of the current through single acetylcholine receptor ion channels, *Nature,* 294, 464-466. (The full version of this paper is in *J. Physiol.,* 369, 501-557, 1985.)

del Castillo, J. and Katz, B. (1957), Interaction at endplate receptors between different choline derivatives, *Proc. R. Soc. London B,* 146, 369-381.

Edmonds, B., Gibb, A.J. and Colquhoun, D. (1995), Mechanisms of activation of muscle nicotinic acetylcholine receptors and the time course of endplate currents, *Annu. Rev. Physiol.,* 57, 469-493.

Katz, B. and Thesleff, S. (1957), A study of the 'desensitization' produced by acetylcholine at the motor end-plate, *J. Physiol.,* 138, 63-80.

Lingle, C.L., Maconochie, D. and Steinbach, J.H. (1992), Activation of skeletal muscle nicotinic acetylcholine receptors, *J. Membr. Biol.,* 126, 195-217. (Excellent review of much of the evidence concerning the mechanism of receptor activation.)

MacDonald, J.F. and Nowak, L.M. (1990), Mechanisms of blockade of excitatory amino acid receptor channels, *TIPS,* 11(4), 167-172.

Neher, E. (1983), The charge carried by single-channel currents of rat cultured muscle cells in the presence of local anaesthetics, *J. Physiol.,* 339, 663-678. (Deviations from simple channel blocking mechanism.)

Rang, H.P. and Ritter, J.M. (1970), On the mechanism of desensitization at cholinergic receptors, *Mol. Pharmacol.,* 6, 357-382.

Triggle, D.J. (1980), Desensitization, *Trends Pharmacol. Sci.,* 14, 395-398.

Unwin, N. (1993), Neurotransmitter action: opening of ligand-gated ion channels, *Neuron,* 10 (Suppl. 1), 31-41.

7.7 SOLUTIONS TO PROBLEMS

PROBLEM 7.1

Notice that the question states that the distribution of open times is a single exponential. This implies that a mechanism containing a single open state of the receptor can describe the data. Using the above hint, the channel closing rate (call this α) is therefore the reciprocal of the mean open time. Thus at -60 mV $\alpha = 1/5$ ms or 200 s^{-1} and at -120 mV $\alpha = 1/10$ ms or 100 s^{-1}. This indicates that the channel closing conformational change is affected by the electric field across the membrane.

In the presence of drug B, the mean duration of the blockages (assuming a single blocked state) will be the reciprocal of the rate for leaving the blocked state (k_{-B} say). Thus at -60 mV $k_{-B} = 1/1.0$ ms or 1000 s^{-1} and at -120 mV $k_{-B} = 1/2.0$ ms or 500 s^{-1}. Apparently the rate of dissociation of drug B from the channel is slowed when the membrane potential is made more negative. For a positively charged drug this is a common finding and suggests the drug is binding within the membrane electric field. However, it could also be that the change in membrane potential has altered the receptor protein conformation and so affected the binding of the drug to the receptor.

To calculate the microscopic association rate for drug B, use the hint above to show that the mean open time in the presence of drug B will be equal to $1/(\alpha + [B]k_{+B})$. Thus the reciprocal of the mean open time in the presence of drug B will be equal to $(\alpha + [B]k_{+B})$ and so $(\alpha + [B]k_{+B}) = 400$s^{-1} at -60 mV and 500s^{-1} at -120 mV; α was 200 s^{-1} at -60 mV and 100 s^{-1} at -120 mV so $[B]k_{+B} = 200$ s^{-1} at -60 mV and 400 s^{-1} at -120 mV. Dividing these numbers by the [B] gives $k_{+B} = 2 \times 10^7$ M^{-1} s^{-1} at -60 mV and 4×10^7 M^{-1} s^{-1} at -120 mV. The equilibrium constant is therefore 50 μM at -60 mV and 12.5 μM at -120 mV.

If the voltage dependence of k_{+B} is described by Equation 7.48 then a plot of $\ln(k_{+B}(V))$ vs. membrane potential (V) will be a straight line of slope $-\delta zF/2RT$. In this case, the slope of this plot is -11.6 and the reciprocal of this indicates an e-fold increase in k_{+B} for every 0.086 V hyperpolarization (86 mV) of the membrane potential. At room temperature (293 K) F/RT = 39.6, so for a drug with a single positive charge $\delta = 11.6/19.8 = 0.59$, suggesting that when at its binding site the drug has passed through 59% of the membrane electric field (note that this is probably not the same as 59% of the distance across the membrane since the membrane electric field is unlikely to fall linearly across the channel protein).

Notice that the slope of the relationship between membrane potential and $\ln(k_{-B})$ is equal in magnitude but opposite in sign to that for k_{+B}, as expected if the blocker traverses the same path when exiting from the channel as when blocking the channel. A shallow voltage dependence for the unblocking rate could suggest that unblocking occurred by permeation of the blocker to the other side of the channel.

PROBLEM 7.2

(a) Assume: the system is at equilibrium, and the Law of Mass Action holds. Use the procedures described in Chapter 1 to derive an expression for p_{AR*} at equilibrium. At equilibrium, the forward and backward rates for each reaction in the mechanism must be equal. The forward and backward rates are defined using the Law of Mass Action.

$$p_R[A]k_{+1} = p_{AR}k_{-1}, \quad p_{AR}k_{+2} = p_{AR*}k_{-2}, \quad p_{AR*}[A]k_{+3} = p_{ARA}k_{-3} \tag{7.54}$$

Each expression is rearranged to give an expression in p_{AR*}

$$p_{AR} = \frac{k_{-2}}{k_{+2}} p_{AR*}, \quad p_R = \frac{k_{-1}k_{-2}}{k_{+1}[A]k_{+2}} p_{AR*}, \quad p_{ARA} = \frac{k_{+3}[A]}{k_{-3}} p_{AR*} \tag{7.55}$$

The proportions of the receptor in each state must add up to 1.

$$p_R + p_{AR} + p_{AR*} + p_{ARA} = 1 \tag{7.56}$$

Substituting into this equation and then rearranging the result gives the desired expression.

$$p_{AR*} = \frac{[A]}{\dfrac{k_{-1}k_{-2}}{k_{+1}k_{+2}} + [A]\left(1 + \dfrac{k_{-2}}{k_{+2}} + \dfrac{[A]k_{+3}}{k_{-3}}\right)} \tag{7.57}$$

(b) Expressions for the mean open time and mean duration of the blockages are:

$$\tau_o = \frac{1}{k_{-2} + [A]k_{+3}}, \quad \tau_b = \frac{1}{k_{-3}} \tag{7.58}$$

(c) $1/\tau_o = 5000 \text{ s}^{-1}$ when $[ACh] = 300 \text{ }\mu M$, and $1/\tau_o = 10{,}000 \text{ s}^{-1}$ when $[ACh] = 800 \text{ }\mu M$. From the answer to (b) we know that $1/\tau_o = (k_{-2} + [A]k_{+3})$. This has the form of a straight line of slope k_{+3} and intercept k_{-2} when $1/\tau_o$ is plotted against $[A]$. Thus, $k_{+3} = $ slope $= (10{,}000 - 5000 \text{ s}^{-1})/(800 - 300 \text{ }\mu M) = 10^7 \text{ M}^{-1}\text{s}^{-1}$. The intercept $= k_{-2} = 2000 \text{ s}^{-1}$. The dissociation rate for the blocker, $k_{-3} = 1/40 \text{ }\mu\text{sec} = 25{,}000 \text{ s}^{-1}$. The equilibrium constant for block of the channel is therefore $K_3 = k_{-3}/k_{+3} = 2.5 \text{ mM}$.

(d) Substituting into Equation 7.57 allows the equilibrium occupancy of AR^* to be calculated at 300 and 800 μM ACh. The results are 0.503 and 0.565, respectively. Therefore at 300 μM, the calculated p_{AR*} is close to that observed experimentally. However at 800 μM, the calculated p_{AR*} is higher than observed. Reasons: possibly desensitization is affecting the p_{open} at higher $[A]$. In addition, the mechanism used to derive Equation 7.57 may not be correct (as would be the case if a desensitized state must be added to the mechanism).

PROBLEM 7.3

(a) The derivation of an expression for p_{AR} in the presence of the antagonist, B, is achieved using standard procedures. The result is given in Equation 7.59.

$$p_{AR} = \frac{[A]}{[A] + \dfrac{k_{-A}}{k_{+A}}\left(1 + \dfrac{[B]k_{+B}}{k_{-B}}\right)} \tag{7.59}$$

(b) A plot of the reciprocal of τ_{on} vs. $[B]$ will be a straight line of slope $p_{free}k_{+B}$ and y-axis intercept k_{-B}. Using the data in the table, the slope is found to be $2 \times 10^5 \text{ M}^{-1}\text{s}^{-1}$ and intercept 1 s^{-1}. p_{free} is $1 - p_{AR}$ in the absence of antagonist. Thus $p_{free} = K_A/([A]+K_A) = 0.1$. As $p_{free}k_{+B} = $ slope, $k_{+B} = $ slope$/p_{free} = 2 \times 10^6 \text{ M}^{-1}\text{s}^{-1}$. The equilibrium constant $K_B = k_{-B}/k_{+B} = 0.5 \times 10^{-6} \text{ M}$. Finally, calculate p_{AR} in the absence of antagonist and then in the presence of each $[B]$ and then use these to calculate the percentage block produced at equilibrium by each antagonist concentration. When $[A] = 100 \text{ }\mu M$, $K_A = 11 \text{ }\mu M$, $p_{AR} = 0.9$ in the absence of antagonist and with $K_B = 0.5 \text{ }\mu M$ and $[B] = 7.5 \text{ }\mu M$, $p_{AR} = 0.36$; %Block $= (0.9 - 0.36)/0.9 \times 100 = 60\%$. When $[B] = 20 \text{ }\mu M$, $p_{AR} = 0.191$, and %Block $= 79\%$. When $[B] = 45 \text{ }\mu M$, $p_{AR} = 0.098$, and %Block $= 89\%$.

The calculated values for %Block are close to those observed at low blocker concentrations, but at higher concentrations the observed block is greater than predicted. Possible reasons for this may lie in the measurement of the onset time constants, in the assumption about the agonist equilibrating much faster than the antagonist, or the mechanism may be wrong perhaps because the receptor has more than one binding site, or binding of the antagonist promotes desensitization of the receptor.

8 G-Proteins

Annette C. Dolphin

CONTENTS

8.1 CLASSIFICATION OF G-PROTEINS

Signal transducing G-proteins are GTPases that can be broadly divided into two classes: the heterotrimeric G-proteins; and the small G-proteins such as p21-*ras,* which consist of a single α-subunit, and only some of which play a role in signal transduction. This chapter will largely deal with the heterotrimeric G-proteins.

Heterotrimeric G-proteins are molecular switches that transduce signals across cell membranes. When a cell membrane receptor is occupied by an agonist, the conformational change produced in the receptor acts as a signal to activate the associated G-protein, and this then activates the relevant effector. The G-protein-mediated signal transduction systems involve amplification of the signal because of the catalytic G-protein step, whereas other signal transducing systems such as ligand-gated ion channels do not have any possibility of signal amplification. Receptor occupation can, through G-proteins, activate many effector systems.

The heterotrimeric G-proteins comprise α, β, and γ subunits. There are more than 20 different α subunits, four β subunits, and seven γ subunits.

8.2 SUBTYPES OF G-PROTEIN α SUBUNIT

Figure 8.1 shows the relationship between the Gα subunits by comparing the percentage homology in their amino acid sequences. Presumably there was a primeval α subunit from which the different subclasses, including G_s, G_i/G_o, and G_q, have arisen during evolution. Different Gα subclasses subserve different functions, although a number of additional Gα subunits have now been cloned for which the function remains obscure. For example, the existence of $Gα_z$ was not known before the cDNA was cloned, and the function of the protein is still unclear. Similarly, the function of the $G_{12}–G_{16}$ subgroups remains undefined.

0-8493-9227-6/96/$0.00+$.50
© 1996 by CRC Press, Inc.

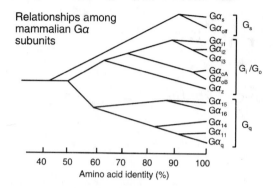

FIGURE 8.1 Relationships between mammalian Gα subunits. The percentage amino acid identity is compared between the different subunits, allowing them to be grouped into subgroups according to similarity. $G\alpha_{12}$ and $G\alpha_{13}$ have been omitted for clarity.

TABLE 8.1

SUBTYPES OF HETEROTRIMERIC G-PROTEIN α SUBUNITS

	MW kDa	Subtypes	Toxin substrate	Function
α_s	45, 52	4	CTX	Stimulates AC
				Activates Ca channels in heart (?)
α_i	40, 41	At least 3	PTX	Inhibits AC
				Activates K⁺ channels
α_o	39	At least 2	PTX	Activates receptors that inhibit neuronal calcium channels
α_z	39	—	—	Couples to same receptors as G_i and G_o
α_Q/α_{11}	40	At least 5	—	Activates PLC
α_T (transducin)	39	At least 2 in rods and cones	CTX, PTX	Activates PDE in retina
α_{OLF}	45		CTX	Increases cAMP in olfactory neuroepithelium
α_{GUST} (gusducin)	39		CTX, PTX	Activated in taste buds involved in bitter taste transduction

---

   Table 8.1 includes only the types of heterotrimeric G-proteins for which functions are well-established. They are defined by their α subunits. The α_s protein shows two bands on gel electrophoresis: one of 45 and one of 52 kDa. The four different subunits are encoded by two separate genes, and alternative splicing during transcription produces two long and two short forms of α_s subunits. The main function of α_s is to <u>stimulate</u> adenylyl cyclase.

   The α_i subunit was discovered through the ability of some hormones to <u>inhibit</u> adenylyl cyclase, and by using a mutant S49 lymphoma cell line, lacking α_s, known as cyc⁻. Activation of the β-adrenoreceptor on these mutant cells does not stimulate adenylyl cyclase, but receptors which inhibit this enzyme (e.g., somatostatin receptors) remain functional. This result implied the existence of a G-protein different from G_s and this was isolated and called G_i. The α_i subunit is ADP-ribosylated by pertussis toxin, and shows two, or sometimes three, bands on gel electrophoresis of 40 and 41 kDa. There are three genes which encode the proteins: α_i 1, 2, and 3. In addition to inhibition of adenylyl cyclase, α_i may activate K⁺ channels, although there is some dispute concerning the type of K⁺ channel involved.

The α_o subunit has a molecular weight of about 39 kDa and constitutes about 1% of brain membrane protein. It is found predominantly in neuronal tissue, although some is also present in other electrically excitable tissues such as heart muscle. There are two genes coding for α_{o1} and α_{o2}. The one suggested function of these G-proteins is to inhibit Ca^{2+} channels.

The subunit α_z is similar in molecular weight to α_o and is also alike in other respects except that it has no N-terminal cysteine for ADP-ribosylation by pertussis toxin. $G\alpha_z$ is thought to be able to associate with the same receptors as $G\alpha_o$ and $G\alpha_i$.

The α_q and α_{11} subunits have a molecular weight of 40 kDa and function to activate phospholipase C. The receptors with which they associate are generally different from those that activate $G\alpha_o$ and $G\alpha_i$.

The α_t subunit is also known as transducin and has a molecular weight of 39 kDa. Two of these subunits have been identified: rod and cone transducin. They activate cyclic GMP phosphodiesterase in the retina. Transducins are substrates for both cholera and pertussis toxins.

There are also specific G-proteins mediating signal transduction in the olfactory and gustatory systems. $G\alpha_{olf}$ has a molecular weight of 45 kDa and is similar to $G\alpha_s$: it was cloned by homology with $G\alpha_s$. It increases the activity of adenylyl cyclase but has a higher signal to noise ratio: the very low basal activity increases upon $G\alpha_{olf}$ activation to much higher levels than with $G\alpha_s$. $G\alpha_{gust}$ (gusducin) was cloned from taste-buds and is a substrate for both cholera and pertussis toxins. There may be more than one of these α subunits.

8.3 G-PROTEIN STRUCTURE

The model in Figure 8.2 shows the predicted secondary structure of "α average", which is derived from the known structures of p21-*ras* and EF-Tu (ribosomal GTPase). In the center is the GDP/GTP binding domain, with binding sites for two or three phosphates, ribose, guanine, and a magnesium ion. Magnesium is essential for the binding of the nucleotide. The C-terminus of the protein contains the receptor binding region for the seven-transmembrane domain type of receptor. The cysteine residue, when present, is the substrate for ADP ribosylation by pertussis toxin. In contrast, cholera toxin ADP-ribosylates the arginine residue near the GTP binding domain, when this is present. The actions of pertussis and cholera toxins are discussed further below. The N-terminal domain of the G-protein α subunit is the region where the β and γ subunits bind. The N-terminus itself is, in many classes of G-protein, post-translationally modified by myristoylation or other fatty acylation. The function of this group is to anchor the α subunit, which is hydrophilic, to the cell membrane; α subunits are also confined to the inner surface of the cell membrane by association with $\beta\gamma$ subunits. Except in the retinal rhodopsin-transducin-phosphodiesterase system, the α subunit remains associated with the membrane, even when activated and dissociated from $\beta\gamma$, because of its fatty acylation.

Effectors, such as the enzymes adenylyl cyclase and phospholipase C, or certain ion channels, are thought to bind to a diffuse domain on the opposite surface of the protein from the GTP binding domain.

8.4 ADP-RIBOSYLATION MECHANISMS

Several bacterial toxins ADP-ribosylate GTPases at different sites. Such toxins include: pertussis toxin, cholera toxin, diphtheria toxin, and *Escherichia coli* heat-stable toxin. These toxins all have a similar A-B subunit structure. The B subunits bind to a cell surface receptor which permits the internalization of the whole toxin by the cell. The A and B subunits are linked together by a disulfide bond and once inside the cell this bond is hydrolyzed to release the A protomer which has enzyme action. The A protomer uses NAD^+ to ADP-ribosylate any

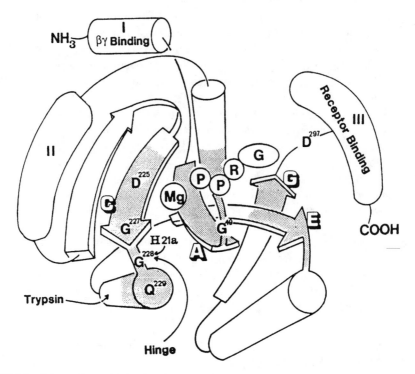

FIGURE 8.2   Schematic model for the predicted secondary structure of "α average". This shows the guanine nucleotide binding domain and other relevant domains. (Reproduced from *G Proteins*, R. Iyengar and L. Birnbaumer, Eds., Academic Press, Orlando, FL, 1990, chap 2. With permission.)

substrate protein that it recognizes. For pertussis toxin the substrates are the $G\alpha_i$ and $G\alpha_0$ subtypes and also transducin and gustucin, whereas for cholera toxin the substrates are $G\alpha_s$, $G\alpha_{olf}$, transducin, and gusducin. The effect of cholera toxin on $G\alpha_s$ is manifest as prolonged activation of adenylyl cyclase and a consequently large rise in intracellular cyclic AMP, which explains how cholera infection causes diarrhea, since elevated cyclic AMP in cells lining the gastrointestinal tract promotes fluid and electrolyte secretion. ADP-ribosylation by pertussis toxin maintains the G-protein in the GDP-bound state, preventing the interaction between G-protein and receptor. However, this can result in an elevation of intracellular cyclic AMP because G_i normally inhibits adenylyl cyclase. For diphtheria toxin, the substrate is not a signal transducing G-protein but the mammalian equivalent of the ribosomal GTPase, EF-Tu.

These toxins are useful tools for identifying G-protein function (see later), and also to determine how much of these G-proteins is present in a particular tissue. For example, the addition of pertussis toxin together with $[^{32}P]$-NAD^+ will label the α subunit of its substrate G-proteins, and following separation by gel electrophoresis, will permit estimation of the amount present by autoradiography.

8.5   MECHANISM OF ACTION OF G-PROTEINS

The essential function of the α subunit is to recognize specific receptors and to couple these to specific effector systems. There is a high degree of specificity: for example $G\alpha_s$ recognizes the β-adrenoreceptor but not the α_2-adrenoreceptor (unless the G-protein or receptor is massively overexpressed). There is similar specificity for effectors: $G\alpha_s$ activates adenylyl cyclase but not K^+ channels.

Let us consider the functioning of G_s. Figure 8.3 shows the β-adrenoreceptor which, when it is not occupied by an agonist, is not associated to any great extent with G_s. The G-protein

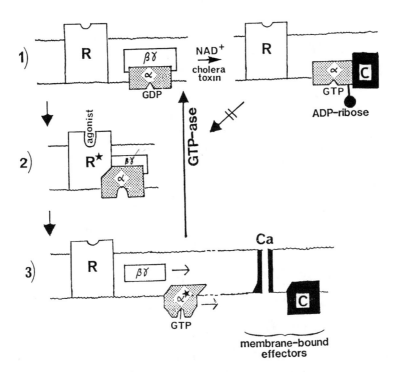

FIGURE 8.3   Signal transduction occurring via G_s.

exists as a heterotrimer, and the α_s subunit binds GDP with high affinity in the resting condition. When an agonist such as isoprenaline binds to the receptor, a conformational change occurs in the receptor which causes it to have a high affinity for G_s. As the receptor, with agonist bound, associates with G_s, the G-protein also undergoes a conformational change causing GDP to leave the binding pocket. There is a relatively high concentration of GTP in the cytosol and so it enters the binding site in place of GDP. A further conformational change then occurs in the G-protein so that the α subunit becomes activated, and may dissociate from the $\beta\gamma$ heterodimer; however, this dissociation has not been shown conclusively to occur in the case of G_s. The activated α_s subunit influences the effector, in this case adenylyl cyclase, and causes the enzyme to become active. Certain G-proteins such as G_s appear to be permanently closely associated with their effectors, and this can be shown by the copurification of G_s and adenylyl cyclase. In contrast, others probably diffuse laterally in the membrane to encounter their specific effector proteins. The α subunit has an inbuilt clock which determines for how long the effector will be activated. Termination of the signal is brought about by the intrinsic GTPase activity of the α_s subunit, which hydrolyzes the GTP to GDP and returns the subunit to its basal state.

It is well known that the effector for G_s is adenylyl cyclase. More recently, however, there has been debate about whether G_s can also directly activate cardiac calcium channels. The interaction of isoprenaline with the β-adrenoreceptor on a cardiac muscle cell enhances the voltage-activated calcium current across the cell membrane. There is an initial rapid effect of isoprenaline which appears to occur too rapidly to result from adenylyl cyclase activation. It has been argued that the small rapid increase in the calcium current results from a direct coupling of G_s with the calcium channels while the subsequent slow enhancement of calcium current arises from the activation through G_s of adenylyl cyclase, a rise in intracellular cyclic AMP, and the phosphorylation of the calcium channels. The direct effect of G_s on cardiac calcium channels has not been detected by some research workers and may be species specific, or may reflect a local rapid rise in cyclic AMP.

8.6   THE GTP BINDING DOMAIN

Figure 8.4 shows the primary structure of a generalized G-protein α subunit. There are common highly conserved regions depicted by the open boxes, which represent the GTP binding pocket. Certain pituitary tumors contain a mutant form of G_s which is constitutively active, and many other mutations have now been made artificially to explore the function of different parts of the receptor. Activating mutations either decrease GTPase activity or increase the off-rate of GDP, so that the mutant G_s binds GTP in the absence of any agonist and is, therefore, constitutively active. Figure 8.5 shows the GTP-binding domain of p21-*ras*, indicating the large conformational change in the protein when GTP is hydrolyzed to GDP. Assuming a similar arrangement in heterotrimeric G-proteins, when the G-protein encounters an agonist-bound receptor there is a conformational change promoting GDP release and GTP binding. Two loops of the G-protein come together to associate with the third or γ-phosphate on GTP, in the presence of Mg^{2+}, which is closely associated with the two terminal phosphates. The conformational change associated with its activation is transferred to the effector binding region of the α subunit. It is, therefore, a multistep process. Then, after a certain time, there is a conformational change which pulls the two loops apart and the γ-phosphate of GTP is hydrolyzed.

8.7   G-PROTEIN-RECEPTOR INTERACTIONS

How can we show that a particular G-protein interacts with a particular receptor? As an initial screen, one may look at the sensitivity of the process to pertussis toxin or cholera toxin. If the process is sensitive to pertussis toxin, which inhibits $G_{i/o}$-protein function, then it is possible to conclude that either G_i or G_o is involved. In contrast, if a process is mimicked by cholera toxin, which permanently activates G_s, then G_s may be involved. It is subsequently necessary to use purified or recombinant receptor together with specific purified or recombinant G-proteins and to measure the increase in binding of the nonhydrolyzable analogue of GTP, GTPγS to the G-protein, or the stimulation of GTPase activity, or GTP-induced affinity shift in agonist binding to its receptor in cell-free systems. All these are measures of productive coupling between receptors and G-proteins.

Cellular reconstitution experiments can also be made in cells from which endogenous G-protein is functionally removed by pertussis toxin treatment. Then either G_i or G_o can be used for reconstitution, to examine which G-protein restores effector activation. Alternatively, antibodies can be used to knock out particular G-proteins, or antisense oligonucleotides can be employed to reduce the synthesis of G-proteins; this will then pinpoint which G-protein is involved in a particular response.

A surprising recent finding is that there is a very high degree of specificity in the system with regard to activation by particular receptors and to effector interaction. There are at least three different α_i, four different β, and seven different γ protamers, allowing for a large number of different combinations. Nevertheless, it has been found that interaction of G_i with a particular muscarinic receptor, for example, will only be effective for one combination of $\alpha\beta\gamma$ subunits. Further specificity in terms of interaction with effectors is revealed by the finding that numerous receptors, such as the α_2-adrenoreceptor, can activate both G_i and G_o, but it is apparently only G_o and not G_i that inhibits voltage-activated calcium channels.

Until relatively recently, the α subunit was considered to be the only primary determinant of G-protein specificity. The $\beta\gamma$ heterodimer was seen as having a "housekeeping" role and acting as an anchor for the α subunit to the membrane. It is now recognized that different $\beta\gamma$ subunits aid α subunits to recognize specific receptors and also turn off free α subunits. So, when the α subunit with bound GTP reassociates with $\beta\gamma$, the GTPase activity of the α subunit is stimulated. Furthermore, it is now becoming clear that free $\beta\gamma$ can itself activate or inhibit a number of enzymes (see later).

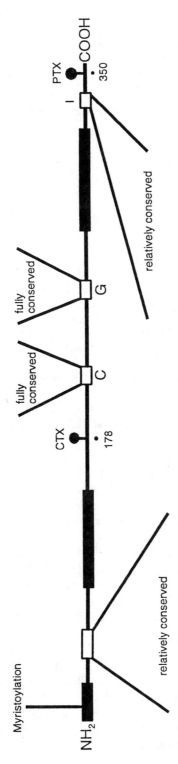

FIGURE 8.4 The distribution of sequence specificity among the α subunits. The empty boxes represent the largely conserved domains found in all α subunits, which are thought to be involved in guanine nucleotide binding. The solid boxes represent regions of greatest amino acid sequence diversity.

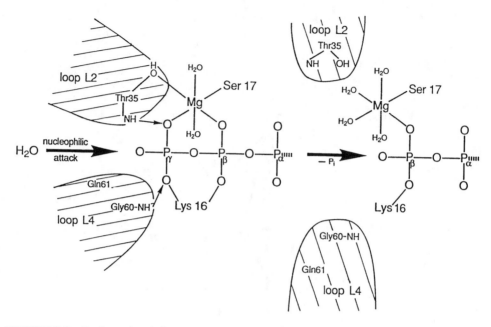

FIGURE 8.5 Conformational change in p21-ras triggered by the hydrolysis of the γ-phosphate. The loss of the terminal phosphate releases loop L2 and loop L4, which are bound to the terminal phosphate via a threonine and a glycine residue, both of which are conserved in all G- proteins. (Reproduced from *The GTPase Superfamily,* J. Marsh and J. Goode, Eds., John Wiley & Sons, Chichester, 1993, p18. With permission of the Ciba Foundation.)

If one considers the effect of noradrenaline on adenylyl cyclase activity, the traditional view is that it will activate both β-adrenoreceptors associated with G_s, and α_2-adrenoreceptors associated with G_i. Stimulation would occur via α_s and inhibition via α_i. However, when adenylyl cyclase was purified, it was found that that the βγ dimer could also activate the enzyme in some cases (Figure 8.6). In fact, when certain adenylyl cyclase subtypes are stimulated by α_s, then βγ will produce further stimulation. In contrast, in type 1 adenylyl cyclase, βγ causes inhibition of the enzyme activity. It is likely that βγ from any G-protein can stimulate or inhibit the different adenylyl cyclase isoforms, and this may explain some of the "cross-talk" between receptors that occurs in intact cell systems. Free βγ from G_q could also interact with adenylyl cyclase, providing a link between two different signal transduction systems (Figure 8.6).

At least six types of adenylyl cyclase have been identified (Figure 8.6), all of which are activated by $G_s\alpha$ in a 1:1 coupling ratio. However, βγ will stimulate G_s-activated type 2 and type 4 adenylyl cyclase but inhibit type 1 (calcium/calmodulin-dependent) adenylyl cyclase. This action of βγ on adenylyl cyclase occurs in the low nanomolar range of concentration. $G\alpha_i$ does inhibit adenylyl cyclase (types 2, 3, and 6) but interestingly it is much less potent than βγ.

Other effector systems affected directly by βγ dimers are calcium channels, inwardly rectifying K^+ channels in heart and brain, β-adrenoreceptor kinase, and phospholipase C-β. Thus G_i, G_o, and G_q can all generate βγ dimers which can alter the function of phospholipase C-β and adenylyl cyclases. For this reason, the final signal depends on the number and type of G-proteins activated at any one time, and there is the possibility of complex and tissue-specific interplay between phospholipase- and adenylyl cyclase-linked receptors. An added complication would be the additional interaction that can occur following the elevation of intracellular calcium, as this can stimulate adenylyl cyclase type 1 and may be promoted by a number of mechanisms.

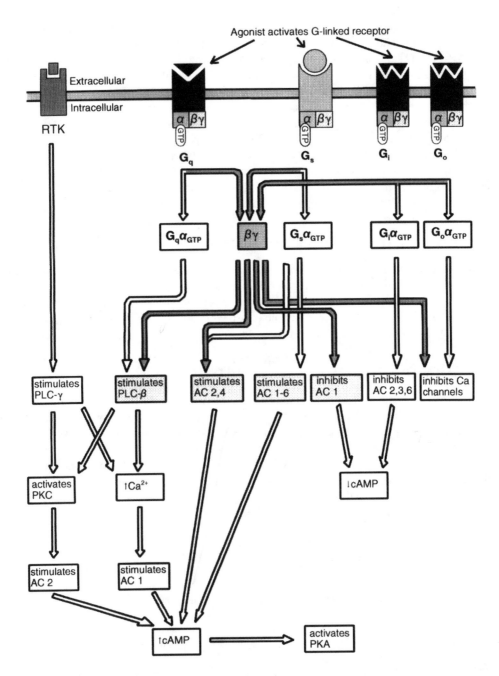

FIGURE 8.6 A schematic diagram of signaling pathways that can regulate the activity of adenylyl cyclases. Pathways involving βγ subunits are shaded. AC 1-6, adenylyl cyclase types 1-6; RTK, receptor tyrosine kinase; PLC, phospholipase C; PKC protein kinase C; PKA, protein kinase A. (Reproduced with modification from Pieroni, P. et al., *Current Opinion in Neurobiology*, 3, 345 1993. With permission.)

8.8 CONTROL OF GDP-GTP EXCHANGE AND GTPᴀꜱᴇ ACTIVITY

The rate of GDP-GTP exchange is normally low but is enhanced by agonist occupation of a receptor. Small G-proteins such as p-21 *ras* have guanine nucleotide exchange proteins which perform a similar function to the agonist-receptor complex in increasing GDP-GTP exchange;

these proteins are specific for each G-protein. Small G-proteins also have a very low intrinsic GTPase activity, which is elevated by association with specific GTPase activating proteins or GAPs. The GTPase activity of signal transducing G-proteins also has a low basal rate: too low to explain the off-rate of certain effectors. For example, there is an obvious need in the visual system for a rapid off-rate of the response to light to permit the temporal discrimination of photons arriving at the retina. The signal transduction system involves activation of the G-protein transducin by rhodopsin, and the G-protein, in turn, activates a cyclic GMP phosphodiesterase, but the response must turn off rapidly to permit readiness for the next photon-generated signal. The GTPase activity of transducin is not fast enough to explain the observed rate at which the signal decays. In fact, it seems that cyclic GMP phosphodiesterase or an associated protein may be acting as a GAP. Thus, the effector may also control the rate of GTPase activity. K^+ channels and phospholipase C-β may also function as GAPs.

8.9 SIGNAL AMPLIFICATION BY G-PROTEINS

Again using the visual system as an example, a single photon can activate one molecule of rhodopsin. One activated rhodopsin molecule can interact during its lifetime with 100 transducins, and the resultant activation of 100 phosphodiesterase molecules causes 10^5 molecules of cyclic GMP to be hydrolyzed before the transducin molecules are returned to their GDP-bound state. G-proteins thus serve as part of an amplification system in signal transduction.

8.10 MODULATION OF G-PROTEIN ACTIVITY

G-proteins can be phosphorylated and thereby their activity can be modulated. For example, the activity of some G-proteins can be turned off when the α subunit is phosphorylated by protein kinase C. There is some evidence for the endogenous ADP-ribosylation of G-proteins. Phosphorylation of the receptor itself by specific receptor kinases activated by $\beta\gamma$ can prevent interaction with the G-protein, hence reducing further G-protein activation. Modulation of the genes encoding G-proteins can alter both the type of G-protein and the amount of G-protein expressed, and this adaptive response mechanism appears to come into play in some clinical situations, such as congestive heart failure.

8.11 FURTHER READING

Clapham, D.E. (1994), Direct G protein activation of ion channels? *Annu. Rev. Neurosci.,* 17, 441-464.
Hescheler, J. and Schultz, G. (1993), G-proteins involved in the calcium channel signalling system, *Curr. Opinion Neurobiol.,* 3, 360-367.
Milligan, G. (1995), Signal sorting by G protein linked receptors, *Adv. Pharmacology,* 32, 1-129.
Pieroni, J.P., Jacobowitz, O., Chen, J. and Iyengar, R. (1993), Signal recognition and integration by G_s-stimulated adenylyl cyclases, *Curr. Opinion Neurobiol.,* 3, 345-351.
Simon, M.I., Strathmann, M.P. and Gautam, N. (1991), Diversity of G proteins in signal transduction, *Science,* 252, 802-808.

9 Phospholipases and Phosphokinases: Sources of Lipid-Derived Second Messengers

Shamshad Cockcroft

CONTENTS

9.1 INTRODUCTION

Phospholipids are a rich source of "second messengers". Receptor-mediated hydrolysis of cellular phospholipids is an ubiquitous event of fundamental importance in signal transduction. The hydrolysis of membrane lipids is catalyzed by different classes of phospholipases having distinct specificities (Figure 9.1). In many cells, it is common to observe activation

0-8493-9227-6/96/$0.00+$.50
© 1996 by CRC Press, Inc.

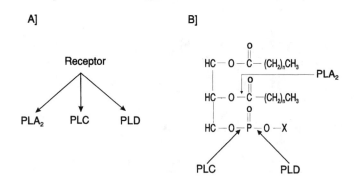

FIGURE 9.1 [A] Receptor activation of cells can activate three phospholipases, [B] site of hydrolysis by the different phospholipases. X represents a phospholipid headgroup, e.g., coline, inositol.

of assorted phospholipases, e.g., phospholipase A_2 (PLA$_2$), inositol lipid-specific phospholipase C (PLC), and phosphatidylcholine-specific phospholipase D (PLD), giving rise to multiple second messengers. In addition to the phospholipases, there is a phosphoinositide-3-kinase (PI-3-kinase) pathway which phosphorylates inositol lipids. These 3-phosphorylated inositol lipids are hardly present in resting cells but are rapidly generated on cell-surface stimulation.

These signaling pathways provide "second messengers" released in the cell interior and they, in turn, control the physiological responses of the cell. Regulated events include cell proliferation, cell differentiation, secretion, contraction, and metabolic processes. The potential second messengers that are derived from the activation of the phospholipases and PI-3-kinase are summarized in Figure 9.2. The first of the lipid signaling pathways to be appreciated was the PLC pathway. It causes the hydrolysis of phosphatidylinositol (4,5) bisphosphate (PI(4,5)P$_2$) leading to the generation of two second messengers, the water-soluble product, inositol(1,4,5)trisphosphate (I(1,4,5)P$_3$), and a membrane-associated product, diacylglycerol (DAG) (Figure 9.2). I(1,4,5)P$_3$ mobilizes Ca^{2+} from intracellular stores localized in the endoplasmic reticulum. Diacylglycerol activates the enzyme, protein kinase C (PKC), which then phosphorylates target proteins.

The I(1,4,5)P$_3$ receptor and PKC activated by these two second messengers have been well characterized. The IP$_3$ receptor has been cloned and sequenced. It has a transmembrane domain near the C-terminus, with a long N-terminal and short C-terminal portions in the cytoplasmic compartment. Four receptor molecules form a Ca^{2+} channel which is in the open state when IP$_3$ is bound to its recognition site localized at the N-terminal. DAG activates PKC in the presence of the phospholipid, phosphatidylserine (PS), and Ca^{2+}. There are nine isozymes known in the protein kinase C family to date, which differ in their specific requirements for activation (see Chapter 11). The majority of the PKC enzymes can be activated by a phorbol ester, PMA, a known tumor promoter derived from croton oil which is used extensively in studies of PKC action.

The activation of phospholipase D (PLD) by cell-surface receptors has only been recognized since 1984 as a signal transduction system. PLD promotes the breakdown of phosphatidylcholine (PC), resulting in the increase in the membrane concentration of phosphatidate (PA) and the water-soluble product, choline. PA could act as a second messenger in its own right or it could be further metabolized to generate DAG, and so activate protein kinase C (Figure 9.2).

The third phospholipase that is also stimulated by many receptors is PLA$_2$ and here the hydrolysis of membrane phospholipids results in the release of arachidonic acid. This fatty acid contains 20 carbon atoms and 4 double bonds (C$_{20:4}$) and is the substrate for two enzymes, cyclooxygenase and lipoxygenase. These enzymes give rise to a multitude of products

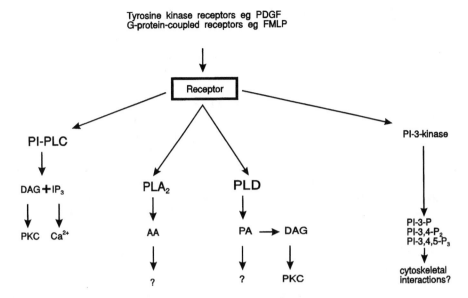

FIGURE 9.2   Scheme illustrating potential second messengers derived from phospholipase and phosphokinase activation by receptors. Multiple second messengers can be derived from signaling pathways triggered by the G-protein-coupled receptors and tyrosine kinase receptors. Rapid activation of three phospholipases and phosphatidylinositol-3-kinase are known to be switched on receptor activation. The products of the individual pathways which are potential second messengers are indicated as well as the downstream events that they regulate.

collectively referred to as eicosanoids. Eicosanoids are bioactive compounds such as prostaglandins, thromboxanes, prostacyclin, and leukotrienes which act as local hormones. Increasingly, evidence is accumulating that arachidonic acid itself may also function as a second messenger. For example, in neutrophils it may be the activator of NADPH oxidase, the enzyme responsible for generating the superoxide required for killing microbes. In brain, arachidonic acid has been suggested as a second messenger for long-term potentiation at the synapse.

The PI-3-kinase pathway has been identified relatively recently, and here the substrate(s) for the kinase are the inositol-containing lipids, phosphatidylinositol (PI), PI(4)P, and PI(4,5)P$_2$. The 3-kinase phosphorylates the inositol ring specifically at the D3-position of the inositol ring, generating a set of unique lipids which are not substrates for phospholipase C. The function of these lipids is unknown.

9.2   FUNCTIONAL SIGNIFICANCE OF MULTIPLE SIGNALING PATHWAYS

The presence of multiple signaling pathways invoked by a single ligand may reflect either a built-in redundancy in the signaling cascade, or individual second messengers may allow functional responses to be triggered at thresholds which can be modulated by the presence of second signals. For example, an increment in Ca^{2+} may set the system to a receptive state, but does not actually trigger a response. A small change in a second parameter, e.g., an increase in DAG or PA, is then sufficient for the system to pass a threshold for a physiological response. The use of multiple signaling pathways permits a sophisticated means of controlling output and fine-tuning cell responses. In practice, different agonists switch on these pathways to varying degrees, and this presumably defines the efficacy of the different agonists. *In vivo*, cells will be responding to a multitude of agonists, and the final outcome will be determined by the net sum of the signals.

9.3 RECEPTORS

Receptors can be classified into G-protein-linked receptors, receptors that possess intrinsic tyrosine kinases, and receptors that regulate tyrosine kinases. G-protein-coupled receptors have a well-defined structure: they traverse the plasma membrane seven times with three cytoplasmic loops and a cytoplasmic tail. The second and the third loop determine which G-protein that the particular receptor will activate. Receptors for some agonists such as platelet-derived growth factor (PDGF) and epidermal growth factor (EGF) possess intrinsic tyrosine kinase activity while many receptors activate extrinsic tyrosine kinases, e.g., the src family of kinases. A number of these receptors stimulate either all three phospholipases, C, D, and A_2, and PI-3-kinase, or a selection of these activities. PDGF and the chemotactic peptide, fMetLeuPhe, are known to stimulate all the three phospholipases and PI-3-kinase in fibroblasts and neutrophils, respectively. In contrast, interleukin 2 or colony stimulating factor only stimulates PI-3-kinase, and the T cell receptor stimulates PLC, PLD, and PI-3-kinase.

9.4 MEMBRANE PHOSPHOLIPIDS AS A SOURCE OF SECOND MESSENGERS

The main substrates for the different phospholipases are phospholipids which are generally resident in the cell membrane. The biological membrane is organized as a bilayer consisting of several phospholipids, mainly phosphatidylcholine (PC), phosphatidylethanolamine, phosphatidylserine, phosphatidylinositol (PI), and sphingomyelin. It is the lipids on the cytoplasmic face which will be degraded by the intracellular phospholipases.

The substrate for PLC and PI-3-kinase is the inositol-containing lipid, $PI(4,5)P_2$. There are three principal inositol-containing lipids in mammalian cells, PI, PI(4)P, and $PI(4,5)P_2$. The fatty acid composition of the inositol lipids has a characteristic pattern whereby the sn-1 position normally contains stearic acid (C_{18}) and the sn-2 position contains arachidonic acid ($C_{20:4}$). PI is present as approximately 5 to 8% of total cellular lipids and, although it represents the bulk of the inositol lipids, it is not a substrate for the PLC. PI can be specifically phosphorylated by PI-4-kinase to PI(4)P and, in turn, it is specifically phosphorylated to $PI(4,5)P_2$ by PI(4)P-5-kinase. The ratio of PI:PI(4)P:$PI(4,5)P_2$ in most cells is approximately 90:6:4. Although $PI(4,5)P_2$ is the main substrate for both the PLC and PI-3-kinase in cells *in vitro*, it is possible for these enzymes to utilize all three inositol lipids as substrates. Since the concentration of $PI(4,5)P_2$ in cells is limited, the lipid kinases play a significant role in maintaining a supply of substrate for the PLC during cell stimulation.

PC is the main substrate for both PLD and PLA_2. PC accounts for nearly 40% of the total phospholipid pool and can be present in two forms. The fatty acid present on the glycerobackbone at the first position can be linked with either an ester bond or the more stable alkyl bond. In many cells, up to 50% of the PC is present in the alkyl form. The significance of this is that alkyl-PC, when degraded by PLA_2, will release arachidonic acid as well as lyso-alkyl-PC, which is further acetylated to produce PAF (platelet activating factor). PAF is a potent receptor-specific agonist and has powerful effects on many cells. However, PLD does not appear to distinguish between the alkyl form of PC and the acyl form of PC.

9.5 INOSITOL LIPID SIGNALING PATHWAY

9.5.1 BREAKDOWN AND RESYNTHESIS OF INOSITOL LIPIDS

The hydrolysis of $PI(4,5)P_2$ (PIP_2) generates two second messengers, $I(1,4,5)P_3$ (IP_3) and DAG (Figure 9.2). Both DAG and IP_3 are rapidly metabolized within cells, as would be expected for molecules that function as second messengers. Figure 9.3 outlines the sequence

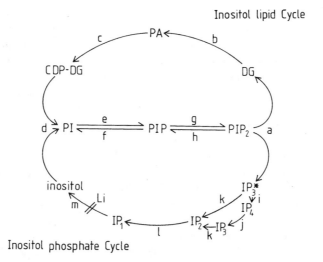

FIGURE 9.3 Cycle of reactions that interconnect the products of receptor-stimulated inositol lipid metabolism. $PI(4,5)P_2$ is initially hydrolyzed to generate diacylglycerol (DG) and inositol-1,4,5-tris-phosphate (IP_3^*) by phospholipase C. The top half of the cycle (inositol lipid cycle) illustrates how the DG is removed. The DG is phosphorylated to phosphatidate (PA) by DG kinase and this is recycled back to phosphatidylinositol (PI) via cytidine diphosphate-diacylglycerol (CDP-DG). The bottom half of the cycle (inositol phosphate cycle) illustrates the metabolism of $I(1,4,5)P_3$ (IP_3^*). (IP_3^*) can be metabolized by two separate routes: dephosphorylation to $I(1,4)P_2$ or phosphorylation to $I(1,3,4,5)P_4$. $I(1,3,4,5)P_4$ is then dephosphorylated to $I(1,3,4)P_3$, an inactive isomer of $I(1,4,5)P_3$. Sequential dephosphorylation of the inositol phosphates leads to the release of free inositol, and this combines with CDP-diacylglycerol to regenerate PI. Key to symbols: (a) phospholipase C; (b) DG kinase; (c) CTP phosphatidate cytidyl transferase; (d) PI synthase; (e) PI-4-kinase; (f) PI-4-P phosphatase; (g) PI-4-P 5-kinase; (h) $PI(4,5)P_2$ 5-mono-esterase; (i) $I(1,4,5)P_3$ kinase; (j) phosphatase specific for removing the 5'-phosphate from either $I(1,4,5)P_3$ or $I(1,3,4,5)P_4$; (k–m) phosphatases with differing specificities for the different inositol phosphates. The site of lithium ion inhibition is shown.

of reactions involved in the removal of the second messengers and the recycling of the breakdown products back to the inositol lipids. Both production and removal of the second messengers is tightly regulated. Resynthesis of the phospholipid is also important, otherwise the cell will run out of substrate in the long term. Figure 9.3 illustrates how the cells replenish their supply of the inositol lipids. At least 13 reactions can be identified in the metabolism of the inositol lipids. In some cases, the enzymes catalyzing these reactions exist as isoforms expressed in a species- and tissue-specific manner and are themselves subject to regulation.

The reactions can be divided into two cycles; the inositol lipid cycle which occurs in the membrane and the inositol phosphate cycle which occurs in the cytosol (Figure 9.3). Examination of the inositol phosphate cycle shows that $I(1,4,5)P_3$ can be metabolized by two separate routes. It can be either phosphorylated by IP_3-kinase to form $I(1,3,4,5)P_4$ or it can be dephosphorylated to $I(1,4)P_2$. Neither of these products interact with the $I(1,4,5)P_3$ receptor to mobilize intracellular Ca^{2+}. Since ATP is used for the phosphorylation reaction, it would imply that $I(1,3,4,5)P_4$ may fulfil some important function.

Current speculation is that $I(1,3,4,5)P_4$ allows influx of Ca^{2+} into the cells from the external medium. Most cells when stimulated with an agonist initially mobilize intracellular Ca^{2+} from the stores but then subsequently depend on Ca^{2+} influx. The role of IP_4 in promoting Ca^{2+} influx remains an area of contention, and until the IP_4 receptor is identified, it will remain so.

$I(1,3,4,5)P_4$ is dephosphorylated to $I(1,3,4)P_3$, an inactive analogue of $I(1,4,5)P_3$. Sequential dephosphorylation reactions of the inositol polyphosphates lead back to inositol monophosphates. The final dephosphorylation of inositol monophosphate is catalyzed by a monophosphatase which is inhibited by lithium ions. This property of lithium ions is widely used as an experimental tool to trap the inositol phosphates, which can be analyzed easily and are, therefore, an indicator of inositol lipid hydrolysis. This inhibition of inositol recycling may explain why lithium carbonate has profound clinical effects. It is used for controlling manic depression and it has been suggested that its effects may be explained by its interfering with the recycling of inositol. While peripheral tissues are able to obtain inositol from plasma, the brain does not have this capacity. Hence, the brain is dependent on recycling inositol phosphates for the resynthesis of the inositol lipids or resynthesizing them by a pathway that is inhibited by lithium ions.

DAG is retained in the membranes because of its hydrophobic nature. Its half life is short, being rapidly phosphorylated to form PA by the enzyme, diacylglycerol kinase. Hydrolysis of PIP_2 occurs at the plasma membrane and the PA is also found at the same location. The PA is then recycled back to PI through the intermediate, cytidine diphosphate-diacylglycerol (CDP-DG) (also known as cytidine monophosphate-phosphatidate), which is formed from PA and CTP at the endoplasmic reticulum. CDP-DG and inositol are then converted to PI by the enzyme PI synthase. The unanswered question is how the PA produced at the plasma membrane is transferred to the endoplasmic reticulum for resynthesis to PI.

9.5.2 PHOSPHOLIPASE C AND ITS REGULATION BY RECEPTORS

In 1985, it became clear that PLC was regulated by receptors through a hypothetical protein, a G-protein designated as G_p. G-proteins, as intermediaries for coupling receptors to effectors, were well established as a concept, e.g., the G-protein, G_s, coupling adenylate cyclase to receptors. G-protein activation of PLC could be observed in plasma membranes, but neither the G-protein nor phospholipase C had been characterized as molecular entities. By 1991, this situation had changed dramatically as a result of the identification, purification, and cloning of both the PLC and the G-protein. Both belong to a multigene family.

Purification and molecular cloning established that PLCs fall into three distinct families in mammalian cells: PLC-γ (150 kDa), PLC-β (145 kDa), and PLC-δ (85 kDa) (Figure 9.4). Within each family there are subtypes designated by Arabic numerals after the Greek letters, as in PLC-β1 and PLC-β2. To date, two members of the PLC-γ family have been identified, PLC-γ1 and PLC-γ2. The PLC-β and PLC-δ family each have four members, PLC-β1, -β2, -β3, and -β4, and PLC-δ1, -δ2, -δ3, and -δ4. All these enzymes are separate gene products. The PLC-γ and PLC-δ family are mainly located in the cytosol while the PLC-β family can be membrane associated. The membrane association is not very strong and, depending on the conditions, the PLC-β enzymes can readily dissociate from the membranes.

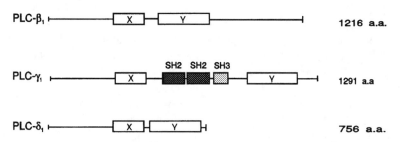

FIGURE 9.4 A linear representation of phospholipase C iosforms: PLC-β1, PLC-γ1, and PLC-δ1.

Figure 9.4 compares the linear display of the sequences of members of the PLC-β, -γ, and -δ families. Although the overall amino acid sequence homology between the different PLC types is low, significant similarity is apparent in two regions which are designated the

X and Y regions. The X and Y regions comprise 170 and 260 amino acids, respectively. These regions are thought to constitute, separately or jointly, the catalytic domain. The PLC-γ isoforms also contain two domains, the src homology domains, SH2 and SH3. These domains govern protein-protein interactions. The SH2 domain targets the molecule to tyrosine phosphorylated sequences present in other proteins, and the SH3 domain is targeted to cytoskeletal components. These domains are found in a large number of unrelated proteins such as GTPase activating protein (GAP), PI-3-kinase, tyrosine phosphatases, and tyrosine kinases. The presence of the SH2 domain, in particular, provided the clues as to how this family of PLCs were regulated.

9.6 REGULATION OF PLC-β AND PLC-γ BY RECEPTORS

The regulation of PLC-β and PLC-γ families is now well understood. That of PLC-δ remains to be established. The PLC-β family is regulated by G-proteins while the PLC-γ family is regulated by tyrosine phosphorylation.

9.6.1 REGULATION OF PLC-β FAMILY BY G-PROTEINS

The G-proteins of the G_q family and the G_i family are involved in the regulation of the PLC-β isoforms. The G_q family comprises at least five G-proteins, G_q, G_{11}, G_{14}, G_{15}, and G_{16}. G_q and G_{11}, which are 88% identical, are both capable of activating PLC-β1. These two G-proteins are ubiquitously expressed and can selectively activate PLC-β1 but not PLC-γ1(or PLC-δ1) isozymes. G_{14}, G_{15}, and G_{16} are expressed in a tissue-restricted fashion and, of these G-proteins, G_{15} and G_{16} are specifically expressed in cells of the hematopoietic lineage together with PLC-β2.

Pertussis toxin has been widely used to identify which G-proteins couple to specific receptors. The pertussis toxin targets are G-proteins of the G_i and G_o families. Pertussis toxin is able to inhibit activation of PLC by receptors in some types of cells, notably neutrophils. For example, if neutrophils are pretreated with pertussis toxin for 2 to 3 h and then stimulated with an agonist such as fMetLeuPhe, inhibition of PLC is observed. Since pertussis toxin is only able to ADP-ribosylate the G_i and G_o family of G-proteins, and such modification interrupts the communication with the receptor, this implies that the G_i or the G_o family are involved in regulating the PLC-β family.

While the α-subunit of G_i does not interact with any of the isoforms of PLC-β, the βγ-subunits of G-proteins are potent activators of some of the PLC-β isoforms: notably PLC-β3 and PLC-β2. Figure 9.5 summarizes the mechanism of PLC-β activation: α-subunits of G_q are required in the nanomolar range to produce PLC activation while βγ-subunits activate PLC in the micromolar range. This distinction is important since more G_i proteins will be needed compared to G_q proteins to activate the various PLC-β isoforms.

9.6.2 IDENTIFICATION OF THE GAP ACTIVITY OF PLC-β

Having identified the main components that constituted the G-protein inositol lipid signaling pathway, attempts were made to reconstitute receptors (muscarinic M1-subtype), G_q and PLC-β1 in liposomes containing the substrate, PIP_2. This was entirely successful. An additional feature emerged from this study which was unexpected: PLC-β1 itself is a GAP or "**G**TPase **A**ctivating **P**rotein". The GAP activity of the effector means that it dictates the length of time the G-protein remains active and thus controls its own activity. Thus, when PLC-β1 is activated by the G-protein, the PLC-β1 will now switch off the G-protein by catalyzing the hydrolysis of the bound GTP.

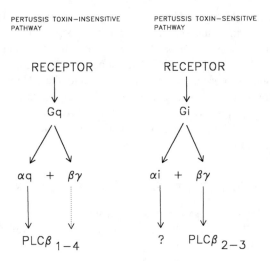

FIGURE 9.5   Activation of PLC-β family by G-proteins.

9.6.3   REGULATION OF PLC-γ BY TYROSINE PHOSPHORYLATION

Binding of PDGF or EGF causes two receptor proteins to cross-link (dimerize) and promotes autophosphorylation of tyrosine residues (Figure 9.6). The tyrosine phosphorylated residues provide recognition sites for SH2 domains of target proteins such as PLC-γ and PI-3-kinase. A physical association of PLC-γ1 or PI-3-kinase with the receptor can be demonstrated experimentally.

Once recruited to the receptor, PLC-γ1 becomes a substrate for receptor protein-tyrosine kinases. Both EGF and PDGF receptors, when activated, phosphorylate PLC-γ1 on tyrosine and serine residues. By virtue of being phosphorylated on tyrosine residues, anti-phosphotyrosine antibodies immunoprecipitate PLC-γ1 from EGF-activated A-431 cells and are, therefore, good tools for studying these events. Four sites of tyrosine phosphorylation in PLC-γ1 have been identified. Purified EGF receptor phosphorylates tyrosine residues 771, 783, 1254, and to a lesser extent, tyrosine 472. By site-directed mutagenesis, it is established that Tyr-783 and Tyr–1254 are essential for PLC-γ1 activation.

PLC-γ2 appears to be present in abundance in hematopoietic cells. It also contains SH2 and SH3 domains, as well as equivalents of the tyrosine residues 771 and 783 of PLC-γ1, but not tyrosine residue 1254. Nonetheless, PLC-γ2 appears to be regulated in a similar manner to PLC-γ1.

9.6.4   IDENTIFICATION OF CYTOSOLIC PROTEINS REQUIRED IN INOSITOL
LIPID SIGNALING

The observation that the three proteins, receptor, G-protein, and PLC-β can be mixed and signaling events reconstituted *in vitro* in model vesicle systems, would suggest that all the components of this signaling pathway are now identified. However, despite the presence of all three components in natural membranes, signaling through receptors is inefficient. This is because there is a lack of cytosolic components which are essential for inositol lipid signaling. In the presence of cytosol, very efficient signaling through the receptor can be observed. The protein in the cytosol that is responsible for efficient signaling is a 35-kDa protein called phosphatidylinositol transfer protein (PI-TP). PI-TP was originally identified as a lipid binding protein that could bind and transfer PI or PC from one membrane

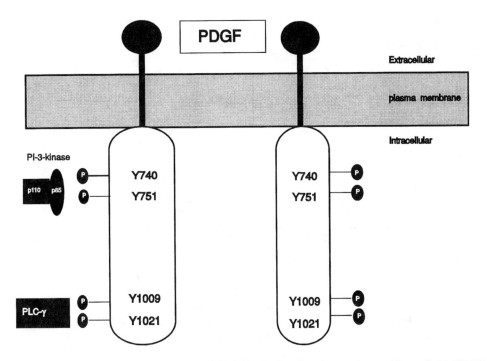

FIGURE 9.6   Recruitment of PLC-γ1 and PI-3-kinase by phosphotyrosine residues of the PDGF receptor. Cross-linking of the PDGF receptor occurs when PDGF binds to its receptor. The receptor contains tyrosine kinase activity which is increased upon cross-linking. Autophosphorylation of specific tyrosine residues occurs. These phosphorylated tyrosine residues can bind to SH2 domains of proteins and forms the basis for recruitment of signaling molecules such as PLC-γ1 and PI-3-kinase from the cytosol.

compartment to another depending on the PI:PC ratio. PI-TP is a highly conserved protein found in all cells and is present at high concentrations.

What role does PI-TP play? The cellular concentration of PI-TP actually dictates the rapid kinetics of IP_3 production in cells upon receptor activation. The mechanism of action of PI-TP is probably related to its ability to bind PI, but since PI is not a substrate for the PLC, it can be speculated that PI-TP presents PI to the inositol lipid kinases for phosphorylation, prior to hydrolysis by PLC.

9.7   PHOSPHOLIPASE D (PLD)

Phospholipase D catalyzes the hydrolytic cleavage of the terminal phosphodiester bond of PC, with the formation of phosphatidic acid and the water-soluble headgroup, choline (Figure 9.7). Also shown in Figure 9.7 is the ability of PLD to transfer the phosphatidyl portion of the PC molecule to ethanol. In this case, the product that is formed is the unusual lipid, phosphatidylethanol (PEt). This lipid is generally absent in cells, but it is relatively metabolically stable in comparison to PA. PA can be converted to DAG by an enzyme known as phosphatidate phosphohydrolase. Transphosphatidylation, in which the phosphatidyl group of the phospholipid is transferred to appropriate nucleophiles such as ethanol, is a unique feature of PLD and, as such, phosphatidylethanol accumulation in the presence of alcohol (0.5%) is routinely used as a marker of PLD activity.

Receptor-mediated formation of PA is a ubiquitous event. Not only do G-protein-coupled receptors stimulate PLD, but also receptors that are tyrosine kinases (e.g., EGF and PDGF

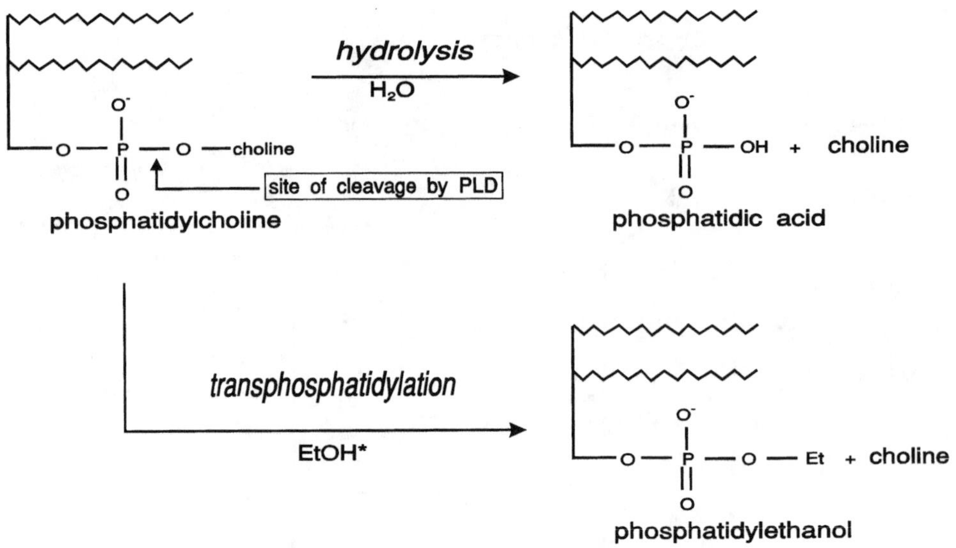

FIGURE 9.7 Hydrolysis of PC by phospholipase D action in the presence and absence of ethanol. Hydrolysis of PC by PLD produces PA and choline. In the presence of ethanol, the products of the reaction are phosphatidylethanol (PEt) and choline. PEt is produced at the expense of PA.

receptors). In addition to agonists, another activator of PLD in intact cells is the protein kinase C activator, phorbol myristate acetate (PMA), a tumor promoter compound widely used in cell signaling studies. In all cells examined, PMA stimulates a prolonged activation of PLD. Similarly, increases in tyrosine phosphorylation are accompanied by PLD activation.

9.8 REGULATION OF PLD

Regulation of PLD has been extensively studied to identify the components that are involved in this signaling process. Multiple mechanisms involving protein kinases and G-proteins have all been suggested (Figure 9.8). Most of our understanding has been obtained by studying the activation of PLD in permeabilized cells where the plasma membrane has been deliberately made permeable to nonhydrolyzable analogues of GTP. These analogues, such as GTP-γ-S, stimulate a robust activation of PLD.

Activation of PLD by GTP-γ-S implies that a G-protein may be required. In addition, direct activators of protein kinase C such as phorbol esters (e.g., PMA) also stimulate PLD. Since, receptor-mediated activation is not sensitive to inhibitors of protein kinase C, this strongly implies that the protein kinase C pathway may not be physiologically relevant. Tyrosine phosphorylation has also been suggested as an alternative pathway for PLD activation.

Although multiple regulation of PLD activity occurs, these pathways are interactive and synergize to provide the full activation of PLD. Thus, activation of PLD by a G-protein pathway is greatly enhanced when PMA is also present. In the absence of any knowledge concerning the molecular details of the PLD enzyme(s), these different regulators may either be operating on different PLD isoforms or on the same enzyme regulated by multiple inputs. A scheme that summarizes the regulatory pathways leading to PLD activation is presented in Figure 9.8. This model encapsulates much of the available information we have about regulation of PLD. These are possible regulatory pathways. What is not known for certain is which mechanism regulates the stimulation of PLD by receptors in intact cells. The stimulation of PLD by the receptor may be exclusively via the G-protein. Such a possibility is suggested by the knowledge that putative inhibitors of the protein kinase C pathway are not inhibitory to receptor-mediated PLD activation.

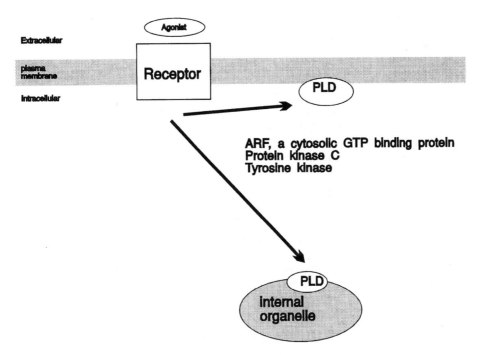

FIGURE 9.8 Potential regulators of phospholipase D. G-protein-coupled receptors and tyrosine kinase receptors when occupied by appropriate agonists activate tyrosine kinase activity as well as phospholipase C. The cell experiences a rise in cytosol Ca^{2+} and activation of protein kinase C (PKC). ARF, a small GTP binding protein is required for activation of PLD. How the receptor triggers the activation of ARF remains to be established. Ca^{2+}, protein tyrosine kinase (PTK), PKC, and the GTP-binding protein, ARF, are potential regulators of PLD individually and in various combinations.

9.8.1 ARF — A SMALL G-PROTEIN PRESENT IN THE CYTOSOL ACTIVATES PLD

Both cytosol and membrane are required for GTP-γ-S-dependent activation of PLD. The cytosol component has been purified to homogeneity and identified by microsequencing to be ARF (**A**DP **R**ibosylation **F**actor), a G-protein of 21 kDa. The membrane compartment contains the PLD.

There are over 40 distinct, low molecular weight G-proteins related to Ras and they regulate a diverse range of cellular processes. These proteins are collectively referred to as belonging to the Ras superfamily and, based on sequence homology, are classified into four subfamilies, Ras, Rho, Arf, and Rab. Ras proteins are essential components of receptor-mediated signal transduction pathways; stimulating proliferation and differentiation. Members of the Rab and Arf subfamily are involved in membrane traffic in the endocytic and exocytic pathway; while members of the rho subfamily participate in cytoskeletal actin organization.

ARF belongs to a family of six members (ARF1–6) found in all eukaryotic cells. ARF was originally identified as a cofactor required for efficient ADP-ribosylation of G_s by cholera toxin, hence its name. Subsequently, it was shown to be a G-protein with structural homology to both the monomeric as well as the heterotrimeric G-proteins.

ARF is myristoylated at the N-terminus. Despite this lipid modification, ARF is mainly present in the cytosol in the GDP-bound form. However, it can translocate to membranes when bound to GTP. ARF is an unusual G-protein in that it will only bind GTP in the presence of a lipid.

9.8.2 PHYSIOLOGICAL ROLE OF PLD

The physiological significance of PLD activation in cells is not apparent, but its role is likely to be related to providing an intracellular signal for a specific cellular event. The time-course for PA formation coincides with the time-course of secretion from intact human neutrophils stimulated by fMetLeuPhe. PA production can be diverted to PEt in the presence of ethanol and this leads to inhibition of secretion in many cell types; examples include secretion from mast cells, platelets, and neutrophils. Moreover, addition of exogenous PLD also stimulates physiological responses in many cell types including insulin release from pancreatic islets and aldosterone secretion from adrenal glomerulosa cells. It seems likely that PLD activation may be related to secretory events.

The ARF connection supports this line of thinking. ARF proteins are thought to participate in a number of membrane trafficking events, in particular traffic through the secretory pathway. What are the consequences when PC is hydrolyzed to PA by PLD? This remains a matter of debate and several possibilities have been suggested:

1. PA may function as a second messenger. For example, it may regulate a protein kinase or a lipid kinase.
2. PA may be converted to DAG, which may be the true messenger. DAG, would then activate protein kinase C.
3. Hydrolysis of PC would increase the ratio of PI:PC in membranes and this may be essential for secretory function.

Clearly, PLD is important in some aspect of cell function. There remain many unanswered questions and identification of PLD function will shed new light on cellular signaling pathways.

9.9 PHOSPHOLIPASE A$_2$ — LIBERATION OF ARACHIDONIC ACID

Many cell types release arachidonic acid from their phospholipids on cell stimulation. Although the main function of arachidonic acid is as a precursor for the biosynthesis of the potent extracellular mediators, the eicosanoids, it may also have a role as an intracellular second messenger.

Most arachidonic acid stored in mammalian cells is esterified at the sn-2 position of glycerophospholipids. PLA$_2$ directly cleaves arachidonic acid from the sn-2 position of the phospholipid, releasing the corresponding lyso-phospholipid. The predominant pools of endogenous arachidonate are distributed between phosphatidylethanolamine (60%), phosphatidylcholine (18%), and phosphatidylinositol (18%). These three phospholipids are the probable source of arachidonic acid in stimulated cells. The enzyme does not appear to be specific for the phospholipid headgroup but specificity resides in cleaving arachidonic acid.

PLA$_2$ enzymes are classified into two groups. One group is represented by the closely related secretory phospholipases A$_2$ that are prevalent in digestive processes (e.g., in pancreas, snake venoms, and secretory granules of neutrophils and platelets). Characteristic of their extracellular location, these secretory phospholipases A$_2$ contain seven disulfide bonds. This is of particular significance since the secretory phospholipases A$_2$ would be inactivated if they came into contact with the reducing environment of the cytosol. Moreover, the secretory phospholipases A$_2$ do not demonstrate any selectivity among the fatty acids in the sn-2 position of phospholipids.

Many ligands that couple to G-proteins or activate tyrosine kinases have been shown to stimulate PLA$_2$, leading to a specific release of arachidonic acid. A phospholipase A$_2$ which has a molecular weight of 85 kDa has been identified in the cytosol (referred to as cPLA$_2$). The cDNA clone encoding for the enzyme has been isolated, and from the amino acid sequence it is clear that it shares no homology with the secreted forms of PLA_2. $cPLA_2$ selectively hydrolyzes arachidonic acid when a natural membrane is used as the source of substrate.

The most interesting feature of $cPLA_2$ so far identified is its ability to associate with membranes when the Ca^{2+} concentration is increased above 300 nM. The ability of $cPLA_2$ to translocate to membranes in a Ca^{2+}-dependent manner appears dependent upon a domain, 45 amino acids long, that delineates a Ca^{2+}-dependent phospholipid-binding motif (referred to as CalB domain). This motif is also present in some other proteins, including protein kinase C, GTPase activating protein (GAP), and PLC-γ1. The biochemical features of $cPLA_2$ strongly suggests that this enzyme may be the target for the hormonally-stimulated phospholipase A_2 activity responsible for mobilizing arachidonic acid in many cell types.

9.9.1 cPLA₂ is Phosphorylated and Activated by MAP Kinase

$cPLA_2$ is substrate for MAP kinase, an enzyme that is rapidly stimulated by growth factor receptor tyrosine kinases, by receptors coupled to G-proteins, and by phorbol ester. Therefore, activation of MAP kinase serves as a convergence point that integrates diverse receptor-mediated signal transduction pathways. Several MAP kinase isoforms (p42 and p44) have been purified and cloned, and the activation of some of these isoforms requires phosphorylation at both tyrosine and threonine residues.

MAP kinase phosphorylates a serine residue (ser^{505}) in a stoichiometric fashion, and this phosphorylation increases the activity of the enzyme twofold. In contrast, mutation of this serine residue to an alanine residue decreases the activity of $cPLA_2$.

Figure 9.9 provides a model of how $cPLA_2$ may be activated by receptors. In this model, the rapid activation of $cPLA_2$ is achieved by synergistic actions of Ca^{2+} and phosphorylation of $cPLA_2$ by MAP kinase. Increased Ca^{2+} causes translocation to the membrane, where the substrate is localized. This step is essential for the activation, and is thought to be mediated by the Ca^{2+}-dependent lipid binding domain (CaLB) located at the amino terminus of $cPLA_2$. MAP kinase activation can occur via a protein kinase C-dependent and -independent pathway. The activated MAP kinase can then phosphorylate $cPLA_2$, and phosphorylation of $cPLA_2$ at Ser^{505} causes an increase in $cPLA_2$ activity.

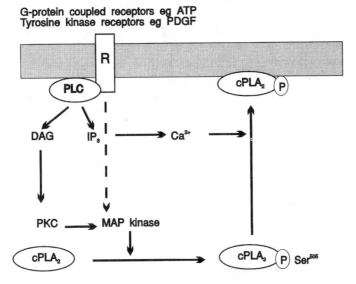

FIGURE 9.9   Mechanism of PLA_2 activation by receptors. Receptors activate the PLC pathway and increase cytosol Ca^{2+} and DAG, leading to PKC activation. PKC activates MAP kinase which can phosphorylate PLA_2 at ser^{505}. Both Ca^{2+} and phosphorylation are required for activation of PLA_2.

9.9.2 OTHER REGULATORY PATHWAYS FOR PLA₂ ACTIVATION

It is unlikely that there is only one mechanism that activates phospholipase A_2. In permeabilized cells, addition of GTP-γ-S stimulates PLA_2. This activation requires the presence of Ca^{2+}, but is not dependent on MgATP, and hence phosphorylation is not essential. The G-proteins responsible for this activation have yet to be identified.

9.10 PHOSPHOINOSITIDE-3-KINASE (PI-3-KINASE)

Ligand binding to a variety of cell-surface receptors leads to a rapid activation of an enzyme known as phosphoinositide-3-kinase (PI-3-kinase). *In vivo*, this enzyme is thought to phosphorylate the headgroup of $PI(1,4,5)P_3$ in the 3-position to yield $PI(1,3,4,5)P_4$, a highly polar lipid. This lipid has been postulated to act as a second messenger in cells, but its putative target(s) are not known. Many agonists activate this pathway; receptors that are tyrosine kinases or indirectly activate tyrosine kinase (e.g., PDGF, insulin, interleukin-2, colony stimulating factor) and G-protein-coupled receptors (e.g., thrombin, fMetLeuPhe) both activate this pathway.

Three forms of PI kinase (I, II, and III) can be distinguished on the basis of size and inhibition by detergents and adenosine. Type I PI kinase phosphorylates the D-3 position of the inositol ring, whereas types II and III enzymes phosphorylate the D-4 position. The products of types II and III PI kinases are substrates for phospholipase C. The PI-3-kinase enzyme has been identified as a heterodimer consisting of a regulatory subunit (p85) and a catalytic subunit (p110) (Figure 9.6).

PI-3-kinase was initially observed in immunoprecipitates of the viral SRC gene product, pp60^{v-src}, in Rous sarcoma virus-transformed cells. Subsequently, PI-3-kinase recruitment to the tyrosine kinase receptors was shown to occur via the SH2 domains of the p85 subunit (Figure 9.6). Since mutant tyrosine kinases, which lack mitogenic or cell transforming activity, fail to associate with PI-3-kinase, it has been suggested that this enzyme may provide cells with some critical signal(s).

In contrast to receptors that act through tyrosine kinases, G-protein-coupled receptors activate a different isoform of PI-3-kinase (γ-isoform). In the case of G-protein-coupled receptors, $\beta\gamma$-subunits of G-proteins activate this isoform of PI-3-kinase (identified in neutrophils).

Wortmannin is a fungal metabolite which binds with high specificity to p110 of PI-3-kinase at nanomolar concentrations. Wortmannin has been used to identify potential pathways where PI-3-kinase may be involved. Wortmannin is a potent inhibitor of several functional responses such as histamine secretion from mast cells, oxidative burst in neutrophils, and membrane ruffling in endothelial cells. In the case of the oxidative burst there is good evidence that another small G-protein, Rac1, is required for assembly of oxidase components at the correct membrane location. Rac1, has also been implicated in the mechanism by which PDGF stimulates membrane ruffling in fibroblasts. Membrane ruffling requires the reorganization of actin filaments. It is, therefore, plausible that the synthesis of $PI(3,4,5)P_3$ may trigger the activation of Rac in cells.

9.11 SUMMARY

The concept that the rather abundant phospholipids are not just structural components that provide the limits of the cell but are sources of a wide variety of second messengers is now widely accepted. Either lipid hydrolysis through phospholipases or lipid synthesis by kinases can generate these second messengers. Hydrolysis of $PI(4,5)P_2$ gives two second messengers, IP_3 and DAG. PLC activation by receptors occurs either via G-proteins or via tyrosine phosphorylation. In addition, PI-TP, a cytosolic protein, is essential for efficient signaling. Activation of PLD is mediated by a small GTP binding protein, ARF. PLA_2, a cytosolic enzyme, is phosphorylated by MAP kinase and this activates the enzyme. In addition, PLA_2 requires Ca^{2+} (300 nM) to migrate to the membrane where its substrate is present. PI-3-kinase phosphorylates $PI(1,4,5)P_3$ to make a highly polar lipid, $PI(1,3,4,5)P_4$, and activation of this family of enzyme can also be regulated by $\beta\gamma$-subunits of G proteins or by tyrosine phosphorylation. The significance of switching on the PLD and PI-3-kinase remains to be clarified.

What should be clear is that the signaling pathways within cells are formed by chains of intercommunicating proteins. Each protein component of a pathway integrates signals from upstream activators (e.g., receptors) and passes them on to various downstream targets or effector proteins. A clear hierarchy emerges when one examines the interconnections between the assorted phospholipases and PI-3-kinase. It should be obvious that PLC and PI-3-kinase are upstream events to phospholipase D and A_2. PLC and PI-3-kinase are coupled to receptors by G-proteins or recruited by phosphotyrosine residues to SH2 domains, while activation of PLD and PLA_2 are consequences of upstream events including the second messengers formed by PLC and PI-3-kinase. The integration of the signaling pathways is summarized in Figure 9.10.

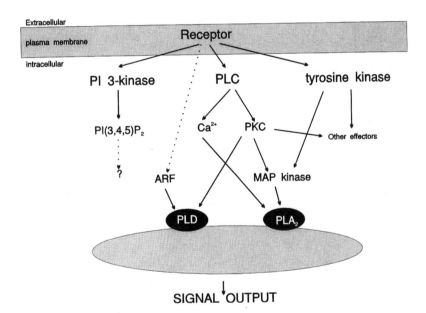

FIGURE 9.10 Communication network involving the phospholipases and PI-3-kinase. PI-3-kinase and PLC are upstream events linked closely to receptors while activation of PLD and PLA_2 are events downstream to PI-3-kinase and PLC. Activation of ARF by receptors is currently not known.

9.12 FURTHER READING

Phospholipase C

Berstein, G., J. L. Blank, D. Y. Jhon, J. H. Exton, S. G. Rhee, and E. M. Ross, 1992. Phospholipase C-β1 is a GTPase-activating protein for Gq/11, its physiologic regulator, *Cell,* 70: 411-418.

Rhee, S. G. and K. D. Choi, 1992. Regulation of inositol phospholipid-specific phospholipase C isozymes, *J. Biol. Chem.,* 267: 12393-12396.

Park, D., D. Jhon, C. Lee, K. Lee, and S. G. Rhee, 1993. Activation of phospholipase C isozymes by G protein $\beta\gamma$ subunits, *J. Biol. Chem.,* 268: 4573-4576.

Thomas, G. M. H., E. Cunningham, A. Fensome, A. Ball, N. F. Totty, O. Troung, J. J. Hsuan, and S. Cockcroft, 1993. An essential role for phosphatidylinositol transfer protein in phospholipase C-mediated inositol lipid signalling, *Cell,* 74: 919-928.

Phospholipase A$_2$

Clark, J. D., L.-L. Lin, R. W. Kriz, C. S. Ramesha, L. A. Sultzman, A. Y. Lin, N. Milona, and J. L. Knopf, 1991. A novel arachidonic acid-selective cytosolic PLA$_2$ contains a Ca^2-dependent translocation domain with homology to PKC and GAP, *Cell,* 65: 1043-1051.

Lin, L.-L., M. Wartman, A. Y. Lin, J. L. Knopf, A. Seth, and R. G. Davis, 1993. cPLA$_2$ is phosphorylated and activated by MAP kinase, *Cell,* 72: 269-278.

Phospholipase D

Billah, M. M., 1993. Phospholipase D and cell signaling, *Curr. Opinion Immunol.,* 5: 114-123.

Cockcroft, S., G. M. H. Thomas, A. Fensome, B. Geny, E. Cunningham, I. Gout, I. Hiles, N. F. Totty, O. Troung, and J. J. Hsuan, 1994. Phospholipase D: A downstream effector of ARF in granulocytes, *Science,* 263: 523–526.

PI-3-Kinase

Stephens, L. R., T. R. Jackson, and P. T. Hawkins, 1993. Agonist-stimulated synthesis of phosphatidyli-nositol-(3,4,5)- trisphosphate: a new intracellular signaling system?, *Biochim. Biophys. Acta,* 1179: 27-75.

Stephens, L. R., A. Smrcka, F. T. Cooke, T. R. Jackson, P. C. Sternweis, and P. T. Hawkins, 1994. A novel, phosphoinositide-3-kinase activity in myeloid-derived cells is activated by G-protein βγ-subunits. *Cell,* 74: 83-93.

10 Calcium and Hormone Action

Ole H. Petersen, Carl C.H. Petersen,
and Haruo Kasai

CONTENTS

10.1 INTRODUCTION

The calcium ion (Ca^{2+}) is now recognized as one of the key cytosolic messengers capable of controlling metabolism, contraction, secretion, growth, and even cell death. Cytosolic Ca^{2+} signals are transient or sustained elevations of the cytoplasmic Ca^{2+} concentration ($[Ca^{2+}]_i$) most frequently occurring as repetitive short-lasting rises in $[Ca^{2+}]_i$ (Ca^{2+} spiking) with a frequency dependent on the stimulating hormone or neurotransmitter concentration. Such signals can either be due to primary opening of plasma membrane Ca^{2+} channels or due to release of Ca^{2+} stored in intracellular organelles. In many cell types, primary release of Ca^{2+} from intracellular stores is followed by secondary opening of plasma membrane Ca^{2+} channels. The best-known plasma membrane Ca^{2+} channels belong to the class of voltage-sensitive ion channels and are usually opened as a consequence of membrane depolarization. This chapter will not deal with such channels, but will concentrate entirely on the processes involved in the control of Ca^{2+} release from internal stores and the events that follow.

It has been known for more than 20 years that hormones and neurotransmitters can evoke release of Ca^{2+} from intracellular stores followed by Ca^{2+} entry from the extracellular fluid. Ten years ago, the discovery that inositol (1,4,5) trisphosphate (IP_3) was the messenger linking hormone-receptor interaction to intracellular Ca^{2+} release marked an important turning point in the development of this subject. Due to the development of methods for high-resolution intracellular calcium measurement considerable insights have recently been obtained into the complex spatiotemporal patterns of hormone-evoked changes in the cytosolic Ca^{2+} concentration ($[Ca^{2+}]_i$). Astonishingly subtle spatial and temporal regulations of $[Ca^{2+}]_i$ can induce ordered sequences of events (dynamic decoding) and agonist-specific $[Ca^{2+}]_i$ signatures.

Hormones and neurotransmitters often act via the same mechanisms. In pancreatic acinar cells both the neurotransmitter acetylcholine (ACh) and the peptide hormone cholecystokinin (CCK) evoke cytosolic Ca^{2+} signals mediated via Ca^{2+} release through IP_3 receptors (IP_3R). The gastrointestinal hormone CCK is also a neurotransmitter. It is therefore not useful to make a sharp distinction between hormone and neurotransmitter actions. This chapter concentrates on the events following the formation of IP_3 which lead to cytosolic Ca^{2+} signal generation. Another chapter in this volume deals with the production and metabolism of IP_3. As a basis for understanding cytosolic Ca^{2+} signal generation we shall first briefly describe the various types of Ca^{2+} transporters known, then proceed to discuss the spatial and temporal aspects of Ca^{2+} signaling, including various oscillator models, and thereafter attempt to explain dose-dependent regulation as well as hormone-specific signal patterns. We shall finally describe some of the molecular targets for Ca^{2+} action as well as the decoding of the signals.

10.2 CELLULAR CALCIUM HOMEOSTASIS

$[Ca^{2+}]_i$ is controlled by the interaction of cytosolic calcium buffers and three categories of transport proteins (channels, carriers, and pumps) expressed differentially on the plasma membrane and on the membranes of calcium stores (Figure 10.1). The resting $[Ca^{2+}]_i$ is maintained low at 0.1 µM, but under hormone stimulation it may rise to 1 µM and in small domains to even higher levels. The most important functional characteristics of the components involved in cellular Ca^{2+} control will be described.

10.2.1 CALCIUM PUMPS

Work on the muscle-relaxing factor led to the discovery of an ATP-linked concentration of Ca^{2+} in a particulate fraction (sarcoplasmic reticulum). It was only later that the role of the endoplasmic reticulum (ER) in controlling $[Ca^{2+}]_i$ became clear. The Ca^{2+} pump in the cell membrane was discovered by Schatzmann in 1966 and the molecular properties of the purified enzyme have been described in some detail. The electrogenic Ca^{2+} pump in the ER, sarcoplasmic reticulum, and cell membrane belong to the P-type of ATPases that are inhibited by orthovanadate. However, from an experimental point of view, it is important that the tumor promoter thapsigargin inhibits the Ca^{2+}-ATPase in the ER but not in the plasma membrane.

Until recently, there has been little precise information about the acute regulation of Ca^{2+} pumps in intact cells. The relationship between $[Ca^{2+}]_i$ and the velocity of Ca^{2+}-pump-mediated Ca^{2+} extrusion has been assessed with the double-fluorescence microdroplet method, which allows simultaneous measurements of Ca^{2+} extrusion and $[Ca^{2+}]_i$ in single cells. During agonist stimulation, the velocity of Ca^{2+} extrusion is directly and acutely regulated by changes in $[Ca^{2+}]_i$ within the range 0.1 to 1 µM. When agonist stimulation evokes repetitive cytosolic Ca^{2+} spikes, each spike is associated with a synchronous increase in Ca^{2+} extrusion velocity.

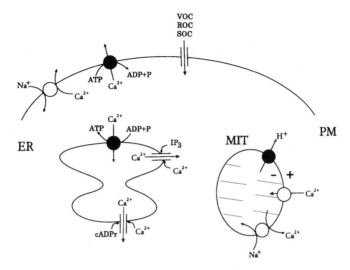

FIGURE 10.1 General outline of Ca^{2+} transport pathways and compartments. The plasma membrane (PM) contains the Na^+-Ca^{2+} exchanger and the Ca^{2+} ATPase and Ca^{2+} entry channels, which can be voltage operated (VOC), receptor operated (ROC), or operated by intracellular store depletion (SOC). The major mobilizable intracellular Ca^{2+} store is in the endoplasmic reticulum (ER) and in ER-derived organelles. These contain Ca^{2+} ATPase and the two types of Ca^{2+} release channels: one activated by inositol trisphosphate (IP_3) and Ca^{2+} and the other by cyclic ADP ribose (cADPr) and Ca^{2+}. The mitochondria (MIT) can accumulate Ca^{2+} via a uniporter because of the intramitochondrial negativity relative to the cytoplasm produced by the electrogenic H^+ pump. The Ca^{2+} exit pathway is provided by a Na^+-Ca^{2+} exchanger.

A large amount of Ca^{2+} is transported since the whole of the mobilizable cellular Ca^{2+} pool can be pumped out within a few minutes. The Ca^{2+} uptake and the Ca^{2+}-ATPase in the ER are half-maximally inhibited when the intravesicular Ca^{2+} concentration is about 300 μM. It is therefore likely that the Ca^{2+}-ATPase of the ER is regulated both by $[Ca^{2+}]_i$ (an increase activating the pump) and the free Ca^{2+} concentration in the lumen of the ER (an increase inhibiting the pump).

In several electrically excitable cell types there is also Na^+-Ca^{2+} exchange. This is an electrogenic process with a stoichiometry of 3 Na^+ per Ca^{2+}. Na^+-Ca^{2+} exchange is not linked to ATP consumption, but does depend on the Na^+-K^+-ATPase (sodium-potassium pump) establishing an adequate transmembrane Na^+ gradient. In many epithelial cells Na^+-Ca^{2+} exchange is insignificant.

10.2.2 Ca^{2+} Channels

There are two types of Ca^{2+} release channels in the ER, namely the ryanodine receptor (RYR) and the IP_3 receptor (IP_3R). The RYR has been characterized at the single-channel level, its amino acid sequence determined, and it is now recognized that there is a family of RYRs. The RYR is activated by a rise in $[Ca^{2+}]_i$, explaining the Ca^{2+}-induced Ca^{2+} release process. The curve relating channel open state probability (P_o) to $[Ca^{2+}]_i$ shows that P_o increases when $[Ca^{2+}]_i$ increases from 0.1 μM to 1 μM, but decreases when $[Ca^{2+}]_i$ increases from 10 μM to 1 mM.

Caffeine potentiates Ca^{2+}-induced Ca^{2+} release via the RYR, and at high enough concentrations the RYR becomes sensitive to the resting $[Ca^{2+}]_i$. Caffeine is a convenient tool because it is extremely membrane-permeant, but unfortunately caffeine inhibits IP_3-evoked Ca^{2+} release and also inhibits agonist-induced IP_3 production, so that the interpretation of caffeine-evoked effects in intact cells can be difficult. There is now substantial evidence indicating that the NAD^+ metabolite cyclic ADP-ribose can enhance Ca^{2+}-induced Ca^{2+} release by sensitizing the RYR to Ca^{2+}.

The IP_3R has been studied at the single-channel level and its amino acid sequence determined. There is a family of IP_3Rs derived from three or four distinct genes with different sensitivities to IP_3. Although the RYR is about twice as large as the IP_3R there are regions of homology, particularly in their C-terminal domains which have the membrane-spanning regions. Binding of IP_3 to its receptor causes channel opening, but cytosolic Ca^{2+} also acts as a coagonist together with IP_3. In the presence of a submaximal IP_3 concentration, a rise in $[Ca^{2+}]_i$ from 0.1 to 0.3 μM evokes a sharp increase in P_o whereas a further increase in $[Ca^{2+}]_i$ to 1 μM markedly decreases P_o. The Ca^{2+} dose-response curve for the IP_3 receptor is thus bell-shaped with a maximum P_o at a $[Ca^{2+}]_i$ of 0.2 to 0.3 μM. We have no single-channel data about the dynamic response to acute changes in $[Ca^{2+}]_i$ and IP_3 concentration.

Heparin competes with IP_3 for binding to the IP_3R, but does not induce channel opening and is therefore a good competitive antagonist. A monoclonal antibody to the IP_3R microinjected into oocytes has been shown to block Ca^{2+} oscillations and Ca^{2+} waves, but such a large molecule cannot easily be applied to small cells via patch-clamp pipettes.

The Ca^{2+} entry channels in the plasma membrane, other than the well-characterized voltage-gated Ca^{2+} channels, seem to be manifold and have not yet been fully characterized. IP_3 directly induces opening of Ca^{2+}-permeable channels in excised inside-out patches from Jurkat T cells, and a recent study shows IP_3 activation of a Ca^{2+} current in human T cells which is inhibited when $[Ca^{2+}]_i$ is elevated. These channels are not activated by the IP_3 phosphorylation product inositol (1,3,4,5) tetrakisphosphate (IP_4), but it has been shown that IP_4 can activate a Mn^{2+}-permeable Ca^{2+} channel in excised patches from endothelial cells. The IP_4-sensitive channels were not activated by IP_3, and IP_4 only opened pathways when $[Ca^{2+}]_i$ was elevated. There is also indirect evidence for Ca^{2+} entry evoked by a combination of IP_3 and IP_4 in lacrimal gland cells.

Depletion of intracellular Ca^{2+} stores in mast cells, as well as in many others, activates a Ca^{2+} current, known as Ca^{2+} release-activated Ca^{2+} current (I_{CRAC}), through channels with a low unit conductance. The ionophore ionomycin and the Ca^{2+}-chelator EGTA can activate I_{CRAC} in the presence of heparin, indicating that IP_3 does not directly control these channels. A recent study of noradrenaline-mediated Ca^{2+} entry in smooth muscle cells suggests that Ca^{2+} store depletion, IP_3, and IP_4, all contribute to the control of Ca^{2+} entry.

10.2.3 Ca^{2+} Stores

The nonmitochondrial Ca^{2+} stores in the ER, or modified portions of the ER, contain Ca^{2+} pumps, Ca^{2+} release channels, and in the lumen, Ca^{2+} binding proteins such as calsequestrin and calreticulin. The distribution of IP_3Rs and RYRs can vary considerably between different cell types, with IP_3Rs and RYRs segregated in separate stores or colocalized. Primary $[Ca^{2+}]_i$ rises have been detected near the nucleus, Golgi apparatus, rough ER, and secretory granules. A rapid exchange of Ca^{2+} can be demonstrated not only in the ER but also in the Golgi apparatus and the nucleus with the ion microscope. There is now also evidence for IP_3Rs in the inner nuclear membrane which may be responsible for nucleoplasmic Ca^{2+} signals.

In the past, mitochondria were thought to play a key role in intracellular Ca^{2+} homeostasis, but this view was modified and a significant involvement of mitochondria in Ca^{2+} homeostasis was proposed only when $[Ca^{2+}]_i$ had risen to pathological levels. It is now clear that agonist stimulation primarily releases Ca^{2+} from the ER and/or ER-derived organelles and it is generally accepted that in the resting state the mitochondria contain little Ca^{2+}, but the role of mitochondria in cellular Ca^{2+} homeostasis is now being reassessed. In intact cells, mitochondria accumulate Ca^{2+} after agonist stimulation, and in permeabilized cells there is a very marked increase in mitochondrial Ca^{2+} content when $[Ca^{2+}]_i$ increases above 0.5 μM. Ca^{2+} uptake into mitochondria is mediated by a carrier, namely a uniporter. The large electrical potential difference created by the respiratory chain H^+ extrusion mechanism provides the driving force. The Ca^{2+} exit pathway from mitochondria is mainly the result of Na^+-Ca^{2+} exchange.

10.2.4 CYTOSOLIC CALCIUM BUFFERS

The cytosol contains slowly diffusible Ca^{2+} binding proteins which are capable of rapidly buffering Ca^{2+}. The effect of these buffers is likely to be highly significant near the Ca^{2+} release channels and the saturation of such buffers may be essential for both initiation of the Ca^{2+} spike and the propagation of the Ca^{2+} wave.

10.3 SPATIAL ORGANIZATION OF CA^{2+} SIGNALS

10.3.1 CALCIUM MICROGRADIENTS

Agonists can induce steep spatial gradients of $[Ca^{2+}]_i$ because Ca^{2+} is buffered and sequestered efficiently. Ca^{2+} gradients formed by this mechanism will be referred to as Ca^{2+} microgradients, since the gradients occur within a spatial dimension of 1 to 10 μm. The Ca^{2+} microgradients can be visualized with currently available methods of Ca^{2+} imaging. Three distinct aspects of the Ca^{2+} microgradients will be discussed separately: the primary site of the $[Ca^{2+}]_i$ rise, the Ca^{2+} spikes, and the spread of the $[Ca^{2+}]_i$ rise.

Several distinct mechanisms for the primary rise in $[Ca^{2+}]_i$ seem to exist. Firstly and most simply, the primary rise in $[Ca^{2+}]_i$ can be triggered at the site of the primary stimulus, for example, sperm triggering the initial rise in $[Ca^{2+}]_i$ at the point of entry in the egg. This mechanism could also account for synapse-specific control of rises in $[Ca^{2+}]_i$ at postsynaptic dendrites. Secondly, if agonist receptors are localized, even homogeneous stimuli could give rise to inhomogeneous rises in $[Ca^{2+}]_i$. Thirdly, the primary Ca^{2+} release site will depend on the spatial distribution and heterogeneity of the Ca^{2+} release channels. For example, in *Limulus* photoreceptors, only the light-sensitive R-lobe is sensitive to IP_3. In *Xenopus* oocytes, flash photolysis of caged IP_3 revealed primary rises in $[Ca^{2+}]_i$ at certain hot spots or foci. More recently, such a mechanism has been proposed to account for the agonist-induced primary rises in $[Ca^{2+}]_i$ in a small trigger zone within the secretory granule area of pancreatic acinar cells (Figure 10.2). IP_3 injected from the opposite side (basal area) of the cells evoked a primary rise in $[Ca^{2+}]_i$ in the trigger zone. This observation indicates that, during agonist stimulation, IP_3 produced at the basolateral membrane could diffuse and primarily act on IP_3 receptors in the trigger zone. In fact, IP_3 could act as a global messenger in small cells. The higher IP_3 sensitivity in the trigger zone is probably due to the localized presence of IP_3 receptors with higher affinity than those in the basal area. Alternatively, the density of IP_3 receptors in the trigger zone may be very high.

10.3.2 LOCAL AND GLOBAL CA^{2+} SPIKES

Rises in $[Ca^{2+}]_i$ induced via Ca^{2+} release channels often occur in the form of repetitive spiking; they exhibit a sharp upstroke from a threshold $[Ca^{2+}]_i$ level and recover to the resting level during sustained stimulation. The mechanisms for spike generation will be discussed later. As typified in the case of pancreatic acinar cells, these Ca^{2+} spikes can occur locally at a specific subcellular domain and form Ca^{2+} microgradients (Figure 10.2). With a sufficiently high IP_3 level and IP_3R sensitivity, the local Ca^{2+} spike can subsequently spread as a wave towards other cellular areas. The global rises in $[Ca^{2+}]_i$ can also be induced transiently, and will be referred to as global Ca^{2+} spikes (Figure 10.2). The cell is thus able to control the spatial extent of the Ca^{2+} signal, which is functionally and energetically important (Figure 10.2).

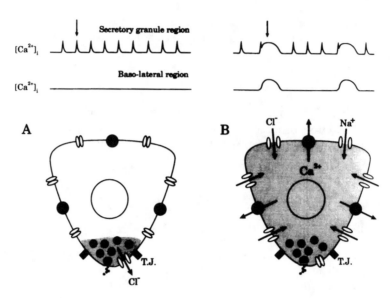

FIGURE 10.2 Local and global cytosolic Ca^{2+} spikes illustrated diagrammatically on the basis of data obtained on pancreatic acinar cells. The cartoons A and B show single acinar cells in which tight junctions (T.J.) separate a small luminal from a much larger basolateral plasma membrane area. Secretory (zymogen) granules are shown in the area close to the luminal membrane (secretory granule region). Ca^{2+}-activated Cl^- and nonselective cation (at physiological membrane potentials, mainly allowing Na^+ influx) channels are shown together with Ca^{2+} pumps. The nucleus is also indicated. The shaded areas represent regions in which $[Ca^{2+}]_i$ is elevated at the times corresponding to the arrows above the $[Ca^{2+}]_i$ traces shown in the top part of the figure. In A the Ca^{2+} signal (for example, generated by a low concentration of ACh or intracellular IP_3 infusion) consists of repetitive Ca^{2+} spikes exclusively in the secretory granule region, whereas in B a more complex signal pattern is shown composed of short-lasting spikes in the secretory granule region followed in some cases by larger global transients generated, for example, by stimulation with the hormone cholecystokinin (CCK).

10.3.3 CA^{2+} WAVES

The coordinated Ca^{2+} activation of many cellular processes is due to waves of Ca^{2+} propagating through the cytosol at velocities of 5 to 100 μm/s. Since the amplitude of a Ca^{2+} wave is nondecremental, active release processes must be triggered by a diffusible factor. Ca^{2+} itself is likely to be the diffusible factor, since positive feedback effects of Ca^{2+} on the Ca^{2+} release channels, IP_3Rs and RYRs, have been discovered.

IP$_3$Rs seem to be responsible for the regenerative Ca^{2+} waves in some oocytes, since they do not have RYRs. Injection of antibodies against the IP$_3$R blocks the IP$_3$-induced, as well as sperm-induced, Ca^{2+} waves in hamster eggs. Many other cells, however, express both IP$_3$Rs and RYRs. For example, smooth muscle cells appear to utilize primarily IP$_3$Rs for the agonist-induced Ca^{2+} waves, despite the fact that they have plenty of RYRs. In sea urchin eggs, on the other hand, RYRs are localized in the cortex, and sperm induces Ca^{2+} waves in the cortical area. In pancreatic acinar cells IP$_3$Rs and RYR-like channels appear to be distributed in different subcellular areas: IP$_3$Rs in the trigger zone and basolateral region, whereas RYR-like channels are in the secretory granule region. The Ca^{2+} wave in the secretory granule region is always induced by the primary rise in $[Ca^{2+}]_i$ in the trigger zone, while at high agonist concentrations the Ca^{2+} wave in the basolateral region is triggered by the rise in $[Ca^{2+}]_i$ in the secretory granule region. The Ca^{2+} wave speed may depend on agonist concentration.

10.3.4 Calcium Nanogradients

A distinct type of Ca^{2+} gradient may be formed by the efficient mobilization of Ca^{2+} through Ca^{2+} channels: if Ca^{2+} mobilization is more rapid than the diffusion of Ca^{2+} in the cytosol, then steep gradients of Ca^{2+} appear close to the inner mouth of open Ca^{2+} channels. This form of Ca^{2+} gradient will be referred to as a Ca^{2+} nanogradient, since theoretical analysis indicates that it decays with a space constant of several tens of nanometers. The nanogradients have two further characteristics. First, the maximum $[Ca^{2+}]_i$ near these nanogradients (Ca^{2+} domain), may be as high as 100 µM. Second, these gradients may appear and disappear within a fraction of a millisecond depending on the state of the Ca^{2+} channels. In the case of Ca^{2+} microgradients, $[Ca^{2+}]_i$ rarely exceeds 1 µM and recovery of the rise in $[Ca^{2+}]_i$ normally takes at least several seconds, because of abundant Ca^{2+} buffering and the slow uptake by pumps. The Ca^{2+} nanogradients may be too small and rapid to be captured with the current state of Ca^{2+} imaging methods.

10.4 CALCIUM OSCILLATIONS

Agonist-evoked cytosolic Ca^{2+} oscillations were first demonstrated in blowfly salivary glands where it was also shown that the frequency of Ca^{2+} spikes increased with increasing agonist concentration. It is now clear that the IP_3R is intimately involved in the mechanism of agonist-evoked cytosolic Ca^{2+} spike generation in very many cell types. Many different oscillation patterns have been described depending on type of cell and stimulus. In an individual cell, the oscillation pattern depends on receptor type, agonist concentration, intracellular Ca^{2+} buffering, and Ca^{2+} influx.

10.4.1 How Much Stored Ca²⁺ is Released per Spike?

There is evidence from many different systems that agonists can evoke Ca^{2+} spikes in the absence of external Ca^{2+}, and the primary event must, therefore, be release of stored Ca^{2+}. The number of Ca^{2+} spikes that can be evoked by a constant hormone level, in the absence of external Ca^{2+}, varies between cell types and also depends on the type and strength of stimulation. In pancreatic acinar cells many short-lasting local Ca^{2+} spikes in the secretory granule region can be evoked by IP_3 or a low ACh concentration when the external Ca^{2+} concentration is very low. In the same cells CCK evokes, in addition, broader global Ca^{2+} transients (Figure 10.1), and in experiments with low external Ca^{2+} concentration only a few (two to eight) such events occur. It is of interest to estimate how much intracellularly stored Ca^{2+} is released during each of these global Ca^{2+} spikes. So far, the only direct data are from pancreatic acinar cells using the droplet method. The amount of Ca^{2+} extruded during a CCK-evoked spike corresponded to about 40% of the total mobilizable intracellular Ca^{2+} pool. The amount of stored Ca^{2+} released during a spike must at least be equal to the amount extruded, and therefore at least 40% of the Ca^{2+} stores are emptied. The Ca^{2+} pumps of the ER are likely to take up a considerable proportion of the primarily released Ca^{2+}. A large proportion of the stored Ca^{2+}, perhaps all of it, is released during each spike and, at least in the pancreatic acinar cells, about 40% of the Ca^{2+} released may be extruded, whereas the remaining 60% is likely to be taken back into the ER. The large Ca^{2+} extrusion highlights the need for compensatory Ca^{2+} entry and explains why only a few global spikes can be fired in the absence of external Ca^{2+}.

10.4.2 What Determines Latency and Interspike Periods?

In hepatocytes there is a linear correlation between the time required to observe the first spike after the start of hormonal stimulation (latency) and the period of Ca^{2+} oscillation. It is not clear exactly what happens during the latent period, but results obtained with confocal microfluorimetry of Ca^{2+} signals evoked by photoreleased IP_3 in oocytes show that there is a substantial dose-dependent latency (about 50 to 100 ms) from IP_3 release to a measurable rise in $[Ca^{2+}]_i$. This is not due to a diffusion delay for IP_3 to reach the IP_3R as $[Ca^{2+}]_i$ in the localized region investigated is flat after the photorelease of IP_3 until a sharp rise in $[Ca^{2+}]_i$ occurs. It seems unlikely that there should be a long delay in IP_3-induced opening of IP_3R channels as ligand-gated channels usually respond within a few milliseconds. Intracellular infusion of the Ca^{2+} buffer, citrate has been shown to increase both the latency and the period between ACh-and IP_3-evoked Ca^{2+} spikes in pancreatic acinar cells. The buffering of the primary IP_3-evoked release of Ca^{2+} may, therefore, be an important point to consider. The relevant buffering undoubtedly has many components including a variety of Ca^{2+} binding proteins in the cytosol and on the surface of organelles, as well as active uptake into ER or ER-derived vesicular structures and possibly also mitochondria. It is characteristic for solutions that buffer H^+ or Ca^{2+} that pH or pCa does not change much upon addition of the relevant ion until a sharp transition point is reached. The active Ca^{2+} buffers may behave in a similar fashion. The lumen of the Ca^{2+} stores contain Ca^{2+} binding proteins and progressive Ca^{2+} accumulation could saturate these buffers and cause a sharp rise in the luminal free Ca^{2+} concentration. This would inhibit the Ca^{2+} pump, inducing a sharp rise in $[Ca^{2+}]_i$. An important reason for the latency as well as the quiet period between Ca^{2+} spikes may therefore be charging of passive Ca^{2+} buffers and Ca^{2+} stores.

10.4.3 OSCILLATION MODELS

Models based on pulsatile IP_3 formation have attracted a lot of attention since they would provide a straightforward explanation for pulsatile Ca^{2+} liberation. The IP_3-Ca^{2+} cross-coupling (ICC) model is based on the idea that Ca^{2+} exerts a positive feedback effect on phospholipase C (PLC), in this way stimulating IP_3 formation. The following sequence is envisaged. Agonist stimulation generates IP_3 which in turn initiates Ca^{2+} release via the IP_3R. The rise in $[Ca^{2+}]_i$ stimulates further IP_3 formation leading to acceleration of Ca^{2+} release. Ca^{2+} activation of PLC can occur, but this process may only operate when the PLC is activated via its G-protein. At a high level of $[Ca^{2+}]_i$, the IP_3R is inhibited and Ca^{2+} release stops, allowing Ca^{2+} reuptake into the ER and/or Ca^{2+} extrusion to occur. The resulting fall in $[Ca^{2+}]_i$ terminates PLC activation and $InsP_3$ formation is reduced to the prespike level. The whole process can now repeat itself.

However, spiking can also be evoked by direct infusion of IP_3 or the nonmetabolizable IP_3 analogue, inositol (1,4,5) trisphosphorothioate (IPS_3), and this is a problem for the ICC model. Digital imaging experiments on pancreatic cells have shown directly that a low concentration of IPS_3 can evoke repetitive cytosolic Ca^{2+} spikes in the secretory granule region, just as in the case of stimulation with low agonist concentrations. Since a constant IP_3 level evokes Ca^{2+} spiking, it is necessary to consider how a steady messenger level can induce pulsatile Ca^{2+} release. Before 1990 it was not known that IP_3R was Ca^{2+}-sensitive and it was natural to consider a two-pool model in which a small primary IP_3-induced Ca^{2+} release would be amplified by Ca^{2+}-induced Ca^{2+} release from RYRs in a separate Ca^{2+} store. Following the discovery that an increase in $[Ca^{2+}]_i$ markedly enhances IP_3-induced Ca^{2+} release through IP_3Rs, one-pool models became attractive.

In a simple one-pool model, IP_3-evoked Ca^{2+} release evokes a modest slow rise in $[Ca^{2+}]_i$, and at a threshold level Ca^{2+} markedly enhances the open state probability of the IP_3-activated Ca^{2+} release channels, leading to a dramatic rise in $[Ca^{2+}]_i$ (Figure 10.3). At a higher level of $[Ca^{2+}]_i$, the negative feedback effect of Ca^{2+} on the IP_3R becomes important and the channels close. At this point, the Ca^{2+} pumps cause reuptake of Ca^{2+} into the ER and extrusion into the extracellular solution. In such a model, the negative feedback initiated by a high $[Ca^{2+}]_i$ should continue for a period after $[Ca^{2+}]_i$ has been reduced below the level necessary to induce the effect in the first place. Since the sensitivity to IP_3 recovers as $[Ca^{2+}]_i$ recovers, it is doubtful whether the direct Ca^{2+} inhibition of the IP_3R is sufficient. An additional effect that may be more long-lasting could be mediated by arachidonic acid, which inhibits both ACh and IP_3-evoked Ca^{2+} release. The phospholipase A_2 inhibitor 4-bromophenacyl bromide prolongs and potentiates IP_3-evoked Ca^{2+} transients. The following negative feedback may therefore occur. The Ca^{2+} spike activates phospholipase A_2 inducing arachidonic acid formation. This, in turn, inhibits the IP_3R and Ca^{2+} release is terminated. However, it is not yet clear whether arachidonic acid formation actually plays any role in the Ca^{2+} oscillation mechanism, and for that reason it is useful to consider two-pool models in which the problem concerning long interspike intervals can more easily be overcome.

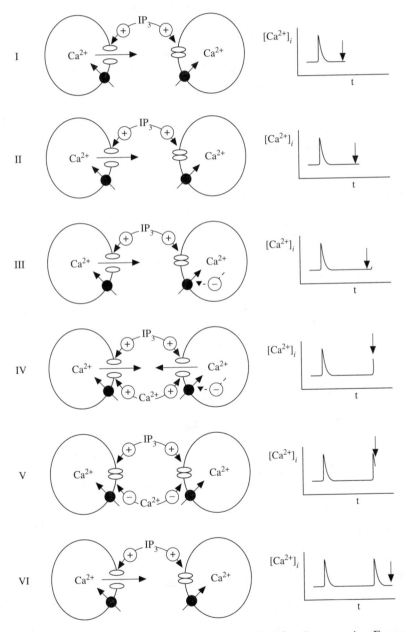

FIGURE 10.3 Two-pool model explaining repetitive cytosolic Ca^{2+} spike generation. For explanation see text ($InsP_3 = IP_3$).

Figure 10.3 illustrates a new form of two-pool model taking into account an apparently fundamental property of IP_3-sensitive stores: quantal Ca^{2+} release. The IP_3-sensitive Ca^{2+} store is probably compartmentalized into vesicular structures and the quantal Ca^{2+} mobilization by IP_3 in single cells may reflect all-or-nothing emptying of stores that differ in their sensitivity to IP_3. This suggests that at a submaximal IP_3 concentration not all IP_3Rs will be open. A subthreshold IP_3 level does not, therefore, primarily activate Ca^{2+} release from all parts of the IP_3-sensitive pool. The small steady Ca^{2+} release is buffered by cytosolic buffers, but also by uptake into stores not initially participating in the Ca^{2+} release process (Figure 10.3, i-ii). This causes a gradual increase in the Ca^{2+} content of these stores and, when the intrastore buffers are saturated, gives rise to a sharp increase in the intravesicular free Ca^{2+} concentration that, in turn, inhibits the Ca^{2+} pump in the membrane of the vesicles (Figure 10.3, iii). Now $[Ca^{2+}]_i$ rises and the channels already participating in the Ca^{2+} release open more frequently. Channels hitherto not responding to IP_3 also open (Figure 10.3, iv). This initiates the explosive Ca^{2+} release that causes the steep rise in $[Ca^{2+}]_i$. Resulting from the now very high Ca^{2+} concentration in the lumen of the vesicles, there will be a substantial driving force for Ca^{2+} release. Soon $[Ca^{2+}]_i$ has risen to a point where the negative feedback on the IP_3R dominates and the channels close (Figure 10.3, v). The intravesicular Ca^{2+} concentration is now low because of the marked release that has taken place and the Ca^{2+} pumps will be fully activated, explaining the falling phase of the Ca^{2+} spike. When $[Ca^{2+}]_i$ is back to the resting level, the whole cycle can repeat itself (Figure 10.3, vi).

The model in Figure 10.3 can be reduced to a single-pool model if all pools are equally sensitive to IP_3. In this case, the Ca^{2+} released (difference between Ca^{2+} release and Ca^{2+} uptake in the same pools) during the interspike period is sequestered exclusively by cytosolic Ca^{2+} buffers. If the IP_3Rs from the less IP_3-sensitive pools are replaced by RYRs, then Figure 10.2 is transformed into the classical two-pool model. It is, of course, also possible that the "second" pool contains both IP_3Rs and RYRs. It cannot be excluded that some agonists may induce fluctuating IP_3 levels that could modulate the basic pattern produced by the mechanism shown in Figure 10.2 (combination of ICC and two-pool model). Several other elements play a role. Substantial amounts of Ca^{2+} are extruded from the cell during each spike, and Ca^{2+} entry is needed to compensate for this loss as otherwise the stores would be unable to reload fully after a spike. The relative importance of passive cytosolic buffering and active buffering by ER Ca^{2+} uptake may vary considerably according to the time course of the oscillating events.

10.5 DOSE-DEPENDENT REGULATION

A physiologically important intracellular messenger such as Ca^{2+} must be regulated in such a way that small changes in the plasma level of the relevant hormone evoke appropriate changes in messenger concentration. In blowfly salivary gland cells, the frequency of Ca^{2+} oscillations increases with increasing 5-hydroxytryptamine concentration in the dose range over which fluid secretion is stimulated. The rate of secretion may, therefore, be a function of second messenger frequency rather than amplitude. In hepatocytes, the frequency but not the amplitude or shape of global cytosolic Ca^{2+} spikes increases with increasing vasopressin or phenylephrine concentration. The simplest explanation is that the cellular IP_3 level is controlled by the intensity of hormone stimulation. An increased level of IP_3 causes a larger primary Ca^{2+} release which, all other factors being unchanged, more rapidly saturates passive and/or active Ca^{2+} buffers, allowing the positive feedback on the IP_3Rs to start earlier in the cycle (Figure 10.3), thereby explaining the increase in spike frequency. Indeed, the shape and frequency of Ca^{2+} spiking evoked by IPS_3 or IP_3 is concentration dependent.

In cells capable of generating both local and global Ca^{2+} spikes the situation is more complex. Pancreatic acinar cells can be stimulated to secrete by the hormone CCK, and the physiological concentration range in plasma after a meal is about 5 to 20 pM. A threshold concentration of CCK of about 5 pM evokes short-lasting Ca^{2+} spikes at a low frequency and only a few of these local spikes in the secretory granule region trigger global Ca^{2+} spikes (Figure 10.2). At a slightly higher concentration (10 to 20 pM), the frequency of local spikes is increased and Ca^{2+} waves are more often triggered. At a pharmacological CCK concentration (for example, 50 pM) every local Ca^{2+} spike triggers a spreading Ca^{2+} wave. The frequency modulation of the local spikes could be explained, as already discussed, by changing IP_3 levels, since an increased IP_3 concentration tends to be associated with a higher spike frequency. A higher IP_3 level may also explain the tendency towards spreading of the Ca^{2+} signal. The local spikes are generated in the secretory granule region either as a result of IP_3Rs having a particularly high affinity for IP_3 or because of a very high density of IP_3Rs in this part of the cell. When the IP_3 concentration is increased by a higher hormone level, the low affinity or low density IP_3Rs in the rest of the cell can also be activated and participate in the Ca^{2+}-induced Ca^{2+} release process, allowing formation of Ca^{2+} waves. In experiments with the nonmetabolizable IP_3 analogue IPS_3, an increase in IPS_3 concentration was associated with a tendency towards generation of broader Ca^{2+} spikes of the global type.

In the case of stimulating pancreatic acinar cells with CCK in the physiological concentration range there is no evidence for regulation of IP_3 production, as it is impossible to detect IP_3 generation in response to CCK concentrations below 100 pM (a toxic level). In this context, it is interesting that the sulfydryl reagent thimerosal can evoke Ca^{2+} spike generation in several cell types, which is dependent on functional IP_3 receptors but without inducing an increase in the IP_3 concentration. The sensitivity of the IP_3R to IP_3 may, therefore, be regulated and it is possible that a hormone, via a mechanism still unknown, can regulate frequency and spreading of Ca^{2+} spikes not only by varying IP_3 levels but also by varying the sensitivity of the IP_3Rs.

There are other mechanisms by which dose-dependent regulation of Ca^{2+} signaling could occur. Hormones may control the Ca^{2+} pumps in the ER and/or the cell membrane. A theoretical model shows that a reduction of the velocity of Ca^{2+} extrusion accelerates Ca^{2+} spiking. There may be messengers that simultaneously control both Ca^{2+} release, channel sensitivity, and the operation of Ca^{2+} pumps. Arachidonic acid can stimulate the Ca^{2+} pump in the cell membrane, but may also reduce the sensitivity of IP_3Rs and IP_4Rs to IP_3 and IP_4, respectively.

10.6 HORMONE-SPECIFIC CALCIUM SIGNAL PATTERNS

Two hormones interacting with separate membrane receptors on the same cell may both use Ca^{2+} as an intracellular messenger, but nevertheless evoke distinct signal patterns so that the information input to the cell is different. In hepatocytes, it has been shown that phenylephrine and vasopressin both evoke cytosolic Ca^{2+} spikes, but the shape of the spikes is receptor specific. The initial phase of the Ca^{2+} spikes (upstroke) are identical, but each vasopressin-induced spike lasts longer because of a slower rate of recovery than in the case of phenylephrine stimulation. Such a relatively simple difference in the Ca^{2+} signal pattern could be explained by different receptor-controlled Ca^{2+}-pump transport rates.

In pancreatic acinar cells the two main agonists ACh and CCK, applied at just supra-threshold concentrations both evoke repetitive local Ca^{2+} spikes in the secretory granule region, but whereas some of the CCK-evoked local spikes trigger global Ca^{2+} transients (Figure 10.2) this is rare for ACh. When the agonist concentration is increased the Ca^{2+} signal pattern, in the case of ACh stimulation, switches to a sinusoidal oscillation (regular fluctuations about a mean elevated $[Ca^{2+}]_i$) whereas in the case of CCK the local Ca^{2+} spike frequency increases and global transients are triggered more often. CCK and ACh therefore evoke very different patterns. The ACh-evoked sinusoidal oscillations cannot be mimicked by any level of CCK and are probably the result of specific stimulation of Ca^{2+} entry, since the sinusoidal oscillations can only be maintained in the presence of external Ca^{2+} whereas the transient spikes can continue for many minutes after removal of external Ca^{2+}. Why low CCK stimuli more easily evoke global Ca^{2+} transients than the equivalent ACh stimuli (dose evoking same local spike frequency) is not clear, but CCK may produce a yet unknown spreading factor. One function of such a factor may be to increase the sensitivity of IP_3Rs and/or RYRs.

10.7 MOLECULAR TARGETS FOR CALCIUM ACTION

Ca^{2+} is different from any other second messenger because it has so many target molecules, namely the Ca^{2+} binding proteins (CaBPs). CaBPs differentially control various cellular processes, such as phosphorylation and dephosphorylation. Coordinated activation of different CaBPs is essential for integrated cellular function.

The coordination is achieved by the spatiotemporal organization of the Ca^{2+} signal and the heterogeneous distribution, affinity, kinetics, and function of CaBPs. Affinities of CaBPs for Ca^{2+} range widely betwen 10 nM and 1 mM, and time courses of activation and deactivation of CaBPs by Ca^{2+} are also different. Although hundreds of CaBPs have been discovered, much work is still required to find further CaBPs and to obtain kinetic data to formulate concrete models for cellular functions. There appears to be a correlation between the affinity and the distribution of CaBPs such that low affinity CaBPs are closely associated with membranes. This can be seen by comparing three major families of CaBPs: EF-hand proteins, the annexin family, and a class of proteins which share the same Ca^{2+}-dependent translocation domain, including cytosolic phospholipase A_2, protein kinase C γ, phospholipase C γ, synaptotagmine, and GTPase activating protein. Many of the EF-hand proteins show high affinity for Ca^{2+} and are distributed in the cytosol. On the other hand, the latter two families of CaBPs display a rather low affinity for Ca^{2+} and are likely to play their roles closely associated with membranes. This may be physiologically relevant, as discussed in the next section.

10.8 CELLULAR FUNCTIONS AND DYNAMICS OF CA^{2+} SIGNALS

Ca^{2+} spikes and oscillations (frequency modulation) have three advantages over a graded amplitude regulation of $[Ca^{2+}]_i$:

1. Ca^{2+} spikes are more resistant to noise than graded rises in $[Ca^{2+}]_i$;
2. A certain frequency of Ca^{2+} spikes could selectively activate CaBPs with particular association and dissociation rate constants for Ca^{2+}; and
3. Local short-lasting Ca^{2+} spikes may have other advantages over a global rise.

A rise in $[Ca^{2+}]_i$ rapidly activates the Ca^{2+} pump in the plasma membrane, but when the Ca^{2+} rise is confined to a small region, only a minor proportion of the plasma membrane will be exposed to an elevated $[Ca^{2+}]_i$ and the amount of Ca^{2+} pumped out of the cell during a spike would be relatively small (Figure 10.2). Apart from this energetic advantage, local spikes may also prevent undesirable Ca^{2+}-dependent activation processes elsewhere in the cell. Ca^{2+} can activate proteases and endonucleases, leading to cell death.

Ca^{2+} microgradients may have considerable physiological significance. For example, a rise in $[Ca^{2+}]_i$ at the postsynaptic membrane is assumed to trigger a synapse-specific modification of synaptic transmission. A polarized rise in $[Ca^{2+}]_i$ of blood cells can modify the direction of migration of these cells. The case of exocrine acinar cells exemplifies the necessity of organized activation of CaBPs in cellular functions. At low agonist concentrations, Ca^{2+}-dependent Cl^- channels are selectively activated by Ca^{2+} spikes in the secretory granule region and Cl^- ions are pushed into the lumen: "push-phase" (Figure 10.2). Outward movement of Cl^- could be driven either by the resting K^+ permeability or by Ca^{2+}-dependent K^+ channels.

Pulsatile fluid secretion expected from the local Ca^{2+} oscillations in the secretory granule region can be optically monitored by digital differential interference microscopy in salivary glands. Exocytotic secretion also appears to be directly triggered by local Ca^{2+} spikes in the granular region (Figure 10.2). Thus, primary $[Ca^{2+}]_i$ spikes within the granular area are necessary and sufficient for triggering both fluid and protein secretion. Spread of Ca^{2+} waves to the basal area at higher agonist concentrations further induces a "pull-phase", where cation and also Cl^- channels in the basolateral membrane are activated (Figure 10.2) and, hence, Cl^- is taken up from blood to cytosol. Thus, the Ca^{2+} microgradients serve as selective switches for the functions of certain areas of the cells in a concentration-dependent manner. In general, temporal sequences of cellular processes activated by Ca^{2+} waves could have a physiological role. Alternatively, spread of Ca^{2+} waves could just be utilized to activate the functions of cells synchronously, as may be the case with smooth muscle cells.

The Ca^{2+} nanogradients beneath Ca^{2+} channels in the plasma membrane could play a role in triggering neurotransmitter release. In this case, CaBPs in the plasma membrane with low affinity to Ca^{2+} may be essential. The functions of many low affinity CaBPs may be influenced by high $[Ca^{2+}]_i$ within the Ca^{2+} nanogradients, and in this context the preferential localization of low affinity CaBPs close to the membrane is physiologically relevant. Ca^{2+} release channels may also be responsible for the Ca^{2+} nanogradient around the mouth facing the cytosolic space. One possible example is the transient activation of Ca^{2+}-activated Cl^- channels in *Xenopus* oocytes and in pancreatic acinar cells, where Cl^- currents decay when bulk $[Ca^{2+}]_i$ measured with Ca^{2+} imaging, reaches its plateau level. This may indicate that the $[Ca^{2+}]_i$ rise and fall that governs the gating of the Cl^- channels is too localized to be captured with Ca^{2+} imaging techniques.

The two distinct forms of Ca^{2+} gradients may offer a way to differentially stimulate distinct CaBPs (dynamic decoding). For dynamic decoding, a lower affinity CaBP must be located close to the Ca^{2+} channels, and another high affinity CaBP distributed in the bulk cytosol. The Ca^{2+} nanogradient is selectively induced at the beginning of a rise in $[Ca^{2+}]_i$ or by a weak stimulus. Thus, weaker stimuli could selectively activate lower affinity CaBPs by high $[Ca^{2+}]_i$ within the Ca^{2+} nanogradients. On the other hand, longer or stronger stimuli cause a Ca^{2+} microgradient, and activate high affinity CaBPs present in the bulk cytosol. Importantly, after the Ca^{2+} channels close, the Ca^{2+} nanogradients dissipate quickly, while the Ca^{2+} microgradients persist for several seconds or propagate to other cellular areas as Ca^{2+} waves. Thus, stronger stimuli could rather selectively activate higher affinity CaBPs because the microgradients influence a larger cellular space and for a longer period than the nanogradients, and their effects thereby dominate the cellular response. One example of dynamic decoding is frequency coding of synaptic efficacy; a single presynaptic spike induces a Ca^{2+} nanogradient and triggers low affinity CaBPs responsible for neurotransmitter release, while tetanic stimulation evokes a Ca^{2+} microgradient and activates high affinity CaBPs which induce posttetanic potentiation. The dynamic decoding could account for alternate openings of luminal and basolateral Cl^- channels in pancreatic acinar cells, if luminal Cl^- channels have lower affinity for Ca^{2+} than basolateral Cl^- channels (Figure 10.1). The notion of dynamic decoding might also apply to other cellular processes where Ca^{2+}-mobilizing stimuli induce distinct or opposing cellular functions, depending on intensity.

Ca^{2+} release from an organelle may serve to regulate that particular organelle. Two intriguing possibilities could be considered. Firstly, the $[Ca^{2+}]_i$ in the lumen of the stores may have a direct regulatory role. Transport of protein in the ER to the Golgi apparatus may be regulated by emptying of Ca^{2+} from the ER. The mitochondrial matrix has a relatively low $[Ca^{2+}]_i$ and agonists can induce a transient rise. There are many matrix proteins that are regulated by Ca^{2+}. Secondly, the functions of organelles could be regulated by Ca^{2+} nanogradients formed just outside the organelles. If secretory granules were provided with Ca^{2+} release channels, the nanogradient could trigger their exocytotic secretion. Hormones may regulate the functions of these organelles in a dose-dependent and hormone-specific manner.

10.9 FUTURE PERSPECTIVE

Recent progress in the Ca^{2+} signaling field has been spectacular, but there are nevertheless many crucial questions that cannot be answered. The subcellular distribution of the different kinds of Ca^{2+} stores is still obscure in most cell types and we have hardly any precise information about total and free Ca^{2+} concentrations in the various stores in the resting or stimulated states. We also have very little useful information about the control of Ca^{2+} pumps in the ER and the mechanisms employed in such a regulation which may be important for a full understanding of the spatiotemporal Ca^{2+} signal patterns. Finally, the nature and regulation of Ca^{2+} entry pathways in electrically nonexcitable cells are still uncertain. Hopefully, the next few years will see substantial progress in these areas.

10.10 FURTHER READING

Berridge, M.J., 1993. Inositol trisphosphate and calcium signalling, *Nature,* 361:315-325.

Bezprozvanny, I., Watras, J., and Ehrlich, B.E., 1991. Bell-shaped calcium-response curves of Ins(1,4,5)P$_3$ and calcium-gated channels from endoplasmic reticulum of cerebellum, *Nature,* 351:751-754.

Bronner, F., 1990. *Intracellular Calcium Regulation,* Wiley-Liss, New York, pp. 480.

Clapham, D.E., 1995. Calcium signalling, *Cell,* 80:259-268.

Endo, M., 1977. Calcium release from the sarcoplasmic reticulum, *Physiol. Rev.,* 57:71-108.

Petersen, O.H., 1992. Stimulus-secretion coupling: cytoplasmic calcium signals and control of ion channels in exocrine acinar cells, *J. Physiol.,* 448:1-51.

Streb, H., Irvine, R.F., Berridge, M.J., and Schulz, I., 1983. Release of Ca^{2+} from a nonmitochondrial intracellular store in pancreatic acinar cells by inositol 1,4,5-trisphosphate, *Nature,* 306:67-69.

Thorn, P., Lawrie, A.M., Smith, P., Gallacher, D.V., and Petersen, O.H., 1993. Local and global cytosolic Ca^{2+} oscillations in exocrine cells evoked by agonists and inositol trisphosphate, *Cell,* 74:661-668.

Woods, N.M., Cuthbertson, K.S.R., and Cobbold, P.H., 1986. Repetitive transient rises in cytoplasmic free calcium in hormone-stimulated hepatocytes, *Nature,* 319:600-602.

ACKNOWLEDGMENT

This chapter has been essentially reproduced from *Annu. Rev. Physiol.,* Vol. 56, 1994 with permission of Annual Reviews, Inc.

11 Protein Kinase C and Diacylglycerol

Ronit Sagi-Eisenberg

CONTENTS

11.1 PROTEIN KINASE C: A CELLULAR TARGET FOR SECOND MESSENGERS

Protein phosphorylation has long been recognized as a key regulatory mechanism to alter the structure and function of cellular proteins. This is achieved by the action of protein kinases and protein phosphatases that act in concert to control their protein substrates' functions.

Protein kinases have been classified mainly into two groups, the serine/threonine kinases and the protein tyrosine kinases, depending on the target amino acid. Among the serine/threonine protein kinases, the pivotal role of protein kinase C (PKC) in mediating cellular responses is well established. This enzyme was first discovered in 1977 by Nishizuka and colleagues, as a proteolytically activated kinase. Its importance was, however, soon appreciated when it was demonstrated that cofactors such as calcium and phosphatidylserine (PS) could reversibly activate the inactive enzyme. A breakthrough in our present understanding of signal transduction

0-8493-9227-6/96/$0.00+$.50
© 1996 by CRC Press, Inc.

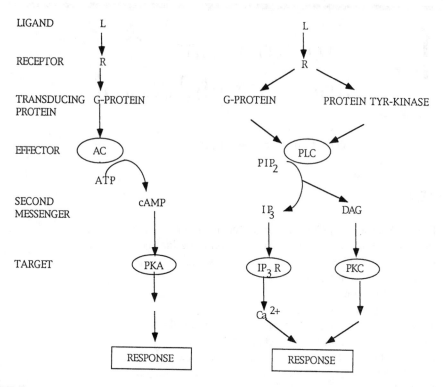

FIGURE 11.1 Schemes showing the roles of protein kinases A (PKA) and C (PKC) in signal transduction following the ligand (L) interaction with the receptor (R). AC is adenylyl cyclase; PLC is phospholipase C; cAMP is cyclic 3′,5′-adenosine monophosphate; IP_3 is inositol(1,4,5)trisphosphate; PIP_2 is phosphatidyl inositol(4,5)bisphosphate; DAG is diacylglycerol; IP_3R is the receptor for IP_3 on the endoplasmic reticulum which mediates calcium release (see Chapter 10).

mechanisms was achieved with the discovery that diacylglycerol (DAG) markedly increases the affinity of PKC for Ca^{2+}, thereby rendering the enzyme active at micromolar concentrations of Ca^{2+}. This important observation provided the first linkage between the process of receptor-induced phosphoinositide breakdown, which produces DAG in a ligand-dependent manner, and a target enzyme capable of changing the function of substrate proteins (Figure 11.1). Furthermore, once Berridge and colleagues had demonstrated that the second product of phosphoinositide breakdown, inositol trisphosphate (IP_3), mobilizes Ca^{2+} from intracellular stores, it became clear that receptors that activate phospholipase C (PLC) leading to phosphoinositide breakdown, produce two second messengers (DAG and IP_3) that concomitantly activate both Ca^{2+} and PKC-dependent pathways (Figure 11.1). This is in contrast to other signal transduction mechanisms where receptor occupancy results in the generation of a second messenger that subsequently binds to and activates one cellular target (e.g., cAMP).

DAG is only transiently produced in response to stimulated phosphoinositide metabolism and can therefore result only in a rapid and transient activation of PKC. Prolonged PKC activation can, however, arise from receptor-stimulated hydrolysis of phosphatidylcholine (PC) by phospholipases C, D, and A_2. Hydrolysis of PC is slower in onset and longer in duration than phosphoinositide hydrolysis and it functions as a major cellular source for DAG. In addition, more recent data have shown that free fatty acids and lysoPC, both products of PLA_2, potentiate DAG activation of PKC. Hence, PKC is a principal cellular target for lipid second messengers (Figure 11.2). This notion is further strengthened by the recent observation that PKC is also activated by phosphatidylinositol(3,4)bisphosphate ($PI[3,4]P_2$) and phosphatidylinositol (3,4,5)trisphosphate (PIP_3), both produced in response to ligand stimulation of PI-3-kinase (PI-3-K) (Figure 11.2; see below).

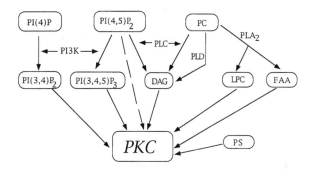

FIGURE 11.2   The various lipid second messengers that have been shown to directly or indirectly activate PKC.

11.2   PKC: A CELLULAR RECEPTOR FOR TUMOR-PROMOTING PHORBOL ESTERS

A major breakthrough in the field of transmembranal signaling was achieved in 1982, when Castagna and colleagues noticed that the powerful tumor promoter 12-O-tetradecanoyl-phorbol acetate (TPA) (TPA is also known as phorbol myristate acetate or PMA) could mimic the action of DAG and activate PKC directly. This discovery has identified PKC as a cellular target for TPA, implicating the enzyme in the control of growth and tumor promotion. It also provided an important pharmacological tool to directly activate PKC independently of the Ca^{2+} pathway and bypassing the need for receptors. These studies with TPA have revealed that PKC is a multifunctional enzyme (see below) and have provided an important clue as to its mechanism of action. Following TPA treatment, the enzyme which is mainly cytosolic, translocates to the plasma membrane where it then encounters its phospholipid cofactors and undergoes activation. Translocation of PKC to the membrane also follows receptor-induced phosphoinositide breakdown.

Subsequent to its translocation to the membrane, PKC becomes susceptible to degradation. The Ca^{2+}-dependent neutral proteases I and II (calpains) cleave PKC producing two distinct fragments; a regulatory domain and a kinase domain that is catalytically active in the absence of activators. Whether the constitutively active PKC fragment plays a physiological role still remains to be determined. In any event, proteolytic cleavage continues and prolonged incubation with TPA results in the depletion of the enzyme from the cell. Prolonged incubation with TPA thus provides yet another important tool to study the cellular function of PKC (see below).

11.3   PKC HETEROGENEITY

The third breakthrough in the research on PKC was undoubtedly achieved when purification protocols, immunological analyses, and most importantly, cloning data revealed the existence of multiple subspecies of PKC. To date, the family of PKC isozymes includes 11 different enzymes that can be classified in 4 major groups. The first group consists of the conventional PKCs (cPKCs): α, β1, β2, and γ, that represent the originally identified Ca^{2+}- and phospholipid-dependent enzymes. These PKCs are the products of different genes, except for the β1 and β2 isoforms that are the products of the same alternatively spliced gene. The second group includes four gene products δ, ε, η, and θ, which are novel Ca^{2+}-independent PKCs (nPKCs). The members of the third group are atypical PKCs (aPKCs), not activated by DAG or TPA. They include the products of the ζ and λ genes. Finally, the fourth group includes a newly discovered PKC, PKC-μ, which has a potential transmembrane domain.

11.4 STRUCTURE-FUNCTION RELATIONSHIPS

Alignment of coding sequences of the first discovered conventional PKC isozymes (α, $\beta 1$, $\beta 2$, and γ) revealed that they are all composed of a single polypeptide chain which consists of conserved, constant (C) and variable (V) regions (Figure 11.3). The related PKCs, identified by screening cDNA libraries at low-stringency conditions (δ, ε, η, and θ), include domains that are similar to the conventional PKCs except that the C2 region is missing (Figure 11.3). PKC-ζ also lacks the C2 domain, but in addition it also differs in its C1 domain (Figure 11.3, see below).

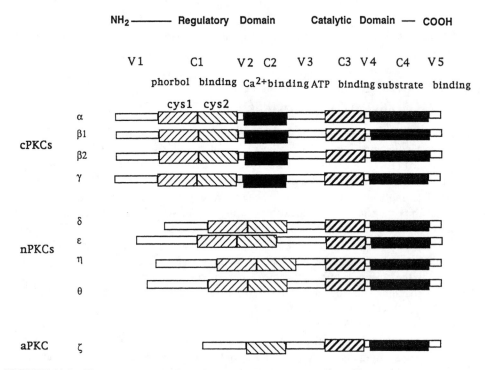

FIGURE 11.3 The structure and related functions of the various domains of the isoenzymes of PKC.

The polypeptide chain can be divided into two functionally distinct domains. The amino-terminal regulatory domain (C1-V3 region) contains interaction sites for calcium, phospholipids, DAG, and phorbol esters. The carboxyl-terminal domain (C3-V5 regions) contains the ATP-binding (C3) and substrate-binding (C4) sites and it possesses the kinase catalytic activity (Figure 11.3). These two regions are separated by the V3 hinge region which is the site of proteolytic cleavage. This region is sensitive to proteolysis by trypsin or by calpains I and II (see above).

11.5 SITES FOR PKC INTERACTIONS

11.5.1 THE PSEUDOSUBSTRATE MOTIF

All PKC isozymes contain a pseudosubstrate motif that resembles a consensus sequence found in many PKC substrates except for an alanine that replaces the serine or threonine residue which serve as targets for phosphorylation (Figure 11.4). This pseudosubstrate sequence, located at the C1 region, interacts with the substrate-binding site within the catalytic region, thereby conferring on the kinase an inactive conformation (see below). This conclusion is based on the findings that a synthetic peptide that replicates the pseudosubstrate sequence

Pseudosubstrate Site

α	RFARKGÅLRQKNVHEVK
βI/II	RFARKGÅLRQKNVHEVK
γ	LFCRKGÅLRQKVVHEVK
δ	TMNRRGÅIKQAKIHYIK
ε	PRKRQGÅVRRRVHQVNG
ζ	SIYRRGÅRRWRKLYRAN
η	TAKRQRÅMRRRVHQING
θ	LHQRRGÅIKQAKVHHVK

FIGURE 11.4   The amino acid sequences of the substrate sites of the various isoforms of PKC.

acts as a potent and specific inhibitor of PKC, whereas the same peptide in which the alanine was replaced by a serine residue promotes kinase activation. The latter is most probably achieved by competition with the endogenous substrate-binding domain for binding to the pseudosubstrate domain. An antibody raised against the pseudosubstrate peptide also activates PKC in the absence of cofactors. It is believed that by binding to the regulatory domain, this antibody, like the lipid cofactors, relieves the catalytic activity from the tonic inhibition exerted by the regulatory domain.

11.5.2 The Phospholipid/Phorbol Ester Binding Domain

The pseudosubstrate sequence within the C1 domain is followed by two tandem repeats of a cys-rich motif (cys1 and cys2; Figure 11.3) whose consensus is $H-X_{12}-C-X_2-C-X_{10-14}-C-X_2-C-X_4-H-X_2-X_2-C-X_7-C$. These sequences, designated the zinc-butterfly motif, share homology with the cysteine-rich "zinc fingers" found in DNA-binding proteins. Whether this putative DNA binding motif plays a role in PKC regulation is presently unclear. Some PKCs were reported to translocate to the nucleus and PKC has been reported to bind DNA, but the physiological relevance of these observations is unclear. Future studies will most probably shed more light on this important point in PKC function.

Using an ultracentrifugation assay, the zinc-butterfly region has been shown to interact directly with liposomes containing phosphatidyl serine and with DAG. Studies with deletion and truncation mutants of PKCs expressed in the baculovirus-insect expression system, as well as with glutathione S-transferase (GST) fusion proteins expressing the cys1 and cys2 domains, have revealed that the zinc-butterfly is also responsible for phorbol ester binding. A PKC truncation mutant, consisting of the regulatory domain, binds radiolabeled phorbol-12,13-dibutyrate ([³H]PDBu) and so does a truncation mutant in which the second conserved region, C2, was deleted. In contrast, a mutant in which the first conserved region, C1, was deleted shows no [³H]PDBu binding. When expressed as GST fusion proteins, each of these domains can coordinate zinc and retain high affinity phosphatidyl serine-dependent binding of [³H]PDBu. Hence, either cysteine-rich sequence could independently bind phorbol ester. Indeed, other proteins (e.g., n-chimaerin and unc-13), that have been shown to contain a single zinc-butterfly motif, were found to manifest high affinity phorbol ester binding. PKC, therefore, appears to contain two phorbol ester binding domains. Nevertheless, the tandem cystein-rich repeat present in the C1 region may be required for PKC regulation by phorbol esters because PKC-ζ that contains only one zinc finger does not bind DAG or phorbol ester. PKC-ζ also fails to translocate or downregulate in response to TPA treatment. Interestingly, this isozyme, which is not stimulated by Ca^{2+}, DAG, or phorbol ester, is selectively activated by PIP_3. Although the physiological role of this phosphorylated inositol phospholipid is still unknown, it is produced in response to the stimulation of cells by growth factors and other agonists. PKC-ζ may thus be the target for PIP_3 and, as such, be involved in the signaling mechanisms for receptors that increase PI-3-K activity.

11.5.3 THE CALCIUM BINDING DOMAIN

The C2 conserved domain is present in all Ca^{2+}-dependent cPKCs but is absent in the Ca^{2+}-independent nPKCs and aPKCs (Figure 11.3). Therefore, it is believed that the C2 domain plays a critical role in Ca^{2+} binding and activation of the cPKCs. Binding studies between Ca^{2+} and GST fusion proteins, expressed in *E. coli* that carry various modifications in the regulatory domain, have shown that the C2 domain confers specificity for Ca^{2+} binding when compared to other divalent cations such as Mg^{2+}. Based on these studies, it has been proposed that in the absence of activating cofactors, cPKCs are in a folded conformation in which the pseudosubstrate region at the amino-terminal end binds to the substrate binding domain in the carboxy-terminus of the catalytic domain, thereby preventing phosphorylation of target proteins. Upon addition of Ca^{2+} and phosphatidyl serine, binding of these cofactors to the C1 and C2 domains causes a conformational change leading to the dissociation of the pseudosubstrate site from the catalytic domain, resulting in the activation of the kinase and phosphorylation of the potential substrates. In the case of nPKCs, in the absence of the C2 domain which confers Ca^{2+} specificity, binding of the phospholipid cofactors and presumably Mg^{2+} most probably results in a similar conformational change also in the absence of Ca^{2+}.

The C2 region of cPKCs shows homology with a Ca^{2+}-binding domain present in several other proteins. These include the cytosolic $cPLA_2$, GTPase activating protein (GAP), phospholipase C, synaptotagmin, and rabphilin. In $cPLA_2$, it is the amino-terminal portion of the enzyme that shows significant homology with the C2 domain. A 16-kDa amino-terminal fragment of $cPLA_2$ that contains the C2-like domain is able to associate with membrane vesicles in a Ca^{2+}-dependent fashion, suggesting that also in $cPLA_2$ it is this region that directs the translocation of the enzyme to the membrane, following stimulation of cells with Ca^{2+}-mobilizing ligands. GAP also binds to acidic phospholipids and this binding modulates its activity. Furthermore, the synaptic vesicle protein, synaptotagmin, facilitates Ca^{2+}-induced fusion of synaptic vesicles with the plasma membrane. Hence, it seems likely that the PKC C2-like domains in all of the above proteins may serve as a Ca^{2+}-binding domain, promoting Ca^{2+}-dependent association with the phospholipids present in the plasma membrane.

11.6 PKC BINDING PROTEINS

The C1 and C2 domains appear to play a role not only in the docking of PKCs to membrane lipids but also in interactions with binding proteins.

A PKC blot overlay assay has led to the identification of several PKC-binding proteins. The proteins identified include known substrates of PKC, such as the myristoylated alanine-rich PKC substrate MARCKS (see below), as well as a class of particulate proteins termed "receptors for activated C kinase" or RACKs. The C1 domain seems to mediate binding of the substrate proteins to PKC whereas the C2 participates in binding the RACKs.

The RACK proteins bind to PKC only in the presence of PKC activators. They appear to contain a consensus sequence that presumably mediates their binding to PKC. Similar sequences are found in annexin I and in the brain PKC inhibitor, KCIP (kinase C inhibitor protein). One of the RACK proteins, termed RACK1, was cloned and found to contain seven repeats of the WD40 motif found in the β-subunit of the heterotrimeric G-proteins. This motif is believed to mediate protein-protein interactions. These results, therefore, suggest that the RACK proteins function in docking PKC to the membrane.

11.7 PKC SUBSTRATES

A large number of putative physiological substrates for PKC have been identified so far. These include numerous receptors, such as the growth factor receptors (e.g., EGF receptor, insulin receptor) and G-protein-coupled receptors (e.g., β-adrenoreceptor, rhodopsin) whose PKC-mediated phosphorylation is associated with their desensitization and downregulation; ion transporters (e.g., Na/Ca^{2+} exchanger, Ca^{2+} ATPase); cytoskeletal proteins (e.g., heavy and light chains of myosin, vimentin); and transcription factors (e.g., c-fos).

One of the major substrates for PKC, whose phosphorylation is often used as a marker of PKC activation *in vivo,* is a calmodulin and actin-binding protein known as the MARCKS protein. This and a related protein (MARCKS/F52) have been implicated in macrophage activation, neurosecretion, and growth factor-induced mitogenesis. PKC-mediated phosphorylation of MARCKS displaces it from the membrane with which it reassociates upon dephosphorylation. This cycle of membrane attachment/detachment represents a mechanism through which PKC might reversibly regulate an actin-membrane interaction. Calmodulin binding to MARCKS is Ca^{2+}-dependent and is also modulated by PKC-mediated phosphorylation.

11.8 METHODS FOR STUDYING PKC FUNCTION

Several methods have been used in studies to elucidate the role of PKC. These include biochemical studies and, more recently, genetic techniques.

11.8.1 INHIBITORS

Two types of inhibitors are widely used to assess the contribution of PKCs to agonist-stimulated responses. These include inhibitors such as H-7, K252, and staurosporine, that act at the ATP-binding site of the enzyme, blocking its catalytic activity. The problem with this type of inhibitors is, however, lack of specificity. Because the ATP-binding site of PKC shares significant homology with the ATP-binding sites of other protein kinases, these inhibitors are likely to bind and inhibit other kinases as well, complicating the interpretation of the experimental data.

More specific are the inhibitors that belong to another class of PKC inhibitors. These are inhibitors that bind to the regulatory domain of the enzyme. Examples include the microbial compound calphostin and the pseudosubstrate peptide. The latter, however, while being most specific for PKC, cannot penetrate intact cells and requires special methods to introduce it into the cells.

11.8.2 PKC DOWNREGULATION

Another approach to study PKC function is to downregulate the enzyme. Following prolonged treatment with phorbol esters, PKC translocates to the membrane where it becomes susceptible to degradation by membrane proteases (see above). As a result, the enzyme is depleted from the cells. This can be detected as a decrease in PDBu binding sites, a decrease in PKC activity, and a decrease in PKC immunoreactivity. Thus, by depleting the enzyme from the cell, its involvement in a particular cellular process can be determined. Moreover, because the kinetics of downregulation of the various PKC isozymes are different, this provides a useful tool to evaluate the contribution of a specific PKC isozyme to a particular process.

11.8.3 INTRODUCTION OF RECOMBINANT PKC ISOZYMES TO PERMEABILIZED CELL

The availability of purified PKC isozymes, produced in the baculovirus-insect expression system, allows the introduction of purified isozymes into permeabilized cells that have lost their cellular function as a result of permeabilization and depletion of endogenous PKCs. The ability of different PKCs to reconstitute the lost function can then be evaluated (see below).

11.8.4 Genetic Manipulations of PKCs

To elucidate the role of specific forms of PKC it is desirable to generate cell lines that overproduce one form of the enzyme, or alternatively, to block the expression of one specific isozyme. This is achieved by transfecting cells with specific PKC cDNAs leading to over-production of the studied enzyme, or transfecting with antisense cDNAs to block PKC expression. The advantage of this method lies in the fact that it allows study of the role of a specific PKC isozyme in intact cells under physiological conditions. This is in sharp contrast to the methods described above which involve the use of either pharmacological reagents, not all of which are specific, or permeabilization of the cells.

11.9 PKC FUNCTION

Several physiological functions have been assigned to PKC. These include involvement in secretion, modulation of ion conductance, modulation of other signaling pathways, control of gene expression, growth, and differentiation. This variety in PKC functions immediately points to the possibility that the individual members of the PKC family may play different biological roles. This concept is supported by the fact that the members of the PKC family differ in their tissue distribution, activation by cofactors, kinetics of downregulation, and substrate specificity. Nevertheless, one of the major unresolved issues in the field of trans-membrane signaling relates to the role of particular isoforms of PKC in mediating cellular responses subsequent to the activation of this enzyme.

11.9.1 The Role of PKC in Regulating Secretion

Early studies have established the role of PKC in regulating secretion. By using phorbol esters to directly activate PKC, and Ca^{2+} ionophores to increase the cytosolic concentration of Ca^{2+}, the synergistic interaction between the Ca^{2+} pathway and that mediated by PKC in triggering the secretory response could be demonstrated in cell types such as platelets, mast cells, endocrine systems, exocrine systems, and neuronal systems. Interestingly, when hista-mine secretion from mast cells was stimulated by a physiological agonist (antigen), PKC activation by TPA resulted in inhibition of the receptor-induced rise in cytosolic Ca^{2+} con-centrations. These studies, reproduced in many other cell types and cellular processes, have indicated that PKC exerts a dual action, exhibiting both positive and negative signals. Inhi-bition of the Ca^{2+} signal is associated with inhibition of phosphoinositide breakdown, implying that PKC acts in a negative feedback control to inhibit its own activation. That the opposing actions of TPA on histamine secretion are indeed mediated by PKC, was illustrated by the fact that depletion of endogenous PKC in mast cells by long-term incubations with TPA led to inhibition of the secretory response, but at the same time resulted in potentiation of IP_3 formation. Two independent lines of evidence suggest that these dual actions are mediated by different isozymes of PKC.

In one study, the rate of downregulation of two different PKC isozymes, following TPA treatment, was compared with the rates by which histamine secretion was inhibited and IP_3 formation potentiated. Under conditions where PKC-β, but not the more resistant PKC-α, is depleted from the cells (following 2 to 4 h incubation with TPA), antigen-induced secretion is completely blocked. However, IP_3 formation remains inhibited. It takes more than 6 h of incubation with TPA to deplete PKC-α from these cells, and this results in relief of the inhibition exerted by TPA, followed by potentiation of the response. This study, therefore, suggests that PKC-β is involved in transmitting the stimulatory signals required for exocytosis, whereas PKC-α plays a negative role by inhibiting phosphoinositide breakdown. In another study, permeabilization of a mast cell line by streptolysin-O resulted in the loss of antigen-mediated secretion because of leakage of critical cytosolic components. Exocytosis could be restored by the addition of PKC-β or PKC-δ, but not by the addition of PKC-α or PKC-ϵ. Furthermore, both PKC-α and PKC-ϵ inhibited phosphoinositide breakdown.

11.9.2 CROSS-TALK WITH OTHER SIGNALING PATHWAYS

Whereas PKC negatively regulates its own activation by inhibiting the activation of phospholipase C, it positively regulates its own activation by phospholipases D and A$_2$. As discussed above, a major fraction of DAG formed in cells is derived from phosphatidyl choline (PC) by the sequential action of PLD, which catalyzes PC breakdown to phosphatidic acid (PA) and choline, followed by the action of PA phosphohydrolase which dephosphorylates PA to yield DAG. PLD activation thereby leads to activation of PKC. The activity of PLD is, however, regulated by PKC. TPA treatment of intact cells results in increased activity of PLD, whereas downregulation of PKC by prolonged TPA treatment abolishes PLD activation in response to agonists. Finally, PLD activity is upregulated in cells overexpressing either the PKC-α or the PKC-β1 isoenzyme. The mechanisms of PLD potentiation involve both activation of the enzyme (presumed in the case of PKC-β1) and increased expression (in the case of PKC-α).

Arachidonic acid (AA) and other fatty acids derived from phospholipase A$_2$-mediated hydrolysis of phospholipids are also involved in the activation of PKC (Figure 11.2). The activity of phospholipase A$_2$ is positively regulated by PKC. Two independent approaches link the PKC-α isozyme with the activation of phospholipase A$_2$. The first made use of the differential downregulation of the PKC isozymes to demonstrate that differential activation of PKC-α is associated with AA release, whereas specific downregulation of PKC-α is associated with a loss of AA release in response to stimulation. A similar conclusion was reached using antisense technology. Inhibition of the expression of PKC-α, but not of PKC-β, caused a loss in phospholipase A$_2$-mediated AA release. The mechanism of activation of phospholipase A$_2$ by PKC is presently unknown.

11.9.3 THE ROLE OF PKC IN THE CONTROL OF GROWTH
AND DIFFERENTIATION

The role of PKC in growth regulation has been evaluated by the generation of cell lines that overproduce specific PKC isozymes. The overproduction of PKC-β1 in rat embryo fibroblasts resulted in multiple phenotypic changes even in the absence of TPA treatment. These included increased growth rate, formation of dense foci in postconfluent cultures, and anchorage-independent growth. Cells overproducing PKC-β1 also became highly susceptible to transformation by an activated H-Ras oncogene. The PKC-overexpressing cells display increased phosphorylation of the MARCKS protein (see above) and after treatment with TPA they display prolongation in the phosphorylation and cytosolic accumulation of this protein. These alterations in MARCKS may thus be responsible for the altered growth characteristics of these cells.

Altered growth regulation associated with enhanced tumorigenicity were also observed in the NIH 3T3 fibroblast cell line transfected with PKC-γ. Transfection of these cells did not induce foci but the cells displayed reduced dependence on serum for growth and displayed enhanced tumorigenicity when inoculated into nude mice. In contrast to these observations, when expressed in a different cell line (C3H/10T1/2 cells), the PKC-β1 could not display anchorage-independent growth. Similarly, overexpression of PKC-α had no effect on the morphology or growth rate of the Swiss/3T3 cell line, and these cells were incapable of growing in an anchorage-independent manner. Thus, it appears that different isozymes are not only associated with different roles, but the same isozymes may exhibit different functions or participate in different signaling pathways, depending on the cell type. Even more surprising is the observation that cells that overproduce PKC-β1 become almost completely resistant to transformation by γ-irradiation. Hence, PKC-β1 seems to play a dual role: while increasing the cell susceptibility to certain oncogenes (e.g., activated Ras), it acts to downregulate the induction or expression of radiation-mediated oncogenes.

The dual role played by PKC is also illustrated in the observation that the incorporation of exogenous purified PKC-β into murine erythroleukemia cells accelerates their differentiation. Hence, PKCs are involved in the control of both cell proliferation and differentiation. That PKCs play a role in cell differentiation is further indicated by the finding that treatment with TPA allows the human leukemia HL-60 cell line to differentiate to macrophages. Differentiation correlates with upregulation of PKC-α, implicating this PKC isozyme in differentiation. Induction of differentiation requires sustained activation of PKC. DAG analogs that only transiently activate the enzyme fail to induce differentiation, which can, however, be achieved by repeated addition of this physiological PKC activator.

The mechanisms through which PKC controls growth and differentiation involve the phosphorylation of growth factor receptors, proteins involved in signal transduction, and proteins involved in gene expression.

In the case of growth factor receptors, as discussed above, PKC-mediated phosphorylation results in inhibition of protein tyrosine kinase activities associated with these mitogenic receptors (e.g., EGF receptor, insulin receptor). In contrast, PKC-mediated phosphorylation of signaling molecules such as the c-raf kinase and S6 kinase appears to result in their activation, thereby stimulating cell proliferation.

By a yet unresolved mechanism, PKC activation also results in phosphorylation of the MAP kinase at both tyrosine and threonine residues. This phosphorylation subsequently results in the activation of the kinase and gene expression.

PKC also directly stimulates gene expression by a mechanism that involves phosphorylation of transcription factors such as c-fos that forms part of the AP1 response element.

11.10 SUMMARY

A great deal of progress on protein kinase C (PKC) has been achieved since its discovery in 1977. Although once considered a single enzyme, it is now clear that PKC consists of a family of related proteins that differ in their tissue distribution, dependence on cofactors for activation, and substrate specificity. The isozymes known today can be classified into the Ca^{2+}- and phospholipid-dependent enzymes that bind and are activated by diacylglycerol (DAG), and the tumor-promoting phorbol esters, the Ca^{2+}-independent isozymes, and those that apparently are not activated by DAG or phorbol esters. PKCs exert a bidirectional control on multiple cellular functions, transmitting both stimulatory signals such as potentiation of secretion and proliferation, and negative signals such as reducing the intracellular concentrations of Ca^{2+}. The different functions of PKC are most probably mediated by different isozymes. The assignment of a particular cellular function to a specific PKC isozyme, however, still awaits future studies.

11.11 FURTHER READING

Bell, R.M. and Burns, D.J. (1991). Lipid activation of protein kinase C, *J. Biol. Chem.,* 266, 4661-4664.

Blackshear, P.J. (1993). The MARCKS family of cellular protein kinase C substrates, *J. Biol. Chem.,* 268, 1501-1504.

Hug, H. and Sarre, T.F. (1993). Protein kinase C isoenzymes: divergence in signal transduction?, *Biochem. J.,* 291, 329-343.

Kikkawa, U., Kishimoto, A., and Nishizuka, Y. (1989). The protein kinase C family: heterogeneity and its implications, *Annu. Rev. Biochem.,* 58, 31-44.

Kiley, S.C. and Jaken, S. (1994). Protein kinase C: interactions and consequences, *Trends Cell Biol.,* 4, 223-227.

Nishizuka, Y. (1992). Intracellular signaling by hydrolysis of phospholipids and activation of protein kinase C, *Science,* 258, 607-614.

Nishizuka, Y. (1988). The heterogeneity and differential expression of multiple species of the protein kinase C family, *Biofactors,* 1, 17-20.

12 Cyclic Nucleotides as Signal Transducers

John C. Foreman

CONTENTS

12.1 INTRODUCTION

The cyclic nucleotides recognized as having a role in signal transduction are cyclic adenosine monophosphate (cAMP) and cyclic guanosine monophosphate (cGMP).

Cyclic AMP is the prototype second messenger, discovered by Sutherland in the late 1950s as a heat-stable molecule formed when adrenaline acted on a particulate cell fraction from rat liver. It was, in fact, Sutherland who produced the hypothesis that the interaction of a hormone with its membrane receptor generated an intracellular "second messenger" which acted upon effectors within the cell to generate a response.

The structure of cyclic AMP is shown in Figure 12.1. It is formed from adenosine triphosphate (ATP) by the action of the enzyme adenylyl cyclase (adenyl cyclase; adenylate cyclase). As with all biological signals, there must be a mechanism for termination of the signal and, in the case of cyclic AMP, this is a phosphodiesterase enzyme which converts cyclic AMP to 5′-adenosine monophosphate (5′ AMP). The effector molecule upon which cAMP acts is a cyclic AMP-dependent protein kinase known as protein kinase A (PKA) and this enzyme, once activated by cAMP, phosphorylates a number of other intracellular proteins needed to generate the overall cellular response. Adenylyl cyclase is a membrane protein that is coupled to receptors by means of heterotrimeric G-proteins. The overall scheme for the formation and control of the cAMP second messenger system is shown in Figure 12.2.

0-8493-9227-6/96/$0.00+$.50
© 1996 by CRC Press, Inc.

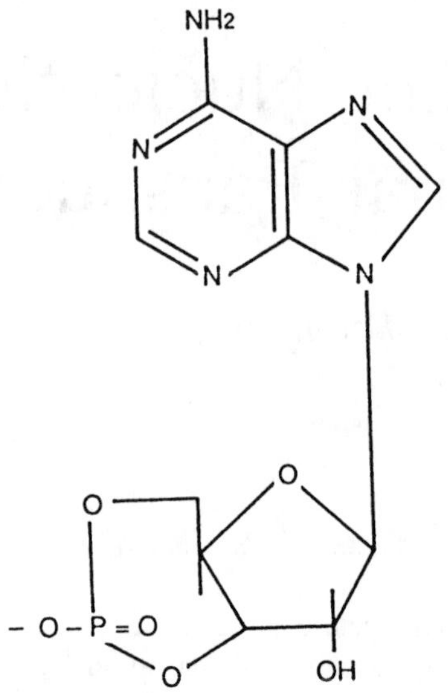

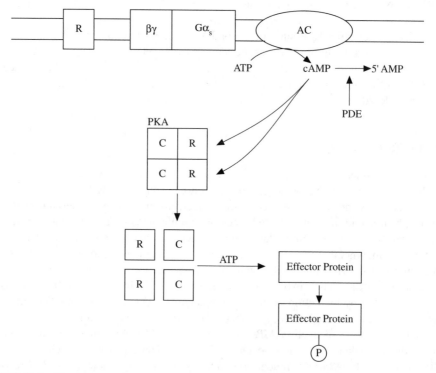

FIGURE 12.1 The structure of cyclic 3′,5′-adenosine monophosphate.

FIGURE 12.2 The scheme for the signal transducing system in which a hormone interacting with the receptor (R) activates adenylyl cyclase (AC) through the G-protein G_s. The adenylyl cyclase converts ATP to cAMP which then causes the regulatory units (R) of protein kinase A to dissociate from the catalytic units. The catalytic units of PKA use ATP to phosphorylate and activate an effector protein.

The formation of cGMP by the enzyme guanylyl cyclase was discovered very shortly after the discovery of cAMP and for many years it was held that cellular activity was controlled by the opposing actions of intracellular cAMP and cGMP. This now seems very unlikely, and there are quite marked differences between the cAMP and cGMP systems. Most importantly, guanylyl cyclase exists as a soluble, cytosolic enzyme and also as membrane-bound enzyme. Attention is focused on the soluble guanylyl cyclase as a target for the action of nitric oxide, whereas the membrane-bound guanylyl cyclase appears to be the receptor for atrial naturietic peptide.

As will be discussed later, receptor-mediated control of cAMP or cGMP levels in cells can occur by alteration to the rate of synthesis of the cyclic nucleotides or the rate of degradation.

The remainder of this chapter will discuss in more detail the components of the cyclic nucleotide signal transduction systems and the interaction of these components.

12.2 ADENYLYL CYCLASE

Adenylyl cyclase has been identified in a very wide variety of prokaryotic as well as eukaryotic cells: even its presence in plants and archaebacteria is disputed. There are three classes of adenylyl cyclase:

- Class I — enterobacterial class
- Class II — calmodulin-activated toxic class
- Class III — universal class

The enzyme which plays a role in signal transduction in mammalian cells belongs to the universal class. The equilibrium dissociation constant for the synthesis of ATP from cyclic AMP:

$$K_d = \frac{[cAMP][PP][H^+]}{[ATP]}$$

is 2×10^{-9} M^2, indicating that the reaction can be readily reversed. The wide distribution of cAMP and this equilibrium dissociation constant for the adenylyl cyclase-mediated reaction has suggested that originally cAMP may have been involved not with signal transduction but with the control of ATP supply for cellular metabolism.

12.2.1 TYPES OF ADENYLYL CYCLASE

Among the mammalian adenylyl cyclases, five subfamilies exist based on amino acid sequence homology, and within these five subfamilies are eight types of adenylyl cyclase. The plant-derived diterpene, forskolin, is known to bind to adenylyl cyclase and to activate the enzyme. Using forskolin linked to the matrix of a chromatography column, the adenylyl cyclase from brain was purified by affinity chromatography. In fact, this method yielded a complex of the enzyme together with the G-protein (G_s) and calmodulin: this close association between adenylyl cyclase and G_s will be discussed further below. The purified enzyme was sequenced and the cDNA prepared was used to express the brain adenylyl cyclase which was referred to as type 1. Using the cDNA for this type 1 as a probe, the other seven types of adenylyl cyclase were identified.

Figure 12.3 shows the sequence homologies of the families and types of adenylyl cyclase. The different adenylyl cyclase types have different tissue distributions and this is summarized in Table 12.1. The adenylyl cyclase type that is involved in the majority of hormone-receptor signal transduction in peripheral tissues is most likely to be type 6.

12.2.2 ADENYLYL CYCLASE STRUCTURE AND ACTIVATION

Perhaps rather surprising is the prediction, from the amino acid sequence, that adenylyl cyclase is a membrane-spanning protein with 12 transmembrane segments arranged in

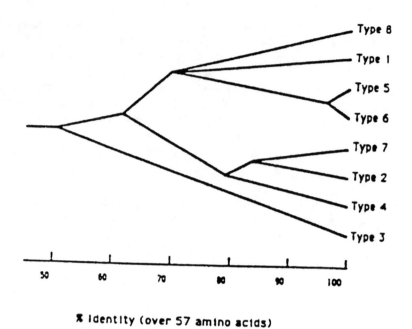

% Identity (over 57 amino acids)

FIGURE 12.3   The types of mammalian adenylyl cyclase showing the degree of amino acid sequence homology among the types.

TABLE 12.1
Distribution of the Types of Mammalian Adenylyl Cyclase

Type of adenylyl cyclase	Tissue					
	Liver	Brain	Heart	Kidney	Lung	Testis
1	–	+	–	–	–	–
2	–	+	–	–	+	–
3	–	+	–	–	–	–
4	(+)	+	(+)	+	(+)	(+)
5	+	+	+	+	+	(+)
6	+	+	+	+	+	(+)
7	–	(+)	(+)	–	–	–
8	–	+	–	–	–	–

Note: Tissue distributions of mRNA for adenylyl cyclase types: – indicates absence; + indicates presence detected by Northern blotting or solution hybridization; (+) indicates presence detected by PCR.

Taken from Iyengar, R., *Adv. Second Messenger Phosphorylation Res.,* 28, 30, 1993. With permission.

2 domains of 6 (Figure 12.4). The two large intracellular loops are believed to contain the catalytic activity of the protein.

The catalytic activity of adenylyl cyclase is stimulated by the GTP-bearing α-subunit of the G_s protein. The G-protein couples the receptor to the adenylyl cyclase and permits a hormone-receptor interaction to activate several adenylyl cyclase molecules, leading to signal amplification. In modeling the interaction between hormone-receptor complex, G_s, and adenylyl

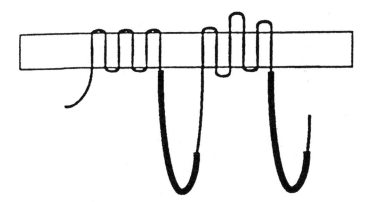

FIGURE 12.4   A model for adenylyl cyclase showing 12 transmembrane segments and 2 long intracellular loops where the catalytic activity of the enzyme is believed to reside.

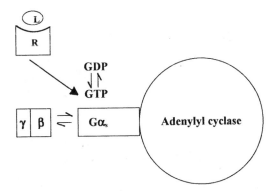

FIGURE 12.5   A model for the interaction of G_s with adenylyl cyclase. Biochemical evidence suggests that the adenylyl cyclase is tightly coupled to $G\alpha_s$. The ligand (L)-receptor (R) interaction increases the rate of exchange of GTP for GDP and the dissociation of the $\beta\gamma$-subunit from $G\alpha_s$. The rate of GTP hydrolysis is also increased. Because the GTPase turnover number is relatively low, the ligand-receptor interaction increases the number of $G\alpha_s$ molecules with GTP bound (active).

cyclase, there is one piece of information that appears to have been frequently confirmed and needs to be taken account of: the α_s-subunit of the G-protein is very tightly associated with the adenylyl cyclase. Figure 12.5 presents a model for the interaction of the hormone-receptor complex with the G-protein and for the interaction of the G-protein with the enzyme. The hormone dissociates from the receptor relatively slowly compared with the rates of association and dissociation of the hormone-receptor complex with the G-protein. This allows a single hormone-receptor complex to activate several G-protein-enzyme complexes. Binding of the hormone-receptor complex to the G-protein increases the rate of exchange of GDP for GTP to promote the activation of $G\alpha_s$ which also requires the dissociation of the $\beta\gamma$ dimer. The binding of the hormone-receptor complex also increases the rate of GTP hydrolysis by the GTPase activity of $G\alpha_s$. Thus, GTP cycling is increased but since the GTPase turnover number is relatively low, the number of $G\alpha_s$ molecules in the GTP-bound state will increase and this, in turn, activates the adenylyl cyclase. Of course the $\beta\gamma$ dimer must dissociate from $G\alpha_s$ before it is activated and then reassociate with it before the next GDP-GTP exchange.

An example of stimulation of adenylyl cyclase by a hormone receptor acting through G_s is the action of adrenaline on the β-adrenoreceptor in the liver cell which elevates intracellular cyclic AMP and ultimately brings about the release of glucose.

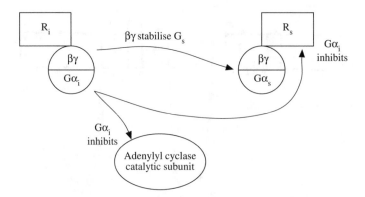

FIGURE 12.6 Different models for the inhibition of adenylyl cyclase by G_i. Interaction of a ligand with an inhibitory receptor (R_i) activates G_i to generate $G\alpha_i$ and $\beta\gamma$. $G\alpha_i$ may inhibit adenylyl cyclase directly or may interact with the stimulatory receptor (R_s) to prevent it from activating G_s. $\beta\gamma$ from G_i may stabilize G_s by driving the equilibrium $G\alpha_s + \beta\gamma \rightleftharpoons G_s$ to the right.

12.2.3 INHIBITION OF ADENYLYL CYCLASE BY G-PROTEIN

In some cells adenylyl cyclase is inhibited rather than activated by the hormone-receptor complex and in this case the adenylyl cyclase is coupled to the hormone-receptor complex by a different G-protein: G_i rather than G_s. An example of a receptor coupled to adenylyl cyclase through G_i is the α_2 adrenoreceptor (see also Chapter 8). There are differing views about the mechanisms for the inhibition of adenylyl cyclase by G_i and these are summarized in Figure 12.6. The most straightforward mechanism is that $G\alpha_i$ interacts directly with adenylyl cyclase to inhibit the catalytic activity of the enzyme. However, not all data are compatible with this model and other explanations for the action of G_i exist. G_i is present in cells in greater quantities than G_s and it has been suggested that when G_i is activated by a hormone-receptor complex, the large quantity of $\beta\gamma$ dimers derived from G_i can inhibit the activation of G_s by driving the equilibrium $\beta\gamma + \alpha_s \rightleftharpoons G_s$ to the right. The inhibition of adenylyl cyclase by α_i and the "stabilization" of G_s by $\beta\gamma$ dimers from G_i are not necessarily mutually exclusive mechanisms. The possibility that α_i interacts directly with the stimulatory receptor and inhibits its ability to stimulate adenylyl cyclase has also been suggested from experimental evidence.

12.2.4 REGULATION OF ADENYLYL CYCLASE

Apart from the regulation of adenylyl cyclase by G_i and G_s, it has been known for some time that the enzyme in some tissues is regulated by calcium, the calcium-calmodulin complex, and adenosine. With the identification of the different types of adenylyl cyclase, the regulation of the different types has been investigated, and Table 12.2 shows how the different types of adenylyl cyclase are regulated. In addition, adenylyl cyclase has been shown to possess a number of protein kinase A phosphorylation sites on the intracellular loops of the polypeptide chain where the catalytic activity of the enzyme is believed to reside. These phosphorylation sites are associated with inactivation of the enzyme and phosphorylation at these sites is one mechanism by which desensitization may occur towards a hormone which acts via a receptor linked to a response through adenylyl cyclase, cyclic AMP, and protein kinase A. The only type of adenylyl cyclase which apparently does not possess a protein kinase A phosphorylation site is type 4.

TABLE 12.2
Regulation of Adenylyl Cyclase Types

Regulator	Adenylyl cyclase type	Effect
$G\alpha_s$	1-6	Stimulation
$G\alpha_i$	6,7	Inhibition
$G\beta\gamma$	2,4,7	Stimulation with $G\alpha_s$
$G\beta\gamma$	1	Direct inhibition
$G\beta\gamma$	3,5,6	No direct effect
Ca^{2+}/calmodulin	1,3	Stimulation
Ca^{2+}	6	Direct inhibition
Adenosine and P-site ligands	1,5,6	Direct inhibition
Forskolin	1-6	Stimulation

Taken from Iyengar, R., *Adv. Second Messenger Phosphorylation Res.*, 28, 30, 1993.
With permission.

12.3 PROTEIN KINASE A

Protein kinase A is the effector for cAMP. Structures for a wide variety of protein kinases
are available and comparison of these has revealed considerable similarity in their catalytic
subunits. As might be anticipated, the regulatory and other subunits differ markedly between
different protein kinases. Protein kinase A is a serine-threonine kinase which exists as a
tetramer: two regulatory and two catalytic subunits. There are two holoenzymes referred to
as PKA I and PKA II which differ in the regulatory subunits, but each regulatory subunit has
two binding sites for cAMP. The two binding sites for cAMP on each regulatory subunit are
not identical and have different affinities for cAMP, and PKA I has a higher affinity for cAMP
than does PKA II. Figure 12.7 shows how cAMP activates its effector, PKA.

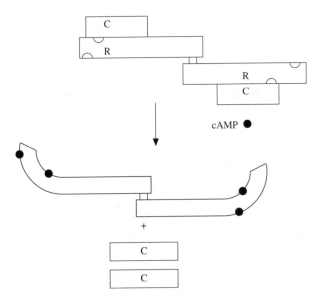

FIGURE 12.7   Protein kinase A comprises two regulatory subunits (R) and two catalytic subunits (C).
Each regulatory subunit has two cAMP binding sites. When cAMP (●) binds to PKA, the catalytic
subunits dissociate and become active.

Interestingly, PKA II regulatory subunits when bound to cAMP exhibit protein phosphatase inhibitory activity. Thus, phosphoproteins formed by the action of the catalytic subunit of PKA may be stabilized by inhibition of protein phosphatases that would otherwise inactivate these phosphoproteins.

12.4 CYCLIC NUCLEOTIDE PHOSPHODIESTERASES

The signal conveyed by cAMP through its effector PKA is terminated by the destruction of cAMP which is brought about by cyclic nucleotide phosphodiesterase. The nomenclature of these phosphodiesterase enzymes in the literature is inconsistent, but on the basis of primary sequence and cDNA data a classification comprising five major families of enzyme has been proposed:

    I. Calcium-calmodulin-dependent phosphodiesterases.
    II. cGMP-stimulated phosphodiesterases.
    III. cGMP-inhibited phosphodiesterases.
    IV. cAMP-specific phosphodiesterases.
    V. cGMP-specific phosphodiesterases.

Within these major families, a number of different subtypes have been identified.

Some phosphodiesterases are activated by hormone-receptor interactions. For example, the action of glucagon on liver cells, which is mediated by a rise in intracellular cAMP, is opposed by the action of insulin on these cells. Part of this effect of insulin results from the activation of a cAMP-specific phosphodiesterase. In the rod cells of the retina, the intracellular level of cGMP is regulated by G-protein (G_t)-induced activation of phosphodiesterase (see below).

12.5 cAMP AS A SECOND MESSENGER

Possibly the best known example of the signal transduction role of cAMP is in mediating the signal generated by the interaction of adrenaline at the β-adrenoreceptor and resulting in breakdown of glycogen and inhibition of its synthesis in the liver and skeletal muscle. There are, of course, many other examples of cells in which cAMP act as a second messenger for the hormone-receptor interaction and these include: secretion of thyroid hormone in response to thyroxine, increase in heart rate in response to noradrenaline, triglyceride breakdown in fat cells in response to adrenaline, and release of cortisol from the adrenal cortex in response to adrenocorticotrophic hormone (ACTH).

12.5.1 CRITERIA FOR ASSESSING THE SECOND MESSENGER FUNCTION OF cAMP

In determining the second messenger function of cAMP, it has been useful to apply a set of criteria for evaluating the experimental evidence for this function of cAMP.

Exogenous cAMP — Exogenously applied cAMP should mimic the action of the hormone-receptor interaction. In fact, in many systems cAMP itself is unable to cross the cell membrane and so it has been common to use more lipid-soluble, membrane-permeable analogues of cAMP such as dibutyryl cAMP or adenosine 3',5'-cyclic-phosphorothioate (cAMPS). Figure 12.8 illustrates this criterion by demonstrating the stimulation of salivary secretion by cAMP in place of the physiological stimulus to the cell which is a 5-hydroxytryptamine-receptor interaction.

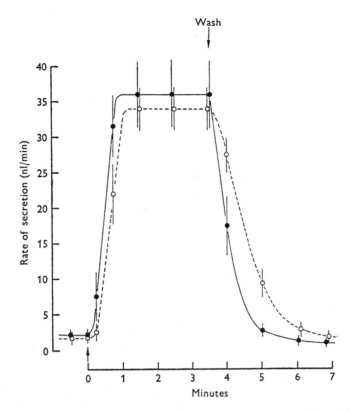

FIGURE 12.8 cAMP 10 mM (○) mimics the effect of 5-hydroxytryptamine 5 nM (●) on the rate of secretion from the fly salivary gland. (From Berridge, M.J., *J. Exp. Biol.*, 53, 171-186, 1970. With permission, Company of Biologists, Ltd.)

Cellular level of cAMP — The hormone-receptor interaction should cause an increase in the cellular level of cAMP with a time course and a concentration-response relationship which are appropriately related to the cellular response.

Inhibition of phosphodiesterase — The presence of a cAMP phosphodiesterase should be demonstrated in the cells responding to the hormone-receptor interaction. It also follows that the cellular response to the hormone-receptor interaction should be potentiated by inhibition of this phosphodiesterase. An example of this can be seen in Figure 12.9 where the methylxanthine inhibitors of phosphodiesterase, caffeine and theophylline, are shifting the concentration-response relationship for 5-hydroxytryptamine and salivary secretion to the left.

Adenylyl cyclase activity — It should be possible to demonstrate the presence of adenylyl cyclase in the cell responding to the hormone and the activity of the adenylyl cyclase should increase when the hormone-receptor interaction takes place. This is one of the most important criteria and it is the one in which pharmacology has played a major role. The use of specific receptor antagonists and the pharmacological application of cholera toxin, pertussis toxin, and forskolin have provided evidence for a role of cAMP in receptor-coupled signal transduction systems.

The relationship between the hormone-receptor interaction and the activation of adenylyl cyclase can be established by the quantitative measurement of the effect of receptor antagonists on these two effects. Precontracted pulmonary smooth muscle in the guinea pig will relax in response to agonists which act on histamine H_2 receptors and this effect may be blocked by selective H_2 receptor antagonists (Figure 12.10). By application of the Schild

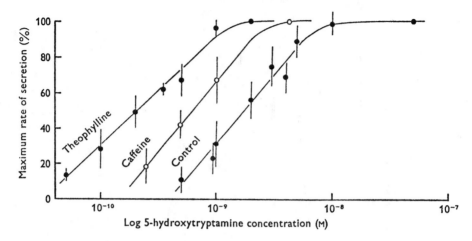

FIGURE 12.9 The phosphodiesterase inhibitors theophylline and caffeine potentiate the action of 5-hydroxytryptamine in stimulating the secretion from the fly salivary gland. (From Berridge, M.J., *J. Exp. Biol.*, 53, 171-186, 1970. With permission, Company of Biologists, Ltd.)

equation (see Chapter 1) to the effects of the H_2 antagonists, the equilibrium dissociation constants for a number of H_2 antagonists can be determined. If the pulmonary tissue is homogenized, the membrane preparation can be used to study the binding of a labeled H_2 antagonist to the receptors (see Chapter 5) and the receptor-mediated activation of adenylyl cyclase can also be measured. Again, the equilibrium dissociation constants for several antagonists can be determined from the binding displacement curves and also from the activation of adenylyl cyclase (Figure 12.11). Comparison of the equilibrium dissociation constants for a variety of antagonists acting at H_2 receptors, obtained from measurements of response, ligand binding, and adenylyl cyclase activity, shows very close agreement of the values for each drug obtained by the three different measurements (Table 12.3) and this provides compelling evidence that in this case, the relaxation of the pulmonary smooth muscle caused by agonists at the H_2 receptor is mediated by the activation of adenylyl cyclase and the subsequent generation of cAMP.

Cholera toxin and forskolin are both pharmacological tools which have been used to activate adenylyl cyclase independently of the hormone-receptor interaction, though they work by different mechanisms. Cholera toxin is a protein consisting of A and B subunits: B is responsible for binding of the protein to the cell and A contains ADP-ribosyltransferase activity which ADP ribosylates, using NAD^+, $G\alpha_s$ as an arginine residue, to maintain $G\alpha_s$ in the active state. Because of the coupling of G_s to adenylyl cyclase, cholera toxin can be used to mimic the activation, by a hormone-receptor interaction, of adenylyl cyclase activation. In broken-cell preparations, nonhydrolyzable analogues of GTP have the same effect as cholera toxin. Forskolin binds directly to the catalytic subunit of adenylyl cyclase and activates it, and so this compound too can be used to mimic the activation by a hormone-receptor interaction of adenylyl cyclase. Pertussis toxin, like cholera toxin, ADP ribosylates G-protein α-subunits, and among those susceptible is $G\alpha_i$. In contrast to cholera toxin, the ADP ribosylation achieved by pertussis toxin causes the G-protein to be maintained in the GDP bound form and hence it is inactive. Such inhibition of G_i will lead to an increase of adenylyl cyclase activity in cells with receptors coupled to G_i and which mediate the inhibition of adenylyl cyclase.

Presence of protein kinase A — The presence of cAMP-dependent protein kinase A (PKA) should be demonstrable in the cells responding to the hormone-receptor interaction.

Protein kinase A substrates as effectors — The presence of PKA-sensitive effector protein(s) should be demonstrable in the cells responding to the hormone-receptor interaction.

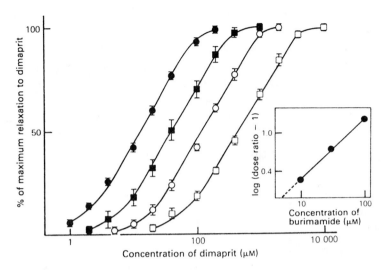

FIGURE 12.10 Concentration-response relationships for the relaxant action of the H_2 receptor agonist, dimaprit, on the guinea-pig lung parenchymal strip. The concentration-response curve for dimaprit alone (●) is repeated in the presence of increasing concentrations of the H_2 receptor antagonist, burimamide (■ 10 μM; ○ 30 μM; □ 100 μM). The inset shows a Schild plot (see Chapter 1) of the concentration-response data. Similar experiments were performed with other H_2 antagonists to generate the data shown in Table 12.3. (From Foreman, J.C. et al., *Br. J. Pharmacol.,* 86, 465-473, 1985. With permission.)

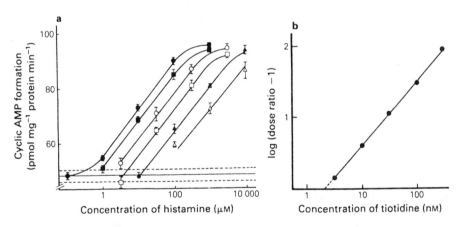

FIGURE 12.11 **a**. Concentration-response relationships for the action of histamine on adenylyl cyclase activity (cAMP formation, pmol/mg protein/min) in an homogenate of guinea-pig lung. The concentration-response curve for histamine alone (●) is repeated in the presence of increasing concentrations of the H_2 receptor antagonist tiotidine (■ 3 nM; ○ 10 nM; □ 30 nM; ▲ 100 nM; △ 300 nM). **b**. Schild plot (see Chapter 1) constructed from the data in a. Similar experiments were performed with other H_2 antagonists to generate the data shown in Table 12.3. (From Foreman, J.C. et al., *Br. J. Pharmacol.,* 87, 37-44, 1986. With permission.)

12.5.2 An Example of cAMP as a Second Messenger

Although some example of the satisfying of the above criteria have been given, the best example, in which all the criteria have been satisfied for considering cAMP as the signal transducer, is the action of a β-adrenoreceptor agonist on skeletal muscle cells (Figure 12.12).

When adrenaline binds to the β-adrenoreceptor on the cell, adenylyl cyclase is activated through G_s and cAMP is formed in the cell within seconds of the application of adrenaline.

TABLE 12.3

Equilibrium Dissociation Constants (K_D) and Inhibition Constants (K_i) for a Selection of Histamine H_2 Receptor Antagonists Obtained by Measuring the Effects of the Antagonists on Smooth Muscle Relaxation, Ligand-Binding and Adenylyl Cyclase Activation

H_2 antagonist	Smooth muscle relaxation K_D (μM)	Ligand binding K_i (μM)	Adenylyl cyclase activity K_D (μM)
Tiotidine	0.004	0.006	0.006
YM11170	0.05	0.04	0.02
Ranitidine	0.4	0.8	0.3
Cimetidine	0.7	0.8	0.8
Metiamide	0.9	0.8	0.8
Burimamide	5.1	4.2	5.7

Note: The K_D values for smooth muscle relaxation and adenylyl cyclase activation were obtained from experiments similar to those shown in Figures 12.10 and 12.11. The K_i values from ligand binding studies were obtained using labeled tiotidine and a membrane preparation from guinea-pig lung parenchymal tissue.

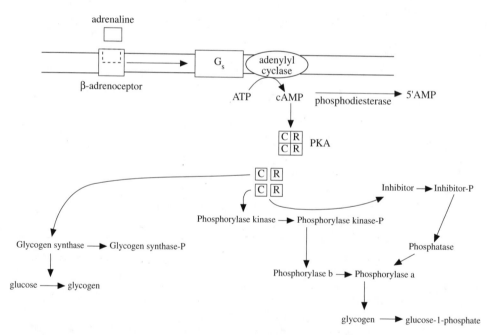

FIGURE 12.12 Cyclic AMP as the signal transducer in skeletal muscle in response to the action of adrenaline at the β-adrenoreceptor. See text for explanation.

The cAMP activates PKA by releasing the catalytic subunits of this enzyme from its regulatory units. The catalytic subunits of PKA phosphorylate the enzyme phosphorylase kinase at serine residues on its α- and β-subunits: it is the phosphorylation of the β-subunit which converts the inactive phosphorylase kinase into its phosphorylated, active form. The active phosphorylase kinase then phosphorylates and activates phosphorylase b, converting it to phosphorylase a, which splits glucose-1-phosphate molecules from glycogen. In addition, there are two other targets for the catalytic subunits of PKA: glycogen synthase and a phosphorylase phosphatase inhibitor protein. Phosphorylation of glycogen synthase inhibits its activity and prevents the synthesis of glycogen from glucose. Phosphorylase inhibitor, when phosphorylated by PKA, inhibits phosphorylase phosphatase whose substrate is phosphorylase a. Thus, dephosphorylation of phosphorylase a by the phosphatase is inhibited and glycogen breakdown is prolonged. The several effector proteins upon which cAMP-dependent protein kinase (PKA) acts work together to inhibit glycogen synthesis and promote glucose release.

12.6 GUANYLYL CYCLASE

Guanylyl cyclase is analogous to adenylyl cyclase but it catalyzes the conversion of GTP to cyclic GMP. In contrast to adenylyl cyclase, two forms of this enzyme have been identified: one which is membrane bound and one which is cytosolic. Also, unlike adenylyl cyclase, neither form of guanylyl cyclase is activated through a G-protein.

The membrane bound form of the enzyme is a large (M_r ~120 kDa) protein which spans the membrane and has a single-transmembrane segment. The membrane protein comprises a receptor domain, a guanylyl cyclase domain, and a protein kinase domain. Thus the receptor and the guanylyl cyclase reside in the same protein. The ligands for this receptor-cyclase system are α-atrial natriuretic peptide (ANP) and brain natriuretic peptide. Genes for two different receptor-cyclase proteins have been cloned: one with a receptor designated ANP_A and the other with a receptor designated ANP_B

Soluble guanylyl cyclase is heterodimeric in structure with subunits of M_r ~70 kDa and ~80 kDa and is a hemo-containing protein. Soluble guanylyl cyclase appears to have no direct membrane ligand-receptor connection but responds instead to the redox state of the cell. It is this cyclase which generates cGMP in response to the free radical nitric oxide (NO·). Nitric oxide is, in many cases, the link between a vasodilator agonist and the relaxation of vascular smooth muscle. An agonist such as acetylcholine acts upon a muscarinic receptor on the endothelial cell to cause a rise in intracellular calcium concentration which, in turn, activates a nitric oxide synthase (NOS) constitutively expressed in the endothelial cell. The NOS converts L-arginine into NO· and L-citrulline and the NO· diffuses into the smooth muscle cell where it activates the soluble form of guanylyl cyclase.

12.7 cGMP AS A SIGNAL TRANSDUCER

In contrast to cAMP, there is little evidence that the effects of cGMP are mediated through the activation of a protein kinase G, although this cGMP-dependent protein kinase has been shown to exist. In fact, relatively little is known, compared with cAMP, about the signal transducing role of cGMP. There now seems little doubt that cGMP is the signal for vascular smooth muscle relaxation in response to the activation of guanylyl cyclase by NO·, but the mechanism of action of cGMP in this context is not known for certain.

One of the best described systems in which cGMP acts as a signal transducing agent is the visual system. An unusual feature of this system is that the signal is relayed by a fall rather than a rise in the intracellular concentration of cGMP The "ligand-receptor" interaction in this system is the photon interaction with rhodopsin which is coupled to the G-protein transducin (G_t). When a photon interacts with rhodopsin, G_t is activated and $G\alpha_t$ interacts with specific cGMP phosphodiesterase (family V — see Section 12.4). This, in turn, causes the phosphodiesterase to become active and the intracellular cGMP is degraded so that the level falls. In the membrane of the rod cell, there is a ion channel which is open in the resting state when the rod cell is receiving no light stimulus: the cell being in a depolarized state. This open state of the ion channel is maintained by cGMP. When under the influence of light, the intracellular cGMP level falls, the ion channel closes, and the cell hyperpolarizes: the hyperpolarization being the signal for neurotransmitter release and the propagation of a nerve impulse (Figure 12.13).

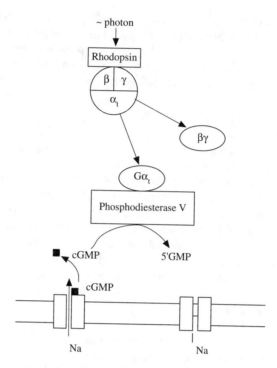

FIGURE 12.13 Cyclic GMP as the signal transducer in the rod cell of the retina in response to the action of a photon on rhodopsin. See text for explanation.

   Another example of the signal transducing role of cGMP is provided by the action of ANP on the kidney. Interaction of ANP with its receptor, which is also the membrane-bound form of guanylyl cyclase, induces a rise in intracellular cGMP which opens a sodium channel in the renal tubular cell and promotes the excretion of sodium. The effects of ANP on sodium excretion and also on intracellular cGMP are both blocked by selective antagonists for the ANP receptor involved.

12.8 FURTHER READING

Adenylyl cyclase — cAMP

Corbin, J.D. and Johnson, R.A. (1988). Initiation and termination of cyclic nucleotide action, *Methods Enzymol.*, 159, 1-815.
Iyengar, R. (1993). Multiple families of G_s-regulated adenylyl cyclases, *Adv. Second Messenger Phosphoprotein Res.*, 28, 27-36.

Protein kinase A

Taylor, S. (1989). cAMP-dependent protein kinase, *J. Biol. Chem.*, 264, 8443-8446.

Cyclic nucleotide phosphodiesterases

Beavo, J.A. and Reifsnyder, D.H. (1990). Primary sequence of cyclic nucleotide phosphodiesterase isoenzymes and the design of selective inhibitors, *Trends Pharmacol. Sci.*, 11, 150-155.

Guanylyl cyclase-cGMP

Goy, M.F. (1991). cGMP: the wayward child of the cyclic nucleotide family, *Trends Neurosci.*, 14, 293-299.

Koesling, D., Böhme, E. and Schultz, G. (1991). Guanylyl cyclases, a growing family of signal-transducing enzymes, *FASEB J.*, 5, 2785-2791.

Anand-Srivastava, M.B. and Trachte, G.J. (1993). Atrial natriuretic factor receptors and signal transduction mechanisms, *Pharmacol. Rev.*, 45, 455-497.

13 Signal Transduction Through Tyrosine Protein Kinases

IJsbrand M. Kramer

CONTENTS

13.1 INTRODUCTION

13.1.1 PHOSPHORYLATION AS A SWITCH IN CELLULAR FUNCTIONING

Phosphorylation of protein was discovered in the era of "allosteric regulation". Regulation of enzyme activity could be explained by the concentration of substrates, the presence of cofactors, and the concentration of the end product (allosteric effectors). One of the pathways thus analyzed was the glycolysis pathway. The first step in this pathway is the conversion of glycogen to glucose-1-phosphate which is mediated by an enzyme called phosphorylase.

0-8493-9227-6/96/$0.00+$.50
© 1996 by CRC Press, Inc.

Enzyme activity could be regulated through allosteric interactions by adenosine-5'-mono-phosphate (stimulatory) and glucose-6-phosphate (inhibitory). This enzyme could be isolated in two forms, an active form designated with an *a*, and a less active form designated with a *b*. In 1956 it was discovered by Krebs and Fischer that the enzyme phosphorylase *b* (inactive) could incorporate one organic phosphate molecule on a serine residue, a process that was accompanied by a change in activity. Through the incorporation of a phosphate, phosphorylase *b* was converted into phosphorylase *a*. Thus, apart from allosteric regulation, a covalent modification such as phosphorylation could also affect enzyme activity. This phosphorylation reaction was catalyzed by a protein kinase called phosphorylase kinase. Later it was discovered that a phosphorylase phosphatase catalyzed dephosphorylation and brought the enzyme back into the phosphorylase *b* state. By 1970 it was clear that almost all enzymes were regulated by phosphorylation/dephosphorylation, and investigators began to question why it was "necessary" to have two broad systems for controlling enzyme activity: allosteric regulation and covalent regulation. Moreover, in the case of phosphorylase and another enzyme, glycogen synthase, it was clear that allosteric and covalent regulation probably worked through similar conformational changes. A basic difference between these two types of regulation became apparent when it was found that hormone receptors, through the release of intracellular second messengers, in turn controlled the phosphorylase kinase activity. While allosteric control generally reflects intracellular conditions, covalent regulation responds mainly to extracellular signals. Covalent regulation allows the organism to control metabolism in individual cells. Phosphorylation and dephosphorylation reactions, as will be seen in the following paragraphs, are always part of a cascade of reactions. Cascade systems allow for an enormous amplification as well as fine modulation of an original signal. While the field of serine/threonine protein kinases exploded, a new type of protein kinase entered the arena in 1978 with the discovery that the Rous sarcoma virus contained a protein kinase, named v-src, that phosphorylated protein on a tyrosine residue. It was then discovered that growth factor receptors contain tyrosine protein kinases and a new field of research rapidly developed. This chapter deals with the events that follow receptor occupation and activation of tyrosine protein kinases. This chapter shall focus on the signal transduction pathways of receptors that either contain protein tyrosine kinase activity in their cytoplasmic domains or associate with cytosolic protein tyrosine kinases.

13.1.2 GROWTH FACTORS, INTERLEUKINS, INTERFERONS, AND CYTOKINES

Research on tyrosine kinase-containing receptors was initiated in the area of cell biology. Factors that could support growth of cells in culture were isolated and named after (1) the cells they were isolated from, (2) the cells they stimulated, or (3) the principal action they performed; for example, platelet-derived growth factor, epidermal growth factor, or transforming growth factor. In the area of immunology, factors were studied that directed maturation and proliferation of white blood cells. The factors discovered were named interleukins or colony stimulating factors. In virology, factors were studied that interfered with viral infection: interferons. And in cancer research, factors were studied that could influence the growth of solid tumors; for example, tumor necrosis factor. Each area of research believed that the factors functioned by and large only in the category in which they came to light. It was also believed that each factor had a set of additional actions that were related to each other in some obvious way. With progress, it became apparent that growth factors, for instance, also acted on cells of the immune system and also had totally unrelated actions. Moreover, it was shown that the context in which the cells were studied (presence of other factors, presence of other cells, attached or in suspension, type of substrate) also determined the outcome of the cellular response. A good example is transforming growth factor β, a factor initially shown to enhance cell transformation, hence its name. Later it was found that this factor was a strong growth inhibitor of transformed epithelial cell lines and that it was a very potent chemotactic factor for neutrophils. It has been proposed that a common name for these factors should be cytokines. The definition for a cytokine is *"a soluble (glyco)protein, non-immunoglobulin in nature, released by living cells of the host, which acts non-enzymatically in picomolar to nanomolar concentrations to regulate host cell function."* This information is not directly relevant for understanding the action of tyrosine protein kinases but it illustrates that various areas of research are coming together and introducing new insights in cell functioning. It also illustrates that tyrosine phosphorylation is not limited to growth-inducing cytokines. Tyrosine phosphorylation has been shown to regulate cell-cell and cell-matrix interactions through integrin receptors and focal adhesion sites. It is also involved in stimulation of the respiratory burst in neutrophils. Occupation of the B-cell IgM and high affinity IgE receptor as well as occupation of the T-cell and interleukin-2 receptor results in tyrosine phosphorylation. Lastly, it is also involved in selection of transmitter responses induced by neuronal contact.

13.1.3 Receptor Classification

Tyrosine protein kinase-linked receptors belong to a family of receptor proteins with a single transmembrane segment. In some receptors the tyrosine protein kinase is an integral part of the receptor, but in others the tyrosine protein kinases associates with the receptor after activation (Figure 13.1). A full account of receptor structure is given in Chapters 2, 3, and 4; Chapter 4 deals with protein kinase receptors.

13.2 TYROSINE KINASE-CONTAINING RECEPTORS

13.2.1 Cross-Linking of Receptors Is Essential for Activation

An essential feature of activation of the tyrosine kinase-containing receptors is that binding of the ligand results in dimerization of the receptors. Platelet-derived growth factor (PGDF) is a dimeric ligand and can cross-link two receptors; epidermal growth factor (EGF), on the other hand, is a monomeric ligand and two molecules are needed to bring two receptors together. In the case of EGF, it is believed that ligand binding changes the conformation in the extracellular domain of the receptor such that the one receptor recognizes the other. The binding of the ligand and subsequent dimerization results in yet another conformational change which unveils the dormant tyrosine kinase activity. The active protein kinase is now able to phosphorylate the neighboring receptor (interphosphorylation) on a number of tyrosine residues (Figure 13.2). The tyrosine-phosphorylated dimeric receptor complex is the active EGF receptor and a similar mechanism applies for the PDGF receptor. At this stage, the receptor is able to phosphorylate and activate enzymes, and is also able to interact with adaptor proteins.

13.2.2 Formation of Receptor Signaling Complexes

The dimerized, phosphorylated receptor initiates a series of signal transduction cascades through association with a number of other proteins (Figure 13.3). The receptor associated with these proteins is called a *receptor signaling complex*. Essential in this association are the various phosphorylated tyrosine residues and their immediately adjacent amino acids. These interactions have been studied in a number of ways.

1. Through measurement of enzyme activity, the generation of second messengers, and analyzing tyrosine phosphorylated substrates. For instance, the EGF or PDGF

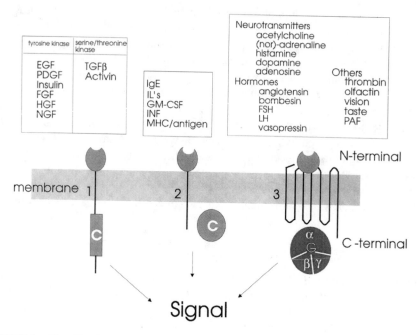

FIGURE 13.1 Classification of cellular outer membrane receptors. Class 1: receptors that span the membrane one time and have intrinsic catalytic (C) activity (tyrosine or serine/threonine protein kinase). Class 2: receptors that span the membrane one time, have no known intrinsic catalytic activity, but may interact with tyrosine protein kinases (C). Class 3: receptors that span the membrane seven times and associate with a heterotrimeric G-protein (G). The column above each receptor class represents examples of ligands that bind to that class of receptors. Abbreviations: EGF, epidermal growth factor; PDGF, platelet-derived growth factor; FGF, fibroblasts growth factor; FSH, follicle stimulating hormone; GM-CSF, granulocyte macrophage-colony stimulating factor; HGF, hepatocyte growth factor; IgE, immunoglobulin-E; IL, interleukin; INF, interferon; LH, luteinizing hormone; MHC, major histocompatibility complex; NGF, neural growth factor; PAF, platelet-activating factor; TGFβ1, transforming growth factor β1.

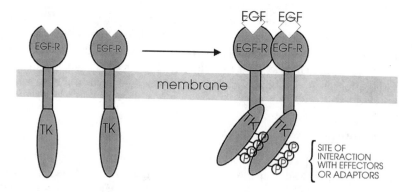

FIGURE 13.2 Occupation of the EGF receptor (EGF-R) results in dimerization, followed by a change in the conformation of the cytoplasmic domain. The change in conformation unfolds the latent tyrosine protein kinase activity of the receptor. The active tyrosine protein kinase phosphorylates the tyrosine residues on the adjacent receptor (interphosphorylation). The dimerized, phosphorylated receptor is the catalytically active receptor. Abbreviations: EGF, epidermal growth factor; P, phosphorylated tyrosine residues; TK, tyrosine kinase domain.

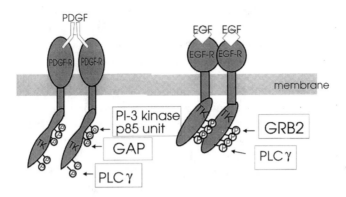

FIGURE 13.3 The activated EGF or PDGF receptors (EGF-R or PDGF-R, respectively) associate with effectors (enzymes such as PLCγ and GAP) or adaptor proteins (such as p85[PI-3kinase] and GRB2) thus forming a *receptor signaling complex*. Abbreviations: GAP, GTPase activating protein; GRB2, growth-factor receptor bound-2; PI-3-kinase, phosphatidylinositol-3-kinase; PLCγ, phospholipase C-γ; PDGF, platelet-derived growth factor; TK, tyrosine kinase domain.

receptors are able to stimulate phospholipase-C-γ (PLCγ) resulting in the generation of diacylglycerol (DAG) and inositol-1,4,5-trisphosphate (IP$_3$). The generation of IP$_3$ explains the initial rise in intracellular free Ca^{2+} which is also seen after receptor activation. In addition, PLCγ is phosphorylated on a tyrosine residue, indicating an interaction with the receptor. Analysis of the phosphoamino acid residues is performed through complete hydrolysis of the polypeptide chain followed by two-dimensional thin-layer chromatography (in the presence of phosphoamino acid markers) and autoradiography. In a similar fashion it was shown that activation of the PDGF receptor results in the conversion of phosphatidylinositol bisphosphate (PIP$_2$) to phosphatidylinositol trisphosphate (PIP$_3$), through activation of an enzyme named phosphatidylinositol-3-kinase (PI-3-kinase). It was also shown that a number of serine/threonine protein kinases were activated, for instance mitogen-activated protein kinase (MAPkinase), ribosomal S6 kinase, and Raf-1 kinase. An important finding was that the monomeric G-protein ras becomes activated upon receptor occupation. It changes from a GDP-bound state (inactive) to a GTP-bound state (active). In a later section the importance of ras will be discussed in more detail. A shortlist of these events are presented in Table 13.1.

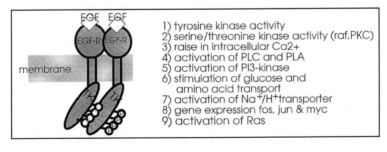

1) tyrosine kinase activity
2) serine/threonine kinase activity (raf,PKC)
3) raise in intracellular Ca2+
4) activation of PLC and PLA
5) activation of PI3-kinase
6) stimulation of glucose and
     amino acid transport
7) activation of Na$^+$/H$^+$ transporter
8) gene expression fos, jun & myc
9) activation of Ras

Table 13.1

2. Through studying physical association of protein with the receptor by immunoprecipitation. To study interaction of proteins with the receptor, cells are labeled with ^{35}S-methionine and stimulated with the appropriate cytokine. At various time

points (in a minutes time-scale) cells are solubilized in a nonionic detergent and the receptor is immunoprecipitated with a specific antibody. After extensive washing, the precipitated complex is dissociated in an ionic detergent and separated by gel electrophoresis. The receptor can be identified by its molecular weight or through detection with antibodies. Using autoradiography, the ^{35}S-labeled proteins that come down with the receptor can by analyzed. Further identification can take place by microsequencing (amino acid sequence), antibody staining (Western blotting), or functional assays. In this way the association of the proteins GTPase activating protein (GAP), Src homology collagen-like protein (Shc), PLCγ, and PI-3-kinase with protein tyrosine kinase receptors has been demonstrated.

3. <u>Through studying protein association in a cell-free system.</u> For this purpose, the receptor is ^{32}P-phosphorylated on its tyrosine residues, its cytoplasmic domain removed through restricted proteolysis, and this domain is used to screen a λphage library expressing a whole variety of cellular proteins. Using autoradiography, the bound ^{32}P-labeled cytoplasmic domain of the receptor can be detected and the relevant λphage clone isolated. This technique has been called cloning of receptor target. The advantage of this approach is that once a selective binding has been established, the identity of the protein can be obtained through DNA sequencing of the λphage insert, followed by screening of sequence libraries for homologies with other proteins in order to unveil its possible function. In this way, GRB-2 and the p85 subunit of PI-3-kinase were discovered to interact with the receptor.

13.2.3 ROLE OF SH2 DOMAINS IN THE FORMATION OF RECEPTOR SIGNALING COMPLEXES

In the search for viral proteins that were able to transform cell lines, a protein named p47[gag-crk] was identified. This protein induced extensive phosphorylation of cellular proteins on tyrosine residues, without itself having protein kinase activity. The 47-kDa protein is a fusion product of the retroviral gag gene and a cellular protein fragment designated as CRK, CT_{10} regulator of kinase. It was shown that the cellular protein fragment consists of 1 domain of 100 amino acids and 2 domains of 50 amino acids and had great homology with parts of the gene isolated from the Rous sarcoma virus which codes for a 60-kDa tyrosine protein kinase called src. The domains were named SH2 and SH3, respectively (SH = src homology). It was then shown that p47[gag-crk] could bind to tyrosine-phosphorylated Src kinase and that the SH2 domains were essential for this binding. In order to explain the increased phosphorylation on tyrosine residues, it was postulated that the p47[gag-crk] protein acts as an adaptor, facilitating the interaction of the Src tyrosine kinase with its substrates. The sequence data that became available from the various proteins that could associate with the tyrosine kinase receptors revealed that all contained one or two SH2 domains. The SH2 domain in the various proteins is able to recognize the phosphorylated tyrosine residues and some immediately adjacent amino acids, and this recognition results in a tight association of the SH2 domain with the receptor (Figure 13.4). The relevance of the SH2 domain is shown by the observation that deletion of this domain prevents association of the p47[gag-crk] with the Src tyrosine protein kinase.

The relevance of this is also illustrated in the case of PLC. This phospholipase consists of a family of isozymes indicated as β, γ, and δ (Chapter 9). Of these phospholipases, only the γ-form contains an SH2 domain, and it is only this form that is directly activated by the tyrosine kinase-containing receptor. The other forms are activated by receptors that have seven membrane-spanning domains and associate with heterotrimeric G-proteins. At this point it should be noted that the proteins that are associated through their SH2 domains with the receptor are also phosphorylated on a tyrosine residue, but it is not clear yet whether or not

Enzymes

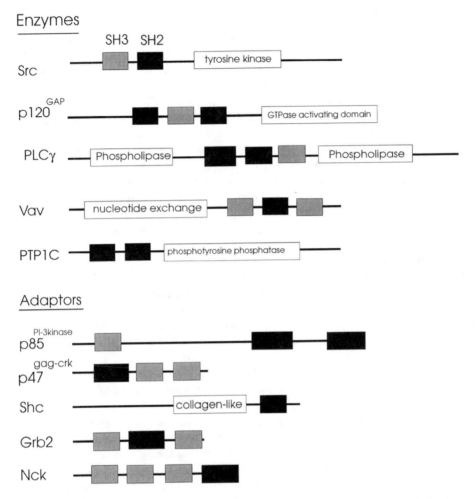

FIGURE 13.4 Sequence analysis of proteins that associate with the phosphorylated tyrosine kinase-containing receptor. This analysis revealed that proteins that associate with the receptors contain a Src homology-2 (SH2) domain. The SH2 domain recognizes specific amino acid stretches around a phosphorylated tyrosine residue. Not all proteins presented in this figure will be discussed in this chapter. The adaptors lack intrinsic enzymatic activity but serve to link the receptor with other effector proteins. Abbreviations: gag-crk, gag-CT$_{10}$ regulator of kinase; GAP, GTPase activating protein; GRB2, growth-factor receptor bound-2; PLCγ, phospholipase C-γ; PI-3-kinase, phosphatidylinositol-3-kinase; PTP1C, protein tyrosine phosphatase-1C; Shc, Src homology collagen-like; Src, sarcoma

this phosphorylation is necessary for the "activation" of these proteins. SH2-containing proteins can be divided into two groups: those that have intrinsic catalytic activity, with PLCγ as a prime example, and those that have no apparent catalytic activity, also called adaptor proteins, with p47$^{gag-crk}$ as an example. From the receptor signaling complex a number of signal transduction pathways branch to transmit the signal into the cell. Four such pathways will be described in the next paragraphs.

Although multiple proteins seem to be able to bind to the phosphorylated EGF or PDGF receptor it is not clear yet if more than one protein at a time can bind to the receptor. It already seems clear that the different proteins show preferential binding to a specific phosphorylated tyrosine residue, which suggests that a given receptor can mediate its signal through a receptor-specific panel of SH2-containing proteins.

13.2.4 The PLC-Protein Kinase C Signal Transduction Pathway

One of the first pathways extensively studied after the activation of EGF or PDGF receptor was the activation of PLCγ resulting in the hydrolysis of PIP_2 into DAG and IP_3. The DAG remains in the membrane and can activate protein kinase C (see Chapter 11). Protein kinase C (PKC) is a serine/threonine kinase that was first characterized on the basis of its activation *in vitro* by Ca^{2+}, phospholipid, and DAG. PKC exists as a still growing family of protein kinases (isotypes), which can be separated in three main families: family I indicated as α, β, γ; family II indicated as δ, ε, η, θ, μ; family III ι, λ, ζ (for further detail see Chapter 11). Through stimulation of PLCγ, a tyrosine signal is transformed into a serine/threonine signal. One of the first substrates of PKC is the EGF receptor itself. It becomes phosphorylated on a serine residue very close to the transmembrane domain. To illustrate substrate specificity of PKC isotypes, it has been shown that the degree of phosphorylation of the EGF receptor has the following rank order: PKCα > PKCβ > PKCγ. This phosphorylation inactivates the receptor in a negative feedback loop. Although numerous proteins have proven to be substrates of PKC, it still is not fully understood how activation of this kinase results in changes in gene transcription as seen after addition of cytokines. One consequence of activation of PKC is dephosphorylation of the transcription factor c-Jun on phosphoamino acid residues thr231, ser243, and ser249. These phosphorylation sites are at the carboxy terminal of the protein, near the DNA binding site. It is likely that the phosphorylated residues negatively interfere with DNA binding. c-Jun can be kept in an inactive, highly phosphorylated state by casein kinase II. On the other hand, an ongoing phosphatase activity shifts c-Jun to an underphosphorylated form. PKCα could theoretically disrupt the balance, either by inactivation of casein kinase II or by activation of the c-Jun phosphatase. Neither of these possibilities have been properly investigated. The dephosphorylated c-Jun homodimerizes and forms an active transcription factor complex. The c-Jun dimer binds to DNA at the TPA (tetradecanoyl phorbol acetate)-responsive element (TRE) (Figure 13.5). Transcription factor complexes that bind to a TRE are also called AP-1, which stands for activator protein-1. However, the physiological role of this PKC pathway has not been confirmed. Protein kinase C is also able to activate, in a cell-free system, the serine/threonine protein kinase Raf-1 through phosphorylation. Raf-1 is part of the ras signal transduction chain, as will be explained in the next section. Whether PKC activation of Raf-1 is a physiologically relevant observation or not is still under investigation. Lastly and surprisingly, PLCγ activation is not necessary for the mitogenic activity of EGF or PDGF.

13.2.5 The Ras Signal Transduction Pathway

13.2.5.1 From Tyrosine Kinase to Ras

Ras has been known for some time as an oncogene (v-H-ras and v-K-ras) that is present in the Harvey and Kirsten rat sarcoma virus strains. Infection with these virus strains causes cell tranformation resulting in a sarcoma. Later it was found that four cellular homologues of the ras gene exists (H-ras, N-ras, K-rasA, and K-rasB) which, when mutated, also cause transformation of cells, i.e., increased division rate, reduced cytokine requirements, growth in nude mice and soft agar. Overexpression of the mutated cellular ras protein can bypass growth signals in cells that would normally be needed for inducing cell division. Conversely, inhibition of ras function through injection of antibodies or by the transfection of a dominant negative mutant can block cytokine-induced cell division. For many years it was known that ras took a central stage in regulation of cell function, but how it would fit into known signal transduction pathways remained unclear. Ras is a 21-kDa G-protein that acts as a binary switch. Like the heterotrimeric G-proteins, it is active in the GTP-bound state and inactive in the GDP-bound state. The ras-GTP complex is able to interact with a downstream effector protein and transmit a signal. However, unlike the heterotrimeric G-proteins, ras has very

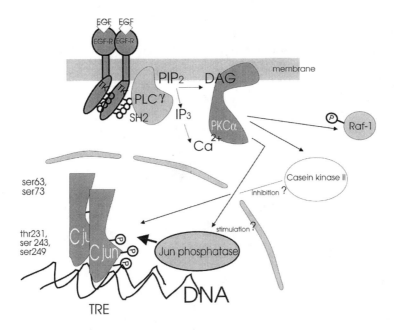

FIGURE 13.5 The protein kinase C (PKC) signal transduction pathway. Activation of phospholipase C-γ (PLCγ) results in the generation of diacylglycerol (DAG) and inositol-1,4,5-trisphosphate (IP$_3$). IP$_3$ causes the release of Ca^{2+} from intracellular stores. Ca^{2+} and DAG activate protein kinase C-α. The active kinase either activates a putative Jun phosphatase or deactivates casein kinase II. Both actions ultimately result in dephosphorylation of the c-Jun carboxy-terminal phosphoamino acid residues (position thr231, ser243, ser249). These events allows a homodimer of c-Jun to bind to the DNA at the TRE site. PKCα has also been shown to phosphorylate the protooncogene Raf-1, thereby opening the MAPkinase pathway (for further details see Figure 13.9). Abbreviations: MAPkinase, mitogen-activated protein kinase; TRE, TPA-responsive element; TPA, o-tetradecanoylphorbol-13-acetate (also called PMA, phorbol-12-myristate-13-acetate) DAG, diacylglycerol; IP$_3$, inositol-1,4,5-trisphosphate; PLCγ, phospholipase C-γ.

little intrinsic nucleotide exchange activity for the replacement of GTP for GDP or GTPase activity, or for the hydrolysis of GTP to GDP + Pi, and yet stimulation of tyrosine kinase receptors results in a rapid shift of ras activity from the GDP-bound to the GTP-bound state. This function is performed by two accessory proteins, one named p120^{GAP} (GTPase activating protein) and one named p155^{GNRP} (guanosine nucleotide release protein) (Figure 13.6). The oncogenic form of ras is in a permanent GTP-bound state due to a mutation that prevents the hydrolysis of GTP. A defect in p120^{GAP} also causes predisposition for tumor formation. Comparison with signal transduction pathways in the eye development of *Drosophila mela-nogaster* and sex organ development in *Caenorhabditis elegans* revealed homologies that helped to elucidate the sequence of events. Through analysis by gene deletion, a series of genes both in *D. melanogaster* and in *C. elegans* could be put in a particular sequence as depicted in Figure 13.7. The genes involved code for a ras-like protein, an SH2-containing protein, and a tyrosine kinase-containing protein. An important finding was that the mammalian GRB2 protein (which binds to an activated tyrosine kinase receptor and was therefore named growth factor-receptor bound-2) could functionally replace the *C. elegans*, Sem5 (sex muscle-5). This finding placed this thus far functionless protein GRB2 between a putative tyrosine kinase-containing receptor (let-23) and ras (let-60). Another important finding was that antibodies against the *D. melanogaster* son of sevenless-gene product (SOS) recognized a protein in mammalian cells that coprecipitated with GRB2. This precipitated protein contained guanine nucleotide replacement activity (conversion of ras-GDP to ras-GTP) and was designated p155^{GNRP}. The sequence was complete. The phosphorylated tyrosine kinase binds an adaptor protein, GRB2, which in turn binds to p155^{GNRP} which in turn brings ras into the GTP-bound state (Figure 13.8). While ras is activated by GRB2/GNRP, the GTPase activating protein, p120^{GAP}, which would inactivate ras through hydrolysis of GTP, temporarily associates with the phosphorylated tyrosine kinase receptor (see also Figure 13.3). The function of this association is not known yet, but it could mean a temporary removal of p120^{GAP} from ras in order to maintain ras in its GTP-bound state.

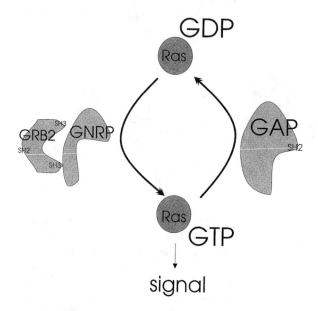

FIGURE 13.6   Regulation of ras. Activation of the GRB2 and GNRP-protein complex removes the GDP from ras, allowing the GTP to bind. The GTPase activating protein (GAP) reverses this action through hydrolysis of GTP. The ras-GTP is the active form of ras. Abbreviations: GDP, guanosine-5'-diphosphate; GTP, guanosine-5'-triphosphate; GNRP, guanine nucleotide release protein; GRB2, growth factor-receptor bound-2; SH, Src homology.

13.2.5.2   From Ras to MAPkinase and Transcriptional Activation

A very early event after activation of a receptor tyrosine kinase is the activation of a serine/threonine kinase designated MAPkinase (mitogen-activated protein kinase), also referred to as extracellular regulated kinase (ERK). After the cloning of the gene it appeared that many variants exist, such as ERK1 and ERK2, and also the three types of Jun N-terminal kinases (JNK1, JNK2, and JNK3). Activation does not occur through second messengers such as cAMP, cGMP, Ca^{2+}, or DAG because after addition of EGF or PDGF to intact cells the MAPkinase can be recovered from cell lysates in an activated state without the presence of any of these second messengers. Activation of MAPkinase cannot be mimicked in a cell-free system consisting of kinase enzyme and the receptor tyrosine kinase alone. It was found that at least two other kinases are involved (Figure 13.9). One is named MEK (MAPkinase ERK-activating kinase) and it phosphorylates MAPkinase on a tyrosine and a threonine residue. MEK has an unusual substrate specificity in that so far no other substrates have been discovered. The second kinase in the cascade is Raf-1, a protein kinase initially discovered as an oncogene. The subsequent finding that activated ras can bind to and activate Raf-1 kinase, connects the MAPkinase activation with the ras pathway. Upon phosphorylation and activation by MEK, MAPkinase translocates to the nucleus. In the case of stimulation by EGF, MAPkinase activation is an absolute requirement for cell proliferation.

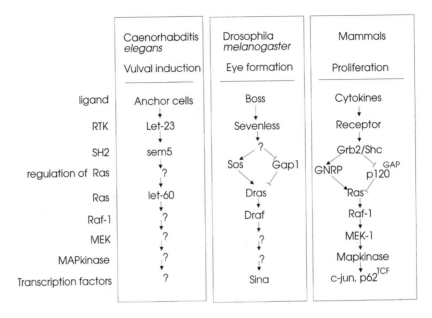

	Caenorhabditis elegans	Drosophila melanogaster	Mammals
	Vulval induction	Eye formation	Proliferation
ligand	Anchor cells	Boss	Cytokines
RTK	Let-23	Sevenless	Receptor
SH2	sem5	?	Grb2/Shc
regulation of Ras	?	Sos Gap1	GNRP GAP p120
Ras	let-60	Dras	Ras
Raf-1	?	Draf	Raf-1
MEK	?	?	MEK-1
MAPkinase	?	?	Mapkinase
Transcription factors	?	Sina	c-jun, p62 TCF

FIGURE 13.7 Comparison of tyrosine kinase-induced signal transduction pathways in *Caenorhabditis elegans*, *Drosophila melanogaster* and mammals. Through comparison with other species, it became possible to arrange the sequence of events from receptor-occupation to Raf-1 kinase activation, with ras as the central switch. Abbreviations: Boss, bride of sevenless; ERK, extracellular regulated kinase; GAP, GTPase activating protein; let, lethal (mutation); MAPkinase, mitogen-activated protein kinase; MEK, MAPkinase ERK kinase; RTK, receptor tyrosine kinase; sem, sex muscle (mutant); Shc, Src homology collagen-like; Sina, seven in absentia (R7 photoreceptor gene product); Sos, son of sevenless; TCF, ternary complex factor.

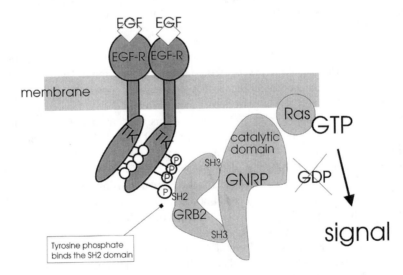

FIGURE 13.8 Activation of ras through tyrosine kinase-containing receptors. Tyrosine phosphorylated residues are recognized by the adaptor protein GRB2 through its SH2 domain. GRB2 is associated with the guanine nucleotide release protein (GNRP) through its SH3 domains. The association of GRB2 with the receptor activates the complex, which in turn removes GDP and allows GTP to associate with ras. Ras-GTP will transmit the signal to a downstream effector. Abbreviation: GRB2, growth factor-receptor bound-2; GDP, guanosine-5′-bisphosphate; GTP, guanosine-5′-trisphosphate.

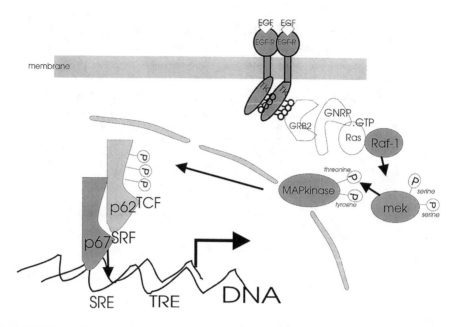

FIGURE 13.9 Activation of mitogen-activated protein kinase (MAPkinase) through Raf-1 and MAP-kinase ERK kinase (MEK). The activated ras interacts with the serine/threonine protein kinase Raf-1 which phosphorylates and activates MEK. MEK in turn phosphorylates MAPkinase on a threonine and tyrosine residue. MAPkinase migrates to the nucleus and phosphorylates the transcription factor p62^{TCF}. This protein associates with p67^{SRF} and together they form an active transcription factor complex that binds to DNA at the serum response element (SRE). The complex is called ternary complex, consisting of SRF, TCF, and DNA. The binding results in increased transcriptional activity of genes containing a serum response element (SRE). Abbreviations: ERK, extracellular regulated kinase (identical to MAP-kinase); GAP, GTPase activating protein; GRB2, growth factor-receptor bound-2; MAPkinase, mitogen-activated protein kinase; MEK, MAPkinase ERK kinase; SRE, serum response element; SRF, serum response factor; TCF, ternary complex factor; TRE, TPA response element.

Activation of the EGF receptor results in a rapid induction of mRNA for the transcription factor c-fos. C-fos was one of the first cytokine-inducible transcription factors discovered, and this transcription factor takes center stage in the regulation of gene expression. The promoter region of the c-fos gene contains a transcription factor-binding domain, called serum-response-element (SRE) and two transcription factors bind to this element: the p67^{SRF} (serum response factor) and the p62^{TCF} (ternary complex factor) proteins. The p62^{TCF} protein is phosphorylated by MAPkinase at various phosphoamino acid residues, and this phosphorylation increases complex formation of the two proteins with the DNA, hence a "promotion" of transcription of the c-fos gene. C-Jun is also phosphorylated and activated after stimulation of the EGF receptor. This phosphorylation takes place at the amino-terminal of the protein (positions Ser63 and Ser73). Cellular overexpression of an oncogenic form of ras (Ha-Ras) activates c-Jun-mediated gene transcription. However, this activation is not via the Raf-1, MEK, and MAPkinase pathway, because the introduction of an active form of Raf-1 into a cell has no effect on c-Jun activation. MAPkinase also only poorly phosphorylates c-Jun. The activation of c-Jun appears to be a consequence of phosphorylation by JNK, another member of the mitogen-activated kinases. Which pathway is followed to link ras with JNK is currently under investigation. Members of the ras family of small G-proteins like Rac1, Rac2, or Cdc42 are potential candidates.

Apart from the role of MAPkinase in transcriptional regulation, its activation also results in the activation of yet another protein kinase, S6kinase, that phosphorylates a small ribosomal particle named S6. This ribosomal particle is part of the ribosomal complex (40S plus 60S) involved in translation of protein. It is not understood how S6 kinase changes the translational machinery, but it is assumed that the mitogenic signal initiated by EFG or PDGF receptor activation requires increased protein synthesis, and maybe even a changed selectivity for translation of mRNAs (not all mRNA that are present in the cell are translated at the same rate). It appears that the ras signal transduction pathway is highly conserved throughout evolution (from yeast to mammals), and that with the increasing complexity of the organism new downstream response elements and effectors were hooked on to create greater diversity. Although each type of cell may respond differently to activation of a tyrosine kinase-containing receptor, the signal will follow a common pathway, only to hit a unique downstream component.

13.2.6 THE PHOSPHOLIPASE A_2 PATHWAY

Activation of the EGF receptor results in rapid activation of voltage-dependent Ca^{2+} channels in the plasma membrane. These channels are activated by hyperpolarization caused by the opening of a K^+ channel, which in turn is opened by the activation of EGF-regulated Ca^{2+} channels (Figure 13.10). The activation of the EGF-regulated Ca^{2+} channels can be prevented by inhibition of PLA_2 or by inhibition of 5-lipoxygenase. These two enzymes are mediating leukotriene release. PLA_2-induced hydrolysis of phospholipids results in the formation of a lysophospholipid and a free fatty acid, of which arachidonic acid is the most prominent. Arachidonic acid, in turn, is a substrate for 5-lipoxygenase which converts it to 5-HPETE which is then converted to leukotrienes. Addition of leukotrienes, in particular leukotriene-C_4 (LTC_4) or arachidonic acid, can mimic the action of EGF, establishing that a PLA_2 pathway initiates the ion-channel cascade. EGF is also able to stimulate the activity of PLA_2 and it is believed that MAPkinase mediates this activation. Introduction of a dominant negative mutant of ras (N17Ras) prevents the activation of MAPkinase and also prevents the activation of PLA_2. Apart from these initial events in the plasma membrane, the generation of leukotrienes is also instrumental in the mitogenic signal of EGF and in the induction of the immediate-early genes c-fos, egr-1, junB, and c-myc. Which signal transduction pathway is involved is not yet studied, but the increase in intracellular free Ca^{2+} can explain some of the events. It should be mentioned that PKC can inhibit the Ca^{2+}-induced opening of the K^+ channel, possibly through phosphorylation. This is another example of a negative feedback loop whereby the EGF receptor quenches it own signal. Lastly, EGF can elicit ruffling of the cell membrane, followed by a rounding up of epithelial cells. These changes are mediated through reorganization of the actin microfilament system, and leukotrienes are instrumental in this response. Leukotrienes cause actin polymerization in the cell cortex (layer adjacent to the plasma membrane). Actin polymerization in the cell cortex is controlled by the activity of two small G-proteins, Rac and Rho (relatives of ras), but it has not been established yet whether or not leukotrienes directly interfere with their activity.

13.2.7 THE Ca^{2+}/CALMODULIN PATHWAY

Tyrosine kinase-containing receptors can evoke a rise in intracellular Ca^{2+} in two ways: (1) through the activation of PLCγ with subsequent generation of IP_3, which in turn causes release of Ca^{2+} from intracellular stores, and (2) through opening of leukotriene-activated Ca^{2+} channels and activation of voltage-sensitive Ca^{2+} channels. Calmodulin is a major Ca^{2+}-binding protein that is able to interact with and control activity of many target proteins, as illustrated in Figure 13.11. A rise in intracellular Ca^{2+} results in an enhanced binding of Ca^{2+} to calmodulin, and hence an enhanced binding of the complex to other proteins. Among these other proteins is the Ca^{2+}/calmodulin-dependent protein kinase II (CaMKII), a broad substrate specific serine/threonine kinase. Also, the highly specific myosin light chain kinase (smooth muscle contraction), phosphorylase kinase (glycogen metabolism liver, muscle), and elongation factor-2 kinase (protein translation) are activated by the Ca^{2+}/calmodulin complex. CaMKII exists as a family, the members of which are designated as CaMKII-α, -β1, or -β2.

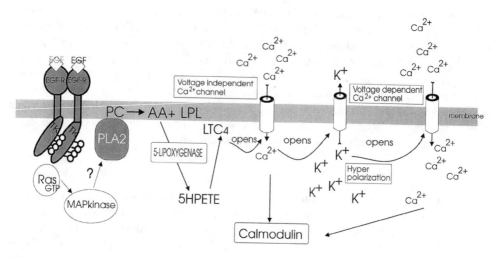

FIGURE 13.10   Activation of ion channels through the phospholipase A_2 pathway. Phospholipase A_2 is activated possibly through MAPkinase, resulting in the release of arachidonic acid. Arachidonic acid is converted to 5HPETE by 5-lipoxygenase. 5HPETE is converted to leukotrienes, e.g., LTC_4. LTC_4 opens an outer membrane Ca^{2+} channel, with a subsequent opening of K^+ channels. The K^+ influx induces hyperpolarization which in turn activates a voltage-dependent Ca^{2+} channel, resulting in a great increase in intracellular Ca^{2+}. The intracellular Ca^{2+} will bind to calmodulin, thereby initiating a large range of cellular events. Abbreviations: AA, arachidonic acid; HPETE, hydroperoxy eicosatetraenoic acid; LPL, lysophospholipid; LTC_4, leukotriene-C_4; MAPkinase, mitogen-activated protein kinase; PC, phosphatidylcholine; PLA_2, phospholipase A_2.

Binding of Ca^{2+}/calmodulin to the catalytic unit of the protein kinase induces autophosphorylation on residue 286 for the α-form and residue 287 for the β-form. Only after autophosphorylation is the protein kinase able to phosphorylate other substrates. Once autophosphorylated the protein kinase no longer requires Ca^{2+}, although its subsequent deactivation is slowed down in a Ca^{2+}/calmodulin bound state. Deactivation occurs through a series of autophosphorylations. The function of CAMKII has been studied mainly in brain, where it is involved in the modulation of neurotransmitter release and neurotransmitter synthesis. Ca^{2+}/calmodulin is required for entry into mitosis of sea urchin eggs, and it may have a role in the regulation of protein kinase p34[cdc2]. This kinase regulates cell cycle progression, especially the transition of cells from G2 into M (mitosis). Other than that, it has been reported that CaMKII is able to affect gene transcription. Ca^{2+}/calmodulin also regulates the serine/threonine protein phosphatase, calcineurin, an enzyme that dephosphorylates proteins and is essential for T-cell activation. The role of calcineurin in T-cell activation was partly discovered by the finding that the immunosuppressants cyclosporin A and FK506 were shown to inactivate calcineurin by complexing the enzyme to immunophilin. Clearly, Ca^{2+} is an extremely versatile second messenger providing numerous signals which can branch off through its binding with calmodulin.

13.2.8   DIRECT TYROSINE PHOSPHORYLATION OF TRANSCRIPTION FACTORS

The most direct way to envision how a plasma membrane-localized receptor could alter gene expression is by a direct phosphorylation of transcription factors. Through studies on the mechanism of cell activation by interferon-α, it became apparent that such a direct pathway exists. Stimulation of cells through the interferon-α receptor leads to activation of associated protein tyrosine kinases called tyk2 and JAK1 (Janus kinase). These two tyrosine protein kinases phosphorylate each other (similar to the receptor-bound tyrosine protein kinases) and

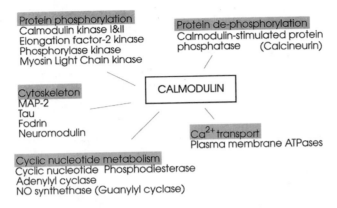

FIGURE 13.11   Calmodulin bound to intracellular Ca²⁺ can interact and activate a number of cellular enzymes. Note the number of protein kinases that are activated by calmodulin. Abbreviations: ATP, adenosine-5′-trisphosphate; MAP-2, microtubule-associated protein-2; NO, nitric oxide; Tau, tubulin assembly unit.

then phosphorylate tyrosine residues on cytoplasmic proteins called p84$^{Stat1\alpha}$, p91$^{Stat1\beta}$, and p113^{Stat2}. These proteins contain an SH2 domain through which they can associate with the phosphorylated tyk2 and JAK1; p84$^{Stat1\alpha}$ and p91$^{Stat1\beta}$ each complex with p113^{Stat2} to form heterodimers. These dimers, in turn, interact with another protein called p48 to form a trimeric transcription factor complex: ISGF3 (INF-α stimulated-gene factor 3). The complex then translocates to the nucleus and forms an active transcription complex that binds to DNA at the interferon-stimulated response element (ISRE). Because the Stat proteins act both as second messengers and as transcription factors, they were given the name Stat, which stands for "signal transducer and activator of transcription". Interferon-γ also induces phosphorylation, but only of p84$^{Stat1\alpha}$ and p91$^{Stat2\beta}$. Recently, it has been shown that such a scheme is operative in EGF-, PDGF-, and nerve growth factor (NGF)-mediated signal transduction. It was first shown for EGF that activation of the receptor results in direct tyrosine phosphorylation of transcription factors. The transcription factor complex that binds the DNA was called Sis-inducible factor (SIF). Sis is an oncogene and the name is derived from simian sarcoma. It now appears that SIF consists of a dimer of p84$^{Stat1\alpha}$ and p91$^{Stat1\beta}$. Thus, upon tyrosine phosphorylation the two Stats dimerize and translocate to the nucleus where they bind to DNA at the Sis-inducible element (SIE) and promote transcription of genes, for example c-fos (Figure 13.12).

13.3 RECEPTORS THAT ASSOCIATE WITH A TYROSINE PROTEIN KINASE

The second class of cell surface receptors to be discussed is the one membrane-spanning receptor with no known intrinsic catalytic activity (see Figure 13.2). The interleukin-2 receptor (IL-2R) and the T-cell receptor (TCR) are two examples that will be illustrated. IL-2 is an important molecule in the regulation of the immune response. IL-2 enhances T-cell proliferation, increases cytolytic activity of natural killer cells, and promotes proliferation of B cells and the release of IgG. The TCR is involved in detection of foreign antigens, together with presentation of a major histocompatibility complex (MHC) molecule, and subsequently regulates the maturation of T cells via thymic selection. The TCR is a complex receptor of six subunits all spanning the membrane (Figure 13.13). Activation of the TCR results in tyrosine phosphorylation of a number of proteins, and it was postulated that a nonreceptor tyrosine kinase must interact with the receptor. In addition, the production of IP$_3$ and DAG

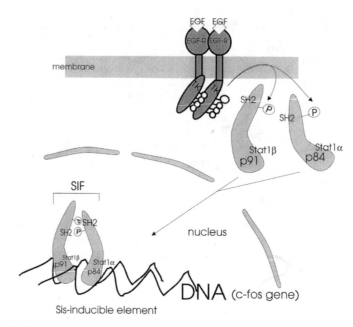

FIGURE 13.12   The activated EGF receptor can directly phosphorylate transcription factors p84$^{Stat1\alpha}$ and p91$^{Stat1\beta}$. Through their SH2 domain, p84$^{Stat1\alpha}$ and p91$^{Stat1\beta}$ can associate with the tyrosine-phosphorylated receptor and are subsequently phosphorylated on tyrosine residues. The p84$^{Stat1\alpha}$ and p91$^{Stat1\beta}$ then form a dimer, also designated as Sis-inducible factor (SIF). The dimer translocates to the nucleus where it binds to a Sis-incducible element (SIE) and activates transcription of, for example, the c-fos gene. Abbreviation: SH, Src homology; Sis, Simian sarcoma, an oncogene that codes for the precursor of platelet-derived growth factor-a; Stat, signal transducer and activator of transcription.

was observed when the ligand bound to the receptors, and the scenario following receptor occupation resembles that observed for the EGF or PDGF receptor. An early candidate for such a nonreceptor tyrosine kinase arose with the discovery of a T-cell-specific member of the src family of tyrosine kinases, called p56^{LCK}. Later, a family of src-related protein kinases, present not exclusively in T cells, was also shown to exist (Figure 13.13). The IL-2R interacts with p56^{LCK} and activates this protein kinase. The TCR receptor ζ-subunit interacts with another src family member, p59^{FYN}. Overexpression of these tyrosine kinases results in antigen and IL-2 hyperresponsive cells. How exactly these protein kinases transmit their signal downstream in the cascade is still under study, but it is believed that adaptor proteins are involved. One such adaptor protein which interacts with src is the src-homology collagen-like protein (Shc) which binds to activated src and after being phosphorylated on a tyrosine residue, allows SH2 domain-containing proteins to dock into the complex, bringing protein kinase and substrate into close proximity and facilitating phosphorylation. One of the substrates can be PLCγ, which in turn generates IP$_3$ and DAG, thereby producing a calcium signal and activating the PKC pathway. Another possible adaptor is p155^{GNRP}, the nucleotide exchange protein that regulates the activity of ras, thereby stimulating the ras pathway.

13.4 ONCOGENES, MALIGNANCY, AND SIGNAL TRANSDUCTION

Malignant cell growth can arise as a consequence of viral infection with certain RNA (retrovirus) or DNA viruses. Certain genes carried along by these viruses were discovered

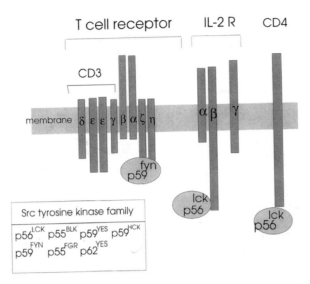

FIGURE 13.13 Receptors that span the membrane only once and have no intrinsic catalytic activity (Class 2) interact with tyrosine kinases from the src tyrosine kinase family. The T-cell receptor is a complex of six subunits from which the ζ-subunit interacts with p59^{FYN}. The interleukin-2 receptor (IL-2R) is made up of three subunits from which the β-subunit interacts with p56^{LCK}. Another example is the CD4 receptor which interacts with p56^{LCK}. The box illustrates the family of src-like tyrosine protein kinases. Abbreviation: CD, cluster of differentiation.

to be responsible for tumor formation and subsequently were called oncogenes. Later, it was shown that nonviral-induced tumors could bear similar genes, for instance ras. Oncogenes "transform" cells, which means that cells lose the capacity to respond to the needs of the organism, continue to divide, require only little growth support from cytokines, often grow without a proper substrate, and have lost their differentiated phenotype. It was an important finding that these oncogenes are in fact gain-of-function mutants of normal cellular genes involved in signal transduction and gene transcription. A large number of oncogenes are mutated components of the upstream part of tyrosine kinase signal transduction pathways. Transformed cells either make active versions of cytokines (growth factors), overexpress a variant form of a tyrosine kinase-containing receptor or nonreceptor tyrosine kinases, over-express SH2/SH3-containing adaptor proteins, overexpress serine/threonine protein kinases, or express variants of the small G-proteins or their accessory proteins. At the downstream end of the signal transduction pathway, variants of certain transcription factors are potent cell transformers (Figure 13.14). Products of normal cellular genes that have the potential to transform cells by gain-of-function mutations are often denoted as "protooncogenes". It perhaps is not surprising that the aberrances in the tyrosine protein kinases themselves, or of one of the components downstream in the signal transduction pathways, result in aberrances in cell growth. After all, tyrosine kinase-containing receptors are "growth factor receptors". Occupation of these receptors, and subsequent activation of the signal transduction pathways, will drive the cell through the cell cycle. Although tyrosine kinase phosphorylation only accounts for 5% of total protein phosphorylation activity in the cell, it occupies a key position in many signal transduction pathways, hence, the incidence of these genes in malignancy is much higher. As an example of the role of oncogenes in cell transformation, ras is found altered in 40% of lung and colon carcinomas, in 90% of pancreas carcinomas, and 30% of all human cancer.

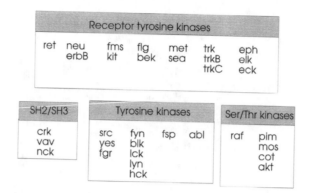

FIGURE 13.14 Upstream components of tyrosine kinase signal transduction cascades are also discovered as cellular or viral oncogenes. These oncogenes are gain-of-function mutants of the "wild type" proteins, e.g., receptor tyrosine kinases, adaptor proteins, nonreceptor tyrosine kinases, and to a lesser extent the serine/threonine protein kinases.

13.5 MAKE YOUR OWN SIGNAL TRANSDUCTION PATHWAY

Use Figure 13.15 to test your knowledge of signal transduction pathways. Connect the enzymes and second messengers with an arrow. Indicate if it is threonine/serine or tyrosine phosphorylation and add protein recognition motifs where possible. After you have drawn the connections, answers to the question are given in Figure 13.16. Abbreviations are explained in the preceding figures.

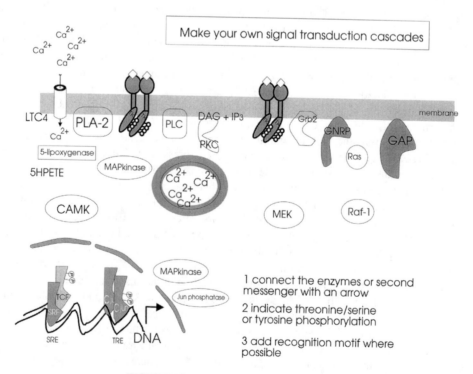

FIGURE 13.15 For legend see section 13.5.

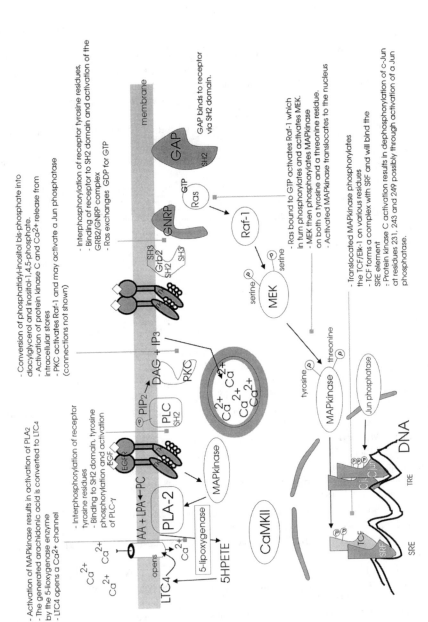

FIGURE 13.16 For abbreviations see preceding figures.

13.6 FURTHER READING

Reviews

Ahn, N.G., Seger, R. and Krebs, E.G. (1992), The mitogen-activated protein kinase activator, *Curr. Opin. Cell, Biol.*, 4, 992-999.

Berridge, M.J. (1993), Inositol trisphosphate and calcium signalling, *Nature*, 361, 315-325.

Crews, C.M. and Erikson, R.L. (1993), Extracellular signals and reversible protein phosphorylation: What to Mek of it all, *Cell*, 74, 215-217.

Egan, S.E. and Weinberg, R.A. (1993), The pathway to signal achievement, *Nature*, 365, 781-783.

Hanks, S.K., Quinn, A.M. and Hunter, T. (1988), The protein kinase family: conserved features and deduced phylogeny of the catalytic domains, *Science*, 241, 42-52.

Karin, M. (1994), Signal transduction from the cell surface to the nucleus through phosphorylation of transcription factors, *Curr. Biol.*, 6, 415-424.

Klausner, R.D. and Samelson, L.E. (1991), T cell antigen receptor activation pathways: The tyrosine kinase connection, *Cell*, 64, 875-878.

Klee, C.B. (1991), Concerted regulation of protein phosphorylation and dephosphorylation by calmodulin, *Neurochem. Res.*, 16, 1059-1065.

Koch, C.A., Anderson, D., Moran, M.F., Ellis, C. and Pawson, T. (1991), SH2 and SH3 domains: elements that control interactions of cytoplasmic signalling proteins, *Science*, 252, 668-674.

Mayer, B.J. and Baltimore, D. (1993), Signalling through SH2 and SH3 domains, *Trends Cell Biol.*, 3, 8-13.

Schaller, M.D. and Parsons, J.T. (1993), Focal adhesion kinase: and integrin-linked protein tyrosine kinase, *Trends Cell Biol.*, 3, 258-262.

Schlessinger, J. and Ullrich, A. (1992), Growth factor signalling by receptor tyrosine kinases, *Neuron*, 9, 383-391.

Thomas, G. (1992), MAP kinase by any other name smells just as sweet, *Cell*, 68, 3-6.

Research Articles

Bar-Sagi, D., Rotin, D., Batzer, A., Mandiyan, V. and Schlessinger, J. (1993), SH3 domains direct cellular localization of signalling molecules, *Cell*, 74, 83-91.

Buday, L. and Downward, J. (1993), Epidermal growth factor regulates p21[ras] through the formation of a complex of receptor, Grb2 adaptor protein, and Sos nucleotide exchange factor, *Cell*, 73, 611-620.

Cararsi, S. and Drapeau, P. (1993), Tyrosine kinase-dependent selection of transmitter responses induced by neuronal contact, *Nature*, 363, 353-355.

Clark, S.G., Stern, M.J. and Horvitz, H.R. (1992), *C. elagans* cell-signalling gene sem-5 encodes a protein with SH2 and SH3 domains, *Nature*, 356, 340-344.

Dickson, B., Sprenger, F., Morrison, D. and Hafen, E. (1992), Raf functions downstream of ras1 in the Sevenless signal transduction pathway, *Nature*, 360, 600-603.

Egan, S.E., Giddings, B.W., Brooks, M.W., Buday, L., Sizeland, A.M. and Weinberg, R.A. (1993), Association of Sos Ras exchange protein with Grb2 is implicated in tyrosine kinase signal transduction and transformation, *Nature*, 363, 45-50.

Kolanus, W., Romeo, C. and Seed, B. (1993), T cell activation by clustered tyrosine kinases, *Cell*, 74, 171-183.

Peppelenbosch, M.P., Tertoolen, L.G.J., Den Hertog, J. and De Laat, S.W. (1992), Epidermal growth factor activates calcium channels by phospholipase A2/5-lipoxygenase-mediated leukotriene C4 production, *Cell*, 69, 295-303.

Waksman, G. et al. (1992), Crystal structure of the phosphotyrosine recognition domain SH2 of v-src complexed with tyrosine-phosphorylated peptides, *Nature*, 358, 646-653.

Warne, P.H., Rodriquez Viciana, P. and Downward, J. (1993), Direct interaction of Ras and the amino-terminal region of Raf-1 *in vitro*, *Nature*, 364, 352-355.

13.7 SOLUTION TO PROBLEM

For solution to problem see Figure 13.16.

Section V

Receptors as Pharmaceutical Targets

14 Receptors as Pharmaceutical Targets

James W. Black

CONTENTS

14.1 HORMONE RECEPTORS

The objective of pharmaceutical research is to discover and develop new substances which can be characterized by their selectivity and specificity. Selectivity describes the particular effects on physiological or pathological states which the substance can produce. These descriptions, such as hypnotic, hypoglycemic, hypotensive, and antiinflammatory, may be wholly empirical. However, this does not impede their therapeutic utility. Thus the clinical utility of drugs such as morphine and digitalis was established long before there were biochemical explanations for their actions. Specificity, on the other hand, refers to the biochemical hypotheses which claim to explain a substance's selectivity. Thus, activation of enkephalin receptors is proposed as the mechanism by which morphine acts, and inhibition of Na^+/K^+-dependent ATPase has been claimed to specify the activity of digitalis. All kinds of biochemical events have been used to specify drug actions. Interactions with enzymes, ion channels, and membrane transporters have been widely used to explain drug actions. However, pharmacological receptors are probably the favorite site of drug action used in explanatory models of their selective activity.

"Receptor" is a much-used term in biology. There are sensory receptors, including telereceptors, mechanoreceptors, baroreceptors, chemoreceptors, T-cell receptors, and so on. Plainly, "receptor" needs an adjective or prefix to be informative. As used here, a receptor is the site of action of hormones, neurotransmitters, modulators of various kinds, and autocoids. As yet, there is no agreed class name for the receptors associated with these agents. However, all of these agents fulfill the role of intercellular messengers and, as this was the concept behind Bayliss and Starling's invention of the term "hormone", it is convenient to think that there is a class of molecules — hormone receptors — which have common features in the same way as the class of enzymes has common features. Thus, enzymes induce chemical changes in substrates without themselves being permanently changed in the process; that is, they are catalysts. By the same token, hormones change the chemical properties of their corresponding receptors without themselves being chemically changed in the process; that is, hormones rather than their receptors are behaving like catalysts. Thus, the hormone receptor both recognizes and responds to its conjugate messenger. For ease of writing, this is the collective sense in which receptors will be referred to in this chapter.

Hormones, broadly defined in this way as chemical messengers, can all be characterized by their selectivity and specificity. The selectivity of hormones describes their role in physiological and pathophysiological regulatory processes. The specificity of a hormone refers to the evidence that they produce their effects by interacting with identifiable protein receptors. Hormones, then, have drug-like qualities, like a natural, physiological pharmacopeia. This is the idea which makes hormone-receptor systems so attractive to pharmaceutical researchers. When new-drug researchers use the drug-like qualities of a hormone as the starting point, they are already a long way to the goal of discovering a protodrug with desirable selectivity and specificity.

The selectivity of a hormone always entails the concepts of *affinity*, the likelihood of hormone and receptor interacting with each other, and *efficacy*, the hormone's response-generating power which derives from activation of the receptors. These concepts are defined by parameters in classical thermodynamic models of hormone-receptor interactions. As these hormone-defining parameters are not readily accessible, even in radioligand binding studies, the industrial pharmacologist usually settles for the empirical parameters of dose-response curves, namely the maximum response and the dose needed for half-maximal response. Modern pharmaceutical research based on hormone-receptor interaction is founded on measuring and interpreting dose-response curves. The target is the ability to manipulate hormonal efficacy as implied in dose-response curves. A significant fraction of a contemporary pharmacopeia is about drugs which mimic, enhance, prolong, or abolish the efficacy of hormones.

14.2 PARTIAL AGONISTS – PROBLEMS IN DETECTING CHANGES IN EFFICACY

The author was introduced to the problems of efficacy and its expression in bioassays within months of starting his first project in pharmaceutical research while using isoprenaline, a fully efficacious analogue of the hormones noradrenaline and adrenaline, to drive the rate of beating of the isolated guinea-pig heart (the Langendorff preparation) via the activation of β-adrenoreceptors. Soon after beginning the project, the dichloro analogue of isoprenaline, DCI, was described as an antagonist of isoprenaline on bronchial muscle. However, in our cardiac preparation, we found that DCI was as efficacious as isoprenaline itself. Subsequently, the Langendorff preparation was replaced with the rate-controlled guinea-pig papillary muscle preparation. On the new preparation, DCI had no agonist activity but was now a competitive antagonist of the catecholamines. The subsequent rapid development of (β-adrenoreceptor antagonists was based on this observation. The tissue-dependence of DCI's efficacy was puzzling so we were not prepared for the second encounter with the phenomenon.

The second encounter occurred several years later when our laboratory switched interests to histamine antagonists. No *in vitro* assays for studying histamine-stimulated gastric acid secretion were known at that time, so we used the anesthetized rat lumen-perfused stomach preparation (the Ghosh and Schild preparation). The guanidino analogue of histamine (IEG) was one of the first compounds tested. For practical purposes IEG behaved like a fully efficacious agonist. Several frustrating years later, it was found that IEG was not quite as efficacious as histamine. When IEG was dosed during a plateau of a maximal secretory response to histamine, a small degree of inhibition was revealed. The subsequent rapid development of histamine H_2-receptor antagonists was based on this observation. It was eventually found that had the rat isolated uterus preparation been used for the screening bioassay it would have immediately shown that IEG was much less efficacious than histamine.

DCI and IEG are now classified as partial agonists. Partial agonist, by definition, is a comparative description. When substance B is unable to produce as large a maximum response as substance A in a particular tissue, and when they can be shown to be producing their effects by acting on the same population of receptors, then substance B is defined as a partial agonist. However, this is a very limited definition. These initial observations with DCI and IEG are now generally recognized. The expression of partial agonism is tissue dependent in a very sensitive way. DCI would have been classified as a full agonist as judged by heart rate changes, and as a simple competitive antagonist as judged by papillary muscle contractions. The variations in the expression of efficacy between closely related analogues of a hormone acting on a particular tissue and the variations in the expression of efficacy by a particular analogue acting on different tissues have both practical and theoretical implications.

Kenakin and Beek published a beautiful data set comparing the activities of isoprenaline (classified as a full agonist) with prenalterol (classified as a partial agonist) on six different tissues. Across the tissues the potency of isoprenaline varied by two orders of magnitude: in tissues where the potency of isoprenaline was very high, the efficacy of prenalterol was also very high — nearly the same as isoprenaline; where the potency of isoprenaline was low, prenalterol had no detectable agonist activity and, indeed, now behaved like a competitive antagonist. From the point of view of pharmaceutical research the implications are clear. Try to find several tissues which will express the activity of the hormone of interest. The relative potencies of the hormone can point to the likelihood that a particular tissue will expose the efficacy of a partial agonist. In pharmaceutical research there is a need in the early stages of a hormone-receptor-based project to be able to detect small changes in the efficacy of hormone analogues. An assay without too much amplification is needed. However, in the later stages of the project, for example, when compounds have been discovered which behave like simple competitive antagonists, there is a need for high-efficacy amplification systems to detect signs of residual agonist activity.

From a theoretical point of view, the efficacy of an agonist in the tissue is dependent on the ratio between the well-understood concept of receptor density and the much more opaque concept of "some kind of coupling factor", the intrinsic ability of bound receptor to generate an intracellular stimulus. The possibility that the same class of receptors might have different coupling efficiencies in different tissues cannot be ignored. However, differences in the density of receptor expression between tissues is now well recognized and is the most attractive way of interpreting the tissue dependence of efficacy. The attractiveness of the concept is not just because of its simplicity, but also because it points to a way in which the new technology of controlling the expression of cloned receptor genes can be harnessed to generate new efficacy-detecting and measuring systems. However, although these new receptor expression systems are an interesting extension to the range of bioassays, they are in no sense a replacement for traditional bioassays based on intact, isolated tissues in *vitro*.

14.3 THE VALUE OF BIOASSAYS

The essence of using intact-tissue bioassays in a hormone-related pharmaceutical project is that the hormone can be used to light up its population of conjugate receptors in a conceptually simple biomolecular interaction. If the resulting events are dominated by this initial binding interaction, as described by the Hill equation, rectangular hyperbolic dose-response curves are likely. Simple hyperbolic dose-response curves are certainly found in *in vitro* bioassays. However, departures from such simplicity are much more common. We are continuing to understand the different events which can lead to complicated dose-response curves. The receptors themselves can be a source of distortion. The dynamics of receptor expression can introduce variation due to internalization or desensitization. However, the commonest receptor-mediated complicating factor occurs when the hormone activates more than one population of receptors. Disclosure of receptor heterogeneity is always interesting and challenging. The problem facing the pharmaceutical researcher is what to do about the discovery. The current climate is that we should always be trying to find more and more specific ligands. However, when a hormone activates more than one set of receptors to produce the same end result, albeit by different processes of transduction, it may be practically more prudent to search for highly nonselective ligands. This may be the best way for reaching the goal of desirable selectivity.

The hormone itself can introduce complexity into bioassays. Many hormones have now to be seen and understood not as chemical entities but as chemical pathways where hormonal activity is distributed across a number of chemical species. The more we learn about the pharmacological properties of members of a pathway the more we are realizing that each one has a mix of common and unique properties. The practical point is that we must be careful about which "hormone" we choose to drive our bioassays. A hormonal chemical pathway may contain sinks as well as sources. Metabolism and uptake of a hormone can introduce significant distortions into bioassays. All of these factors leave their fingerprints on dose-response curves and a pharmaceutical researcher developing a new bioassay has to learn to read the signs.

A particularly exciting challenge to industrial pharmacologists occurs when the cells which synthesize the hormone, with or without storage, are found in the same tissue as their conjugate receptors. For example, these cells can be neurones, mast cells, or enterochromaffin cells. Controlled release of synthesized or stored substances can be achieved by either chemical or electrical stimulation. Intact-tissue bioassay in this mode of indirect agonist offers two exciting opportunities. First, tissue architecture constrains and directs the release of substances to particular cellular targets in a manner which may not be achievable by the hormone diffusing into the tissue uniformly from the organ bath compartment. Second, indirect release may be able to produce a composite of coreleased substances which potentially can interact with each other. Both of these phenomena are clearly recognized now and offer opportunities to the pharmaceutical researcher. Potentiating interactions at the postreceptor level occurring between coreleased substances is a particularly important opportunity for the future of drug research.

14.4   ARE BIOASSAYS VALUABLE IN PHARMACEUTICAL RESEARCH?

So far, I have given an outline of different ways in which complex dose-response curves in intact tissue bioassays can be the result, the pharmacological resultant, of two or more interacting activities. Now, if all that these bioassays achieved was to blur and obscure the underlying activities, they would have to give way to the newer, analytically simpler assays based on chemistry and biochemistry. However, the beauty of intact-tissue bioassays is that they are analytically tractable; by using families of dose-response curves and appropriate mathematical models, the complexity of intact hormone-receptor systems can indeed be interpreted. Bioassay allows them to be studied as systems in ways denied to simple biochemical assays.

Are intact-tissue bioassays capable of being a stand-alone, initial, technology for discovering new drugs in hormone-receptor-directed pharmaceutical projects? The answer, based on our own experience and much published evidence, must be positive. However, there is no doubt that *in vitro* bioassays are slow, resource-intensive, need skilled investigators, and are expensive. The questions today are about whether we can economize on these bioassays or even eliminate them altogether by using more productive chemical screens. Radioligand binding assays are an obvious example. They have been widely used in the industry for many years but we do not know how their use is optimized in relation to bioassay, even after several years of personal experience of radioligand-binding assays running alongside bioassays for both gastrin and cholecystokinin receptors. Every compound we have made has been evaluated in both kinds of assay. Now there is no doubt, not surprisingly, that we have got much more information about new compounds using bioassay. However, in retrospect, could we have economized on bioassay by using binding assays to select out inactive compounds? The judgment at this time is that we would have missed some interesting compounds. To some extent, this is a matter of style more than tactics. In the main, all of the compounds made in our program have been designed to try to answer a question about structure-activity relations. Several thousand dollars will have been spent in making each of them. As a result, a trivial biological evaluation of the binary type, 0 or 1, is inappropriate. At issue is the struggle between biologists and chemists to learn to understand and trust each other. It is not too much of a caricature to see that the chemist believes that every molecule he struggles so hard to make will have interesting properties if only the biologist would evaluate it adequately; the biologist, on the other hand, is convinced that his assays will reveal the desired properties of a molecule if only the chemist would make the right compound. Our experience shows it takes at least two years of continuous collaboration before the chemist and biologist really learn mutual trust!

14.5 THE ITERATIVE PROCESS OF DRUG DEVELOPMENT

The involvement of medicinal chemists in a new hormone-receptor-targeted drug project begins right at the start. To get involved, enough of the structure of the hormone needs to be known to allow all the possible shapes of the molecule to be visualized by physical valence-wire models, or space-occupying CPK nuclear models, or nowadays, by various computerized simulations on a PC computer. Whatever way is chosen, the chemist, in principle, walks around the molecule in his mind as he carries out an imaginative interrogation. What is it about this molecule that interests me as a chemist? Where are the likely sources of noncovalent interactions with its receptor-ionic charges, electron densities on carbonyls and amino groups, pi-electron systems, and so on? Today, the chemist may have additional information from the molecular modeler about conformational probabilities. Whatever the input to his imagination, the medicinal chemist distills out a single first question, a question which he believes he can try to answer by making a simple analogue or derivative of the natural hormone. Of course, the question cannot be answered with surgical precision. Every precise change in the molecule produces many more consequential changes in its conformation, in charge distribution, in electrostatic fields, and so on, which ensure that the chemical question will be liable to have an opaque biological answer first time around.

The answer to the chemist's question is provided by bioassay. Since there is a question to be answered, every biological result including, even especially, that the new molecule is totally inactive, is full of interest. Whatever the result, a new question is raised, a new inquisitorial compound has to be made, a new biological test has to be carried out. This iterative process is, in principle, at the heart of all traditional hormone-receptor pharmaceutical research programs. However, in practice, the process cannot be driven like this as a single logical cycle. Generally speaking, compounds take longer to synthesize than to evaluate in bioassay. On average, a medicinal chemist will produce 15 target compounds per year. So a team of chemists are usually involved, working in parallel on parceled-out parts of the perceived problem. The molecular modelers, who are also part of the iterative loop, also have to work to a different rhythm from either the synthetic chemists or biological analysts. Nevertheless, the principle of the interrogative loop is always in play.

While during our lifetime there have been continuous and extraordinary advances in medicinal chemical technology, in chemical analytical methods, and chromatography, the most spectacular changes seen in about 40 years of pharmaceutical research have been in molecular modeling. The pharmaceutical industry has made a huge investment in this runaway technology. However, I sense a certain amount of industrial disappointment in the yield from this investment, and would agree that molecular modeling has not dramatically shortened the number of iterative loops in going from a hormone to a hormone-based compound with potential clinical utility. However, this is to miss the point. Three features of molecular modeling are no longer in doubt. The technology is allowing us to tackle problems, such as the ubiquitous polypeptide hormones, which would have been logically and imaginatively impossible 20 years ago. The technology continues to advance with breathtaking speed, a speed which would have been impossible without the earlier major investments. The technology is making a greater and greater contribution to the synthetic chemist's imagination. As far as molecular modeling is concerned, this author is a junkie.

14.6 ME-TOOISM

The logical, imaginative and iterative approach to new drugs based on hormone-receptor systems sketched out above stands in marked contrast to the industrial approach we experienced 40 years ago and to the direction in which the industry is now moving compulsively at hectic speed. In the past, industrial research used to be criticized for its practice of random screening and for its generation of me-too drugs. Of course, the biological screening was not random. Far from it, the screening tests were chosen with great care to reflect identified medical needs. Pharmacologists tried to reflect the importance of meeting medical needs by using experimental pathology paradigms for screening tests. Thus, assays were often based on experimentally induced animal pathology such as sterile inflammatory responses to foreign bodies like cotton, wool, or turpentine, or arthritis induced by antigen-adjutant presentation, or stomach ulcers induced by histamine or aspirin, or convulsions induced by leptazol or electricity, and so on. The compounds screened were not chosen at random either. They were chosen by working one's way, systematically, through the company's accumulated compound collection, its database, or by systematically ringing the changes of substituents in a lead molecule epitomized by "methyl, ethyl, propyl, butyl, futile"! The intellectual sterility of the process was not because of randomness but because of the lack of a necessary connection between the chemistry and bioassay.

In parenthesis, the critical charge of me-tooisms was also, we believe, misplaced. To some extent, we can accept the commercial charge of me-tooism. Premium prices have undoubtedly been asked for compounds with clinically insignificant acute differences. However, side effects become recognized on a slow, time-dependent basis. Therefore, inevitably, the older drug has accumulated more reports of side effects on its data sheet and the newer me-too drug can be pedaled by marketing manipulators as "just as good but safer." However, personally, I do not have such a cynical view of me-tooism. There are two reasons for this. Me-too drugs establish the image-challenging thought that compounds having quite different chemical structures can nevertheless have congruent pharmacological properties. The concept of such classes of drugs is the basis of pharmacology. Second, while the different chemical structures have one feature in common, they invariably present often usable and important differences in their pharmacokinetic and toxicological profiles.

14.7 SHORT-TERMISM

As indicated, the development of hormone-receptor-based research programs have changed all that. The logical, imaginative, iterative approach which has been painted has been shown to work regularly and reliably. The record is clear. If you follow John Locke's advice of "steadily intending your mind in a given direction," you will succeed. However, there is a large unknown element: how many iterations or how many years it will take are entirely unpredictable. This has become the problem as the pharmaceutical industry has allowed itself to be pressurized into short-termism as an antidote to exponentially escalating costs of research and development; particularly, thanks to extensions to the drug regulatory requirements, to development costs. Consequently, all the emphasis today is on speed, on what is called high-throughput screening. The potential for high-throughput screening is based on the spectacular advances in immunological and molecular biological technology made in the last 10 years or so. A whole range of procedures are now available which include cloned receptor genes cotransfected with reporter genes in cell lines or, with even greater chemical purity, there are assays such as the scintillation proximity assays where the pure chemical receptors are bound to beads which house the scintillant, thus solving the distance problem. All of these new assays can be executed robotically. All of these new assays have the following features in common. They are ingenious. They are fundamentally chemical and not biological assays. They are highly productive but they express the absolute minimum of information: presence-absence, 0 or 1. Fundamentally, these are automated assays. Important questions are not being asked and so intelligent analysis is compromised. Nevertheless, do these productive, automated, assays provide a greater, faster, yield of chemical leads?

At this moment the question has still to be answered. However, a vital complementary question has also still to be answered. Where are the compounds to come from to feed assays which can consume around 2000 or more chemicals per week? The immediately obvious source are the in-house compound libraries. The major drug research-based companies have now anything between 0.5 and 1 million compounds in their compound libraries. So a research program which can assay about 2000 compounds per week will be kept occupied for at least a few years just working through its own library. The problem with in-house libraries is that they are not an ensemble of randomly structured organic molecules. The distribution is severely lumpy. By that we mean that many of the synthesized molecules will be in closely related groups, having been synthesized for previous programs, successful as well as unsuccessful. Unless one is irredeemably optimistic, this may not be an ideal pool of molecules to trawl for new leads.

14.8 COMBINATORIAL CHEMISTRY

Therefore, the hunger at the heart of the new passion for high-throughput screening has to be satisfied from some other, generous, source of new compounds for screening. Swapping by contract, or purchasing by corporate takeover or amalgamation are obvious approaches, but are very expensive, offer limited strategies, and do not avoid the lumpiness problem. Fortunately, there have also been advances in chemistry as extraordinary as the advances in molecular and genetic biology. Combinatorial chemistry is the name of the new game.

I have no personal experience of combinatorial chemistry, but the technology for making large numbers of molecules coupled to appropriate chemical selection procedures began, we believe, with laboratory experiments to study molecular evolution in purely chemical systems. Spiegelman and his co-workers started with a bacterial phage, one of whose four genes was a replicase enzyme to make copies of itself. They showed that repeated exposures *in vitro* of viral RNA, the replicase, and supplies of the four nucleotides led to wholly new RNA sequences with a 15-fold increase in replication rate; the mutations arose from errors in replication. Subsequently, combination of methods to induce mutations in RNA or DNA, plus repeated steps of amplification by PCR (polymerase chain reaction), has led to the ability to generate up to 10^{13} sequences of single-strand DNA. These can then be screened on columns on which are bound an appropriate protein. A high affinity DNA ligand for thrombin was discovered in this way. When organic chemists took over from molecular biologists, they developed the techniques for generating libraries of 10^6 to 10^7 peptide sequences. The reactions and the assays were carried out on beads. The technology has advanced by introducing control of sequence development plus the ability to tag each sequence for ease of identification. Synthesis of constrained peptide sequences has now been followed by combinations of nonpeptide molecules. As greater constraints are introduced, the numerical productivity falls but presumably the proportion of leads increases.

Combinatorial chemistry is now a rapidly developing activity which, as a technology, is attracting the attention of highly ingenious chemists. At this time, it is impossible to predict where this technology will lead us. We do not know whether some of the basic limitations will be overcome. At this time, all the methods are restricted to binary reactions which take place readily. This is in contrast to the problems facing a synthetic chemist who wants to make a specified molecule. Not only are a number of sequential steps needed, but also many of the stages require demanding conditions for the reactions to occur. Thus, it is difficult to see how combinatorial chemistry can, in the near future, be the basis for the iterative, interrogative approach to hormone-receptor-related ligands.

High-throughput screening of data bases plus input from combinatorial chemistry is designed to generate leads. As we understand the process, leads will then be developed using more conventional methods. The assumption seems to be that finding leads is the rate-limiting step in the drug discovery process. Now, I am not convinced that this is so. Developing and optimizing leads into clinically testable new chemical entities, NCEs as they are termed in the industry, is usually a much slower phase. However, the productivity of the industry, as judged by the discovery of completely new drugs, is limited more by the choice of targets than by the discovery of leads. Care in choosing a target is the most critical decision point in pharmaceutical research.

14.9 SELECTING TARGETS FOR DRUG DEVELOPMENT

My personal approach to choosing targets is to seek answers to six questions:

- Is the project purged of wishful thinking?
- Is there a chemical starting point?
- Are there relevant bioassays?
- Will it be possible to confirm laboratory-defined specificity in humans?
- Is there a clinical condition relevant to this specificity?
- Does the project have a champion?

The wishful thinking criterion is the most important of all. All drug discovery projects begin with a desire to prevent illness or treat sickness. Wishful thinking refers to the tenuousness of the perceived relationship between that desire and the means proposed to satisfy it. The commonest example today is the claim made again and again — once we know the gene product then we will be able to find new drugs. So far, no one has shown that this will be likely or even possible. Fortunately, most hormone-receptor-directed projects are relatively free of wishful thinking as far as discovering a ligand is concerned, although the potential utility of the ligand might well be fanciful. Fortunately, again, a hormone-receptor project has a chemical starting point, the hormone itself. We are inclined here to an assumption which we cannot prove, namely that in seeking new ligands based on the hormone's chemistry we stand a fair chance of retaining the hormone's evolutionarily derived selectivity. Hormone-receptor targets also score well on the bioassay criterion. Very often the bioassay expresses an important feature of the hormone's selectivity. Ideally there are advantages for efficacy detection, for example, in having several bioassays including radioligand binding assays to choose from. Assays based on different species can be very valuable. An important criterion, choose from. Assays based on different species can be very valuable. An important criterion, we believe, is to develop ligands whose activity is not species dependent; the most reliable predictor for extrapolation to humans.

In choosing a target, it is important to imagine how to investigate the proposed new ligand in humans. Will we be able, in practice as well as in principle, to confirm the selectivity of the ligand as defined in the laboratory experiment? This can be particularly challenging in relation to CNS-directed compounds. However, most of the hormones, transmitters, and modulators found in brain are also found in the gut, so perhaps a CNS ligand's specificity can be evaluated in the periphery. It is also important before choosing a target to imagine what clinical disorder might be explored by the new specific ligand. No commercial judgment should be involved at this point. The only test is feasibility. For drugs with a new, previously unavailable, specificity there is plenty of evidence that prior commercial assessment is rarely valid. When a drug is developed with a specified mode of action, physicians will have the opportunity to explore unanticipated disorders.

The last question usually has an obvious answer: the need for a champion. The need derives from the common experience that drug research programs often go through lengthy periods of stalemate. During these periods, passion and conviction are needed to prevent the faint hearts from quitting.

Index

Index

H